Open Wide And Say Moo!

The Good Citizen's Guide to Right Thoughts and Right
Actions under Obamacare

By Richard N. Fogoros

Publish or Perish DBS
Pittsburgh, PA
http://publishorperishdbs.com

Reach the author by email at DrRich@CovertRationingBlog.com

Second Edition
May 15, 2013

Manufactured in the United States of America

Disclaimer: Nothing in this book should be construed as specific or personal medical advice.

ISBN 978-0-9881976-1-9
1.   Health care reform – United States 2. Medical care – United States 3. Medical Policy – United States

DEDICATION

For my children, and yours

TABLE OF CONTENTS

ACKNOWLEDGEMENTS

This book was first produced on-line, in serial fashion (Dickens-like) on my *Covert Rationing Blog*. From March through July, 2012, working as rapidly as I could manage, I posted each successive chapter as I finished it, one chapter roughly every seven to ten days. I attribute my successful completion of this project to two things. First, a schedule like this did not leave much time for introspection, nor for much second-guessing about the practicality or the wisdom of such an undertaking. But more importantly, I was greatly encouraged to keep up the pace by the ongoing exchange I enjoyed with readers, who saw fit to offer their comments and criticisms on this work-in-progress.

I am thus very thankful for the many people who took the time to read the on-line version of this book as it unfolded, and particularly, for those who were moved to let me know what they thought of it (even when those thoughts were of a scatological nature), or to suggest ways I might improve it (or, on occasion, to suggest places I might shove it). I want especially to recognize the efforts of "Sp1ndoctor," who for five months hosted an ongoing discussion about this book on Sermo; I learned a lot from that lengthy exchange. I hope that this, the finished version of the book, accurately reflects how seriously I took all the comments I received, whether favorable or unfavorable.

I also gratefully acknowledge the support of my beloved wife Anne, who always manages to put up with me with far more grace than I deserve, whenever I become distracted for long periods by projects like this one. Even during those times when it cannot possibly seem like it to her, she makes my world go around.

A PERSONAL NOTE ON PROGRESSIVES

I am pretty hard on Progressives in this book. This fact has led a few early readers to declare me a "hater," and to assert that, therefore, all good people are duty-bound to dismiss anything I have to say. This convenient tactic is all too common today, and all too often it succeeds in stifling the open expression of potentially useful ideas.

This tactic is not new. It always accompanies deeply-held ideologies or beliefs which (through revolution, persuasion, or percolation) have insinuated themselves into the official axioms of authority. Whether we're talking about the Communism of Stalin, the Catholicism of Torquemada, or the Progressivism of early 21st Century America, anyone who persistently expresses ideas that are counter to the accepted dogma are routinely condemned to one of three categories – the stupid, the crazy, or the evil. The prescribed remedy (re-education, institutionalization or elimination) depends on the final diagnosis, and on the degree of frustration and anger among those in authority. (Being assigned to irrelevancy as a hater is the kindest form of "elimination," and for this I am very grateful.)

I do not hate progressives. Indeed, in general I love progressives. These are people with whom I gather around the Thanksgiving table; people with whom I work; people with whom I go bicycle riding or running; people with whom I quaff a beer and swap stories; people with whom I mourn a loss or celebrate a union or a birth. While it is difficult to generalize, progressives tend to be especially kind-hearted, altruistic, and empathetic. They are typically pleasant to be around, and often make good friends. They do not, by their very natures, engender hatred.

These everyday progressives – the "small-p" progressives – are progressives because they want what's best for everyone. They are turned off or even disgusted by ideologies that simply accept with seeming equanimity that life will create winners and losers, and that it's the individual's problem not to become a loser. Most progressives have nothing against winners, but simply insist that something must be done for those who do not win. It is easy to understand why these well-intentioned people are attracted to an ideology that purports to know a way to prevent anyone from ever becoming a loser. What's not to like about that?

So I do not hate progressives; quite the contrary.

It's the "capital-P" Progressives – the leadership, the self-proclaimed expert class, the ones who know all the answers, the Philosopher Kings – with whom I have a problem. (This book explains in great depth the nature of this problem.) But I cannot find it in myself to hate even these Progressives. Rather, I recognize that they simply have a particular (though wrongheaded) way of looking at the Universe. Their worldview is mistaken and ultimately very harmful - specifically, as I will show, as it is applied to our healthcare system – but in general even Progressives are attempting to do good, and most of them are not particularly detestable as compared with the rest of humanity.

If Progressives are who they say they are – expounders of an ideology based on scientific and rational thought – one should expect them to answer their critics with logic, rather than simply dismissing them by means of labels. If Progressives think the synthesis described in this book is wrong, then (I appeal to my open-minded readers and my progressive friends) would it not be better for them to engage in a collegial discussion, to explain logically where I have gone awry, thereby convincing me (and any people I may have led astray) of my error? Such an approach would do far more credit to Progressivism than the approach we see them taking far too often – condemning dissenters without a hearing in the modern version of *auto-da-fe*.

My plea for a collegial engagement with Progressives is more than just a device. In my career so far I have had two very close and official encounters with Inquisitors armed with the Truth of the Central Authority. While I emerged from both of these frightening encounters unharmed, I found the experiences to be life-changing; this is not an experience I wish to repeat. It is therefore with a certain amount of trepidation that I release this book into the wild, a book that already has been declared by some to be a vehicle for expressing my supposed hatred for Progressives.

I have no desire to poke Progressives with a stick. I seek understanding, and not confrontation.

It is of little consolation to me that Martin Luther said precisely the same thing as he nailed up his 97 Theses. Just look what came from that.

INTRODUCTION

From a recently discovered fragment, attributed by some to Plato:

Socrates: What have you there, my young friend?

Meno: An ancient volume I have just acquired from Phaedo, the antiquities dealer. It's a curiosity.

Socrates: How so?

Meno: Well, look here at how the author has so badly mishandled his title. It's simply not possible for a person to open their mouth wide while saying moo.

Socrates: Ah, it is a book about healthcare. Likely, then, there is some pretentiously obscure message shrouded in that strange title.

Meno: Obviously the author is attempting to draw a comparison between patients and cattle.

Socrates: Let me see this book for a moment. . . . . Yes, he appears to be complaining that in his land they are establishing a new healthcare system that will treat patients like the interchangeable members of a herd of beeves.

Meno: Well, he would have been better off comparing them to a herd of sheep. After all, one can open one's mouth quite nicely while saying, "Baaa!"

Socrates: True enough. But I get the impression this troublesome fellow chose "Moo" for a particular reason.

Meno: But that doesn't make sense. No doctor who truly wanted to do a thorough examination of a patient's oral cavity would ask the patient to purse their lips in such a manner. (Never mind while asking them to make such a demeaning sound!)

Socrates: Precisely. Does it not follow, then, that for some unfathomable reason the doctor in this case does not actually intend to do a thorough examination? But that at the same time, apparently, he wants to pretend otherwise - possibly to himself as well as to his patient?

Meno: You're proposing that this doctor, by saying "Open wide" as if a full examination is about to take place, is engaging in a purposeful fiction? A fiction which he reveals in the very next moment when he specifies exactly what he means by "wide?" It is absurd.

Socrates: But doctors do something like this all the time. Has no doctor ever said, "This won't hurt much," just before he does something unspeakable to you?

Meno: Certainly. It's how they earn their drachmas. But my doctor is simply trying to get me to hold still long enough for him to violate my person (only in the most professional way, of course). In contrast, the strange doctor imagined by this author is telling his patient, "I'm going to do an extremely inadequate and cursory examination of your oral cavity, and we're both going to pretend I gave you the full bore going-over you ought to expect from a competent professional."

Socrates: I think that's exactly what the doctor is saying. But there's one more thing - a very odd thing, too - implicit in the doctor's command to open wide and say moo.

Meno: You mean that, for such a singular and inappropriate command, it is delivered very matter-of-factly?

Socrates: Yes, my young friend. The attitude of supreme confidence this command carries with it is noteworthy. The doctor clearly expects that his patient will comply fully with the fiction he is proposing to perpetrate, without protest or complaint, even though compliance is to the patient's own detriment, and furthermore that the patient will do so with the most submissive of utterances.

Meno: You give the author too much credit. I think he is simply an ass, and botched the title of his book.

Socrates: Let us see.

The title of this book is not as ill-chosen as you may think at first glance. It is, in fact, a particularly apt illustration of my overall theme.

Under Obamacare, or under any Progressive healthcare system, the Good Citizen must learn to develop the proper mode of thought. When a doctor or some other agent of the healthcare authority informs you with all apparent sincerity that something is true, while their every action indicates that something quite different is true, and you choose to believe what you are told, instead of what your own senses are saying to you, this is called right thinking. Then when you act on what you are told, again in contrast to all the evidence to the contrary, it is called right action.

"Open wide and say moo" is therefore a metaphor that suggests how we as patients are likely to be treated under Obamacare, and it implies how we are expected to respond.

To such an absurd command a skeptic might reply, "What in the hell are you talking about? Do you want me to open wide or not? And what the hell is this 'moo' business?"

This is neither right thinking nor right action.

In contrast, right thinking will allow you to process such a request from your doctor in the proper way. You will recognize that the vague command to "open wide" is a mere courtesy. It is a way for you (and your doctor) to pretend that a thorough oral examination is about to take place, and thus to feel better about the kind of healthcare you are about to receive (or give). The real command, you will recognize, is the more specific one, the one that, in essence, defines what is actually meant by "wide."

And so: Being a Good Citizen (and thus a perfect Obamacare patient), you will purse your lips, just barely wide enough to allow your ObamaDoc (a doctor whose primary interest is in keeping the Central Authority happy) a quick, cursory look at your oral cavity, the kind of look that will certainly preclude discovering anything amiss, and you will simultaneously utter that most placid noise of bovine compliance.

For Obamacare to work, you will need to accept that the quality of healthcare you are receiving is precisely the high quality the Central Authority insists you are receiving, which is to say, the highest quality that can possibly exist - despite the obvious evidence you may notice (if you are of a mind to notice) that it is not.

Most of the people who will run Obamacare, we must realize, will not be lying to us. They actually will believe what they are saying. They fully expect us to believe it, too, and they will become quite exercised if they begin to perceive we do not. Here, an analogy to religion (which will be a recurring theme in this book) is apropos.

When something horrible has happened to you or a loved one, your pastor is likely to tell you that we must all trust that God has a plan, and that in God's plan what seems very bad to us today must always serve God's higher (if hidden) purpose. And we must have faith that someday, when it is all done, we will understand that higher purpose. And we will rejoice.

Similarly, when we think we see something terribly awry with the healthcare we or our loved ones are receiving (or not receiving, as the case may be), we will be exhorted to trust that the Central Authority also has a plan that serves a higher purpose. And just as true believers will be rewarded with God's higher purpose in the end, so will the Good Citizen, by and by, be rewarded by the fruits of the Central Authority's own supreme plan (as long as he or she does not become too disabled or too dead to appreciate it).

It is critical to understand that Obamacare, or for that matter, any Progressive program for societal improvement, simply will not work without your full buy-in and full cooperation - without your right thinking and right action. For this reason the Central Authority is very, very interested in making sure you develop these proper ways of thinking and acting.

Right thinking, in essence, is faith that the enlightened expertise embodied within the Central Authority knows what is best, for us as individuals and for all. And right action is complying, without complaint, with that central judgment. (For practical purposes, of course, right action will suffice all by itself, as long as you refrain from expressing too publicly your not-right thinking.)

The utter inability of most people to comply with these simple (but non-negotiable) requirements is precisely why no Progressive program for societal improvement, anywhere, has ever worked well for a very long time.

The closest that Progressive policies have ever come to realizing the universally beneficial ends which Progressives always promise has likely been in the Scandinavian countries. Here, the trauma of the World War II experience, combined with a homogenous population sharing a deeply-felt common goal, resulted in a generation of citizens who were truly dedicated to the attitudes, thoughts, and actions (specifically, working hard and tirelessly for the good of the whole), which were needed to make their collective society a success. Their children's generation was slightly less dedicated to selfless action for the sake of the collective. Their grand-children's generation seems far less so. Today, even Scandinavian socialism is fraying, at least around the edges.

Perhaps three generations of Good Citizens is the most Progressivism can hope for, even under the most favorable of conditions.

In any case, we in the United States are now committed to Obamacare. And even if some unexpected political upheaval should cause our political leaders to overturn this legislation, odds are high that shortly thereafter we will just end up with Obamacare II (or, more accurately, Hillarycare III), or some other form of Progressive healthcare.

And given the fact that we will all be enjoying our healthcare from now on under Obamacare (or its equally Progressive successor), it behooves us to understand what, exactly, our new healthcare system will require from each of us in order to function as it is intended. These requirements, whether we choose to understand them or not, will turn out to have a major influence over all of our lives (and limbs). But by understanding the requirements which are being placed upon us, then we can each decide whether we will be a Good Citizen - or something else. (While it may not always be easy or pleasant - or perhaps legal - there is always a something else.) So, a main goal of this book is to explore the requirements placed upon all Good Citizens by a Progressive healthcare system - what those requirements are, why they are non-negotiable, and what our options may be, as individuals, relative to them.

If Obamacare is a terrible mistake, as I believe it is, when we chose it (through our confirmatory voting in 2012, if not before) we at least made an explicit recognition that the status-quo is no longer feasible. It is infeasible because even our pre-Obamacare out-of-control healthcare spending promised to trigger societal destruction within a few decades. But the cure we have chosen - moving to a Progressive healthcare system - is likely even worse than the disease. I hope to show why this is so, and perhaps to convince a few people that, before it is too late, we ought to explore a different option for bringing fiscal sanity to our healthcare system.

Unfortunately, our window of opportunity to change paths is closing quickly. Once Obamacare (or any Progressive healthcare system) moves beyond a certain point, entropy will dictate that it cannot be undone, short of the traditional method for un-doing the various massive, elaborate, Byzantine constructions mankind is perpetually inventing, which is to say, via total societal upheaval. So time is of the essence.

This book is divided into three parts.

In Part 1, I will discuss how and why it looks (so far, at least) like we are going to end up with a Progressive healthcare system. I will consider the fiscal black hole our healthcare system has become, and show why some fundamental change in American healthcare has been inevitable for years (whether we take purposeful action to effect such change or not). I will describe the four ways it is possible to get healthcare costs under control. (Yes, there are four.) (And yes, there are only four.) Of these four, we as a nation have chosen the Progressive solution, since its proponents can always make it sound the least painful. For this reason I will end Part 1 by considering the general Progressive program for societal perfection, a program which will determine the chief characteristics of our new healthcare system.

In Part 2, I will survey what we can expect Obamacare to look like once it is fully rolled out. I will examine its basic tenets, and the implications and mechanics of the herd medicine it will impose. I will consider the kinds of things we will experience personally when we seek healthcare (or are ordered to get some) under Obamacare. Finally, I will survey some of the bigger-picture aspects of Obamacare, such as "life-cycle" medicine (i.e., aged-based priorities for healthcare), and how and why Progressives will stifle medical progress.

Part 3 can be entirely skipped by anyone who likes what they've read about Obamacare in Parts 1 and 2. (Your right action, in placing this book aside, should go a long way toward paying your penance for picking this book up in the first place.) Part 3 will examine what we can do, as individuals and as groups, to protect ourselves from some of the hazards of Obamacare, to reverse its most odious parts, and even to begin to construct a replacement healthcare system that might avoid the fatal flaws not only of Obamacare itself, but also of the Pre-Obamacare system of healthcare which has led us to it.

None of this, I understand, constitutes a particularly happy message. So I will try to keep it relatively light, employing along the way a bit of irony, sarcasm, wry humor, perhaps some puns (though very few if I have anything to say about it), and in general my sunny disposition. Just keep in mind, amidst all the merriment, that we are still pretty much screwed, unless we decide to do something about it.

PART 1 - PROGRESSIVE HEALTHCARE, AND WHY WE HAVE CHOSEN IT

CHAPTER 1 - RUN FOR THE HILLS, AS WE ARE ALL DOOMED!

"The good news is that we know more about the economics of health care than we did when Clinton tried and failed to remake the system."
- Paul Krugman

I originally meant to call this chapter, "Healthcare Economics," but I decided that name would frighten people off.

Everyone (that is, everyone with an ounce of common sense) is frightened by economics. Economics is the index case of what happens when you attempt to apply mathematics and the language of science to what is essentially a study of human behavior. (Microeconomics, as I understand it, attempts to study the behavior of one or two guys at a time; macroeconomics purports to study the behavior of everyone, all at once.)

Human behavior will stymie anyone who tries to understand it, let alone predict it, or especially control it. (Even God, according to Genesis, became so frustrated with human behavior that on at least one occasion he was moved to wipe just about everybody out and start over. And all to no avail, one must note.)

And so economists, having dedicated their lives to studying something that intrinsically surpasses all understanding – such that even astrophysicists seem closer to their goal of understanding what happened before the Big Bang than economists are to theirs – are reduced to devising massive, complex and unlikely constructs of mathematical clockwork only they can understand, with which to pummel one another in professional meetings, in peer-reviewed publications, and on CNBC.

Oh, and they also advise our political leaders.

So I have called this chapter by a name that is far less alarming than "Healthcare Economics," and that I hope will not send readers scurrying away. Besides, the name I have chosen is at least partially true. For it seems reasonably likely that we are indeed all doomed, though heading for the hills probably will not help very much.

Assuming that we can avoid the Really Bad doomsday scenarios that are always out there (collisions with asteroids, nuclear war, electromagnetic pulses, sudden ice ages, etc.), then the thing that is most likely to produce among us the renting of clothes, gnashing of teeth, heaping of ashes upon heads, and other behaviors commonly associated with the End Times, is the fiscal black hole we've made of our healthcare spending.

Our healthcare spending is sufficiently out-of-control that it produces a real threat to our survival as a society, and within many of our lifetimes. It was largely the effort to control this runaway spending that led us to adopt

Obamacare in the first place, even though Obamacare (as I hope to demonstrate) promises to be just as destructive itself.

In the first five chapters of this book that comprise Part 1, I aim to show how our healthcare system's dire fiscal problems have led us to choose a Progressive healthcare "solution." Here in Chapter 1, I will describe the astounding magnitude of our healthcare system's financial mess, and how we have created it. In Chapters 2 and 3, I will survey some of the incredibly harmful changes we have made to our healthcare system in an attempt to cope with the fiscal mess. These changes have caused so much damage that, when it was time to try to choose among the four possible methods for bringing the costs of healthcare under control (which are described in Chapter 4), we finally acceded to the Progressive solution for which many of our elected representatives had been pining at least since the time of the Clintons. Accordingly, in Chapter 5 I will discuss the Progressive program in general, and show why control over our healthcare is the lynchpin to the Progressives' overarching plans for all of us.

THE FISCAL GOLDEN AGE OF HEALTHCARE

Once Upon A Time, when people received a service from a physician, they paid for it themselves. Physicians who wanted to maintain a viable practice would keep their prices within the reach of their patients. And if somebody could not pay they would typically accept a reduced fee, or even a couple of chickens in exchange. During this time, healthcare was not considered a crisis, or a right, or even very important in the lives of most people.

I call this the Lancing Boils And Getting Paid In Chickens era of healthcare. It was the dark age of medicine - there was generally very little a doctor could do for you, other than lance those boils, set some but not all broken bones, and hasten your demise with leeches and bleeding. (At this point we must say a prayer of thanks that Progressives care very little about history, and so are relatively unlikely to re-discover the benefits of leeches and bleeding.) But while it was the dark age of medicine, it was the Golden Age of healthcare finance. Healthcare in those times accounted for none of our (or anyone's) national, collective debt.

Even when inhaled anesthesia first came into common usage - making various surgical procedures such as appendectomies and Caesarian sections routinely available for the first time - the cost of healthcare was not considered a major societal problem. Somehow, arrangements were made to reimburse doctors for their services, whether through cash payments, barter, or some sort of Victorian E-Z payment plan, thus allowing the patient to avoid destitution, and most doctors to avoid the sundry nefarious activities that have always been available to cash-strapped medics.

Indeed, right up until World War II, when penicillin was discovered, physicians and their skills could offer relatively little benefit for most serious illnesses beyond the surgical variety. As a result, relatively little money was spent on healthcare. And by the traditional means of barter or negotiated settlements, or the more modern means of charity hospitals, hospitals run for their employees by the big railroad and lumber companies, or in the later years, fledgling Blue Cross plans, all the medical services that were considered useful were somehow paid for on an as-you-go basis. There was no fiscal burden placed upon society. And all was well - at least fiscally.

THE MEDICAL GOLDEN AGE

Conservative Americans can rant and rave about it all they want, but the fact is undeniable that the remarkable advances we've seen in American healthcare over the past 50 - 60 years were ushered in by a new fiscal era - an era in which we began to pay our healthcare costs collectively.

This new era was begun during World War II, when companies began offering health insurance to their employees in order to attract workers during the wage controls then in effect. Health insurance proved so popular that Congress changed the tax laws to make the insurance premiums paid by employers tax-deductible so as to encourage the practice, and before very long virtually every company provided health insurance to their employees as a matter of course.

The tax-deductibility of employer-provided health insurance was the game-changer. Healthcare costs suddenly were no longer borne entirely by individuals, or by individual businesses which paid the insurance premiums. Instead, they were distributed among the American taxpayers, whose taxes had to make up for the insurance deductions taken by businesses. So-called "private" health insurance became publicly subsidized.

The public funding of healthcare advanced by a giant step with the institution of Medicare and Medicaid in 1965, which amounted to direct public funding of healthcare for a large proportion of the population. So, by 1970, most of American healthcare was paid for by the taxpayer either directly, or indirectly through subsidized private insurance. We had largely collectivized the financing of our healthcare.

While most of my conservative friends would like to think otherwise, when you look at the big picture it becomes apparent that this collectivization of healthcare financing has not been the unmitigated disaster they like to claim. There have been substantial benefits, and chief among these is the incredible progress we've made in medical learning and medical technology over the past half century.

In fact, this taxpayer subsidization of healthcare catalyzed an incredible golden age of medicine.

It turns out that, the moment everything that is deemed "healthcare" is "covered" by taxpayer-supplied or taxpayer-subsidized health insurance, and therefore payment is guaranteed for virtually any medical product by the full faith and credit of the United States government, a huge amount of investment money suddenly appears to fund research and development in every aspect of medicine you can imagine. And the next thing you know, you've got medical progress.

Medical entrepreneurs figured out in about a minute and a half that to be successful, all they had to do was to come up with a product that offered a measurable benefit to some group of people with some illness - no matter how marginal that benefit might be, or how expensive their product - and they were certain to have a ready market for their product and a customer who would pay the going rate without complaint. The more products you could develop, the greater your profits. And so R&D budgets went through the roof.

An utter explosion in medical progress, virtually all of it arising in the United States, began in the 1950s and 1960s, and really accelerated in the 1970s when Medicare was up and running full-bore. With a bit of sputtering, it continues until this day. Except for the Manhattan Project and the moon shot (whose fruits medical researchers strongly relied upon in doing their work), the kind of concentrated scientific effort that was applied to advance the science of medicine during this interval is unsurpassed in human history.

And like the Manhattan Project and the moon shot, it was ultimately funded by the taxpayer.

The medical technology that has been developed since the 1950s has done immeasurable good. Uncountable heart attacks and strokes have been prevented or aborted; cancers have been cured or beaten back; people who formerly would have been crippled can conduct normal daily activities without assistance; and some scourges of mankind (such as smallpox and polio) have been nearly vanquished altogether.

But there is a problem. Coincident with this explosion in medical progress has been an explosion in medical spending, spending to such a degree that, unless we bring it under control, we are headed for societal chaos.

THE MAGNITUDE OF THE PROBLEM

A fundamental principle in economics is that when we are buying consumable products that we are consuming ourselves - like Caribbean cruises, sports cars, ice cream, or healthcare - we should spend no more on those products than we individuals are able to pay ourselves.

I realize that by adding healthcare to this list I have probably angered a lot of readers. But I assure you that I am not making a political statement here; I am simply stating an economic principle, which (as is the unfortunate case with principles) is inherently true even if inconvenient.

It is certainly true that some societies, including ours, have decided to purchase some of these consumable products (healthcare, for instance) collectively, so that individuals don't pay for them at all. And the collective purchase of consumables constitutes a somewhat different situation that I will address in a moment.

But for consumable products that everyone agrees ought to be paid for by the individual (let's just take Caribbean cruises as a relatively non-controversial example), the individual must arrange to cover the cost. The reason for this principle is obvious. If individuals could arbitrarily decide to go on a cruise whenever they'd like, but leave the cost to others who have no say in whether the cruise takes place, the economic system would soon collapse.*

---

*Like most laws, principles, and ethical mandates, this one can be systematically violated by certain, small, well-defined groups of people without crashing the whole system, as long as the rest of the population (for whatever reason) decides to overlook, tacitly approve of, and pay for the irresponsible behavior of this elite group. I am referring, of course, to our political leaders.

But what about those societies which have decided to purchase collectively certain products and services (like healthcare) that are consumed by individuals? It turns out that these societies must operate under a very similar economic principle: A society should spend no more on products which are consumed by individual citizens than it can pay without incurring long-term, multi-generational debt.

In the United States as we have seen, we have decided to pay for healthcare collectively. Whether your healthcare is provided directly through government payments or through tax-deductible insurance premiums, to a great extent society is collectively footing the bill.

This would not be a problem, economically, if we were doing it on a pay-as-you-go basis. But we're not. We're running a huge national debt today, and largely because of healthcare obligations that debt will reach stupendous proportions in the foreseeable future.

Reasonable people can argue over whether having a large national debt is good or bad, but the answer lies at least partially in what it is that the debt has been incurred to pay for.

The ability to borrow money, and carry debt, is important to a vibrant economy. Individuals can borrow even large amounts of money as long as they promise to pay it back and their credit rating is sufficiently high. But if a person fails to pay back what they owe according to a predetermined schedule, society takes steps to stop further borrowing and to force them to repay. If they get in too deep, society ushers them into bankruptcy, and allows them to slowly make themselves whole again. But society does *not* allow them to simply keep borrowing indefinitely.

This is because individuals die. If we were to allow individuals to simply accumulate as much debt as they want until they die, leaving it to somebody else to pay it back, the economic system would soon disintegrate. So before people can borrow money, they need to demonstrate their ability to repay it, or to have their estates repay it upon their death. In this way there is a natural limit to how much individuals can spend on consumable products in their lifetime.

Societies, like individuals, must borrow no more than they can eventually pay back. The difference is that, unlike individuals, society lives "forever." That is, the accumulation of debt that cannot be paid off in a single generation is not necessarily alarming, because society will "always" be there to pay it off.

As it turns out, the ability to accumulate even huge amounts of debt is vital for complex societies like ours, as it permits us to maintain a buffer for economic stability, to smooth out boom-bust cycles, and to maintain reasonable predictability and encourage steady growth. The ability to carry multi-generational debt enables the government to borrow the money it needs to make multi-generational investments, things like building up the nation's infrastructure, providing for national defense, advancing medical research, and engaging in other forms of non-commodity spending that will allow society to progress, to grow stronger, and to steadily improve the lives of successive generations of its citizens.

The "right" kind of long-term national debt, then, is a chief enabler of economic growth and prosperity, an investment in the nation's future. It is appropriate to ask future generations of Americans to share the financial burden of that debt, since they will reap the benefits of the investment.

Things go very wrong, however, when we burden society with the "wrong" kind of debt, the kind that represents an open-ended promise to purchase products and services that are consumed by individuals, such as healthcare. There are two problems with this kind of debt.

First, this kind of debt is not an investment in the future, whose fruits will be realized by our children and grandchildren, and whose returns will more than compensate for the overall debt obligation. Instead, it benefits only the individuals currently alive who are the direct recipients of the consumable services, leaving no direct benefits but only an ever-increasing debt burden to those who will be left paying the bills decades later.

Second, while there is a natural limit on how much an individual can spend for products and services they consume during their lifetime, once the responsibility of paying for those consumables shifts to society there is no longer such a natural limit (since societies live forever). The debt can now be borne by multiple generations. Because there is no longer an inherent limit to what an individual can consume, and because it is to the advantage of present and would-be officeholders to eliminate any remaining arbitrary limits, individuals are eventually encouraged to consume as much as they want. And without these limits (either natural or imposed by rules) the provision of such services to individuals rapidly becomes an entitlement, whereupon the natural checks and balances that (in past times, at least) apply to other parts of the federal budget are no longer available.

When society faces an accelerating debt burden that is completely open-ended and is not subject to normal checks and balances, that society is dealing with a "disproportionate economic variable" (DEV) – that is, an economic obligation that grows without limit and completely out of proportion to the growth of the overall economy. Healthcare spending, which unrelentingly consumes an ever-increasing proportion of our GDP, is such a DEV.

DEV's are inherently destructive to a society, and for that reason they are typically rare. Indeed, in viable societies the only commonly encountered DEV is wartime spending, where a disproportionate amount of a society's wealth must be spent in the violent struggle for survival (or, alternatively, in the violent struggle to take away valuable resources of the opponent in order to power future growth, in which case war is sort of like a high-risk start-up). Indeed, the disproportionate spending in wartime is tolerable only because war itself is temporary. It should be noted, however, that one reason war is temporary is that in a prolonged war, a runaway DEV can cause a country to spend itself into oblivion. (See: the multi-decade Cold War and the demise of the Soviet Union.)

Until the time we began to collectivize our healthcare expenditures, healthcare spending in the United States acted like any well behaved economic sector. That is, until the 1950s healthcare spending remained at a steady 4% of the GDP. But by 1960, healthcare spending had become a DEV. Healthcare spending was at 5.3% of the GDP in 1960, 7.3% in 1970, 10.2% in 1980, 13% in 1993, 14.9% in 2002, and 17.6% of the GDP in 2009.

We already cannot afford to pay-as-we-go for all the healthcare we're consuming. Instead, we're violating that economic principle I mentioned earlier, and accumulating massive amounts of federal debt to cover the cost ($16 trillion at last count, enough that we're already flirting with fiscal brinkmanship), which we are leaving to future generations to figure out how to pay off. And it's about to get much worse.

Assuming we survive credit downgrades, the European debt crisis, oil disruptions in the Middle East, and other more routine difficulties, the most immediate fiscal threat to our economic survival becomes apparent when you think about all the expensive medical technology we've managed to accumulate over the last 50 years, and imagine applying it to our rapidly aging population, that is, to the baby boomer generation – which (I can personally assure you) is planning to make exuberant use of all this stuff. The magnitude of this problem is actually pretty easy to estimate.

Consider: All the people who will constitute our population of Old Farts for the next 30 years (a group which claims your humble author as a member) are alive today. We can count them. We can also enumerate with fair accuracy the quantity of many of the various illnesses and ailments they will suffer - the strokes, heart attacks, heart failures, Alzheimer's disease, hip replacements, cancer, drooping body parts and ED. And we can estimate reasonably closely (if our leaders succeed in stifling medical progress, and therefore medical technology is held at its current level) what kinds of drugs, devices, nursing care and other expensive medical appurtenances they will require. And with this information we can add up all the sums and multiply all the multipliers to estimate what it's all going to cost us.

Indeed, the GAO has done this. It's looking like it will cost $30 - 40 trillion over the next several decades, just to cover the medical entitlements which we have promised current and not-too-distant-future older Americans, Americans who have themselves been paying taxes for many years, and who have arranged their affairs according to the expectations created by those promises.

That's way more money than it will take to cause societal collapse.

CAN'T WE JUST ELIMINATE WASTE AND INEFFICIENCY?

In Chapter 4, I will talk about the four ways that are available to reduce this dangerous level of healthcare expenditures. You may be surprised to learn that none of these four methods is to eliminate all the waste and inefficiency in our healthcare system.

I am in favor of eliminating waste and inefficiency, of course, and I applaud most efforts to do so. But eliminating waste and inefficiency did not make the list of four for a simple reason. It will not work. That is, even if we somehow got rid of all the wasted healthcare expenditures taking place today (and there truly is a tremendous amount of it), that won't be enough to rescue us from economic oblivion.

This is not a pleasant thing to hear, nor is it a common thing to hear. Indeed, it is a central assumption of all of the healthcare reform plans ever proposed that we can get our spending under control simply by eliminating - or at least substantially reducing - the vast amount of waste and inefficiency in the healthcare system. Conservatives propose to do this by incorporating the efficiencies of the marketplace, thus eliminating the waste and inefficiency imposed by government bureaucrats. Progressives propose to do it by adopting and enforcing strict, top-down regulations (ideally, through a single-payer system which employs the officially-perfect wisdom of various expert panels) that will control the wasteful and inefficient behaviors of greedy and/or ignorant healthcare providers. But one way or another, schemes for reforming healthcare all propose to bring spending under control by eliminating waste and inefficiency.

Another way of describing what all the reformers across the political spectrum are telling us is: There is so much waste in the system that we can avoid healthcare rationing by getting rid of it. Most Americans believe this. Most policy experts believe this. They have to believe it, because nobody wants to even think about healthcare rationing.

But this is unfortunately false. No matter how much waste and inefficiency you think might be gumming up our healthcare system today, there is not enough to explain the uncontrolled rise in healthcare spending we have been seeing for decades, and therefore, not enough to allow us to avoid rationing altogether in any economically feasible, publicly funded healthcare system.

To understand why this is the case, we must first recognize the fundamental problem with our healthcare spending. The real problem is not simply that we're spending a lot of money on healthcare, or even that we're spending a larger proportion of our GDP on healthcare than any other country. If that's all the problem was, we could with modest difficulty adjust the rest of our spending to accommodate it, and get our national budget under control that way.

Rather, the real problem is that our healthcare expenditures constitute a particularly deadly DEV. Specifically, for decades those expenditures have been growing at double digit rates, several multiples faster than the overall inflation rate, and each year consume an ever-greater proportion of our national spending. Unless this disproportionate rate of growth is stopped, eventually healthcare spending will cannibalize our entire economy. (What will really happen, of course, is that the debt we are accumulating to pay for our healthcare will grow to the point of producing societal upheaval, sending us back to a more typical era for mankind, where healthcare is a little-thought-of luxury, and not a necessity or a right. This will happen well before healthcare consumes 100% of the economy.)

To reiterate, it is not the amount of spending on healthcare that is creating a fiscal crisis, it is the rate of growth of that spending.

Once we understand the problem – that it is the rate of growth of healthcare spending that threatens our society – then demonstrating that waste and inefficiency cannot possibly account for that rate of growth is a matter of simple mathematics.

There are only two things that can possibly account for the excessive growth rate of our healthcare expenditures. Either it is caused by unrelenting growth in wasteful spending (as we are assured by our political leaders), or it is caused by unrelenting growth in useful healthcare spending. If it is the latter, then in order to get spending under control in a collectivized payment system we must cut back on or ration useful healthcare. This is why we all fervently pray, and most of us choose to fervently believe, the excess rate of growth must be caused by wasted spending.

This desired conclusion, unfortunately, leads to mathematical absurdities, and therefore (for anyone who eschews magical thinking) turns out to be utterly false.

I am going to show you some data from a spreadsheet. It is a spreadsheet that illustrates what would have to happen in order for wasteful spending to account for our current level of healthcare inflation. The spreadsheet is based on the following four assumptions:

Assumption 1) The annual growth rate of spending on useful healthcare (discussed further below) is economically well-behaved. That is, it matches the rate of overall inflation. The spreadsheet therefore assumes a 3% annual inflation rate for useful healthcare spending.

Please note that this is the very assumption which politicians invoke whenever they say that all we need to do to control healthcare costs is to eliminate waste and inefficiency. In fact, the whole point of this spreadsheet is to test the logic of this assumption. For, if useful healthcare spending is not economically well-behaved, then eliminating all the wasteful spending would still leave us with disproportionate healthcare inflation.

Assumption 2) 25% of healthcare expenditures at Year 1 of this spreadsheet are wasteful. I have picked 25% arbitrarily, a value that happens to fall within the range of popular estimates. As it turns out, the initial value we choose for the level of wasteful spending at Year 1 in this spreadsheet has very little influence over the outcome. So if you don't like this number, feel free to pick your own.

Assumption 3) The annual rate of growth of overall healthcare spending (i.e., healthcare inflation) is 10%. This is a rough average of what we have actually seen for the last few decades.

Assumption 4) Total healthcare inflation is the sum of healthcare inflation due to the growth of "well-behaved," useful healthcare spending, and the healthcare inflation accounted for by spending on waste and inefficiency. Given that the inflation rate for useful healthcare spending is 3% (Assumption 1), this spreadsheet simply calculates the cumulative annual inflation rate for wasteful spending that would be necessary to account for an overall rate of healthcare inflation of 10% (Assumption 3).

Before I show you the spreadsheet, we should discuss the difference between "wasteful" and "useful" healthcare. In actual practice, this is not a distinction which is straightforward. It depends, for one thing, on who gets to define "wasteful." If I am a 92-year-old man who gets a $12,000 stent procedure to eliminate my angina, I and my doctor might consider it money well-spent, while you might consider it wasteful.

But for the purposes of this present analysis, I am defining "wasteful" healthcare in the way our politicians define it – or at least in the way they want us to think they are defining it. That is, wasteful healthcare is completely wasteful - it is a totally useless expenditure, and is no more beneficial than flushing money down the toilet. In contrast, useful healthcare is that which is likely to provide at least some of its intended benefit to patients.

Any other definition of useful vs. wasteful healthcare would require us to place a value judgment on just how much benefit a healthcare service must provide before we consider it to be useful, and thus worthy of paying for. Another name for such a process is "rationing," and we all know that we're not going to do any rationing. No, sir.

So, the definition we must use for "useful" vs. "wasteful" healthcare, by process of elimination, can only be the definition I have just laid out.

Here is the spreadsheet:

YEAR	INDEX OF OVERALL DOLLARS SPENT	% WASTEFUL SPENDING	% OF ANNUAL INCREASE DUE TO USEFUL SPENDING	% OF ANNUAL INCREASE DUE TO WASTEFUL SPENDING
1	100	25	-	-
5	161	46	17	83
10	259	61	12	88
20	673	80	6	94

We can immediately see several things. First, as expected, the amount of money we're spending on healthcare, assuming a rate of healthcare inflation of 10%, is doubling roughly every 7-8 years. It's this growth rate that threatens our survival as a society.

Second, in order to account for this unsupportable growth in healthcare spending by invoking waste and inefficiency, the proportion of healthcare spending that is caused by waste must increase to ridiculous magnitudes very rapidly, such that (for instance) by the 10th year we will have more than doubled (61%) the proportion of all healthcare expenditures that are wasteful; and by the 20th year, as much as 80% must be wasteful.

Similarly, the proportion of the annual increases in healthcare spending that would have to be due to waste and inefficiency rapidly climbs to equally ridiculous magnitudes. By year 5, wasteful spending will have to account for 83% of the annual increase in healthcare expenditures, and that proportion continues to climb, eventually approaching 100%.

To me, these numbers seem absurd on their face. But if you still need to be convinced, consider that in real life, runaway healthcare inflation has already been taking place in the United States for decades - so our position on such a spreadsheet would not be at Year 1; we are much closer to Year 50. And no matter what value for wasteful spending we might have plugged in at Year 1, by Year 50 wasteful spending would have to be well above 80%, and more likely approaching 100%. In order for waste and inefficiency to account for the situation in which the American healthcare system finds itself today, therefore, one would have to believe that virtually all healthcare spending is wasteful. (And if you believe that, then solving the crisis would be a simple matter of discontinuing all healthcare.)

Now let us illustrate the same point in a slightly different way. This time, let's pretend that as recently as 2009, when President Obama was inaugurated, our healthcare system was 100% efficient. That is, only three years ago there was no waste whatsoever. Then let's allow that the remaining three assumptions given above are still operative. The following table results:

YEAR	INDEX OF OVERALL DOLLARS SPENT	% WASTEFUL SPENDING	% OF ANNUAL INCREASE DUE TO USEFUL SPENDING	% OF ANNUAL INCREASE DUE TO WASTEFUL SPENDING
2009	100	0	-	-
2010	110	7	30	70
2011	121	15	28	72
2012	133	17	26	74

We can see from these results that, even if only three years ago we had a completely efficient healthcare system, in order for waste to account for the excess growth in healthcare spending we've experienced since that time, then after just three years as much as 74% of today's annual increase in spending has to be due to waste and inefficiency.

Any way you cut it, the spreadsheet leads to nothing but absurdities. Assumption 1 - that useful healthcare spending is economically well-behaved - therefore cannot be true.

Wasted spending may and likely does account for a significant proportion of our healthcare expenditures, but it simply cannot account for the sustained, disproportional growth in healthcare expenditures that threatens to collapse the system.

So yes, by all means, let's try to eliminate waste and inefficiency from our healthcare system. But if we hope to survive as a culture, we will, at the same time and as an entirely separate endeavor, have to figure out how to get the growth in useful healthcare spending under control.

SUMMARY

It is critical to understand that a fundamental, nearly intractable, doomsday-magnitude fiscal problem with our healthcare spending preceded Obamacare, and continues today despite Obamacare. Simply getting rid of Obamacare would not fix the underlying problem.

CHAPTER 2 - THE DEMISE OF THE HEALTH INSURANCE INDUSTRY

"The committee's investigation found that WellPoint's Blue Cross targeted individuals with more than 1,400 conditions, including breast cancer, lymphoma, pregnancy and high blood pressure. And the committee obtained documents that showed Blue Cross supervisors praised employees in performance reviews for rescinding policies. One employee, for instance, received a perfect 5 for 'exceptional performance' on an evaluation that noted the employee's role in dropping thousands of policyholders and avoiding nearly $10 million worth of medical care."

- Los Angeles Times, June 17, 2009

I fear that, in Chapter 1, I may have left you with the impression that our healthcare expenses have been piling up for the past 50 years, to the point where our entire culture is about to collapse under the weight, without anyone or any organization doing anything about it.

If so, I apologize, for nothing could be further from the truth. In fact, our healthcare expenses have been piling up for the past 50 years, to the point where our entire culture is about to collapse under the weight, in spite of the heroic efforts on the part of our health insurance companies, our doctors, and our government to stem those costs.

Indeed, their efforts have been little short of astounding. The health insurance industry has driven itself upon the shoals in a daring attempt to rescue our healthcare finances, and lies there today, foundering and needing rescue itself. Doctors have made what amounts to a suicide attack against the rising costs, essentially throwing away the very essence of their own profession in the attempt, and leaving for posterity a signed suicide note. And our government – well, our government of course has tremendous resources, and has spent or pledged the lifetime earnings of the next three or four generations of its citizens in what appears to be an entirely fruitless effort to bring healthcare costs under control. (Our leaders assure us they feel very badly about this, however.)

So it's not for lack of trying. It's that what they have all been trying – namely, covertly rationing our healthcare – not only does not and cannot work, but also intrinsically makes things much worse.

This and the next chapter will demonstrate the sorry state to which such misguided efforts to control costs have reduced our healthcare system and its participants – and well before Obamacare ever came along.

A BIT ON COVERT HEALTHCARE RATIONING

I have been writing a blog for six years about the covert rationing of America's healthcare, so there is plenty I could say about this. However, I will limit myself, with exquisite difficulty no doubt, to just saying what covert rationing is and why it's a problem.

First, let's be clear on the definition of healthcare rationing. *To ration healthcare is to intentionally withhold at least some useful medical services from at least some of the people who would benefit from them.*

To ration covertly is to do the above without admitting to it, and most often while indignantly denying it.

I will not go into an exhaustive argument here to "prove" we're rationing our healthcare covertly, or that covert rationing intrinsically wastes far more money than it can ever save. I have done that elsewhere. Instead, I will simply lay out a 3-point thesis which makes it intuitively obvious that covert rationing is what we're doing, and that by doing it we're compounding the underlying fiscal problem.

Point #1: Healthcare rationing is a fiscal imperative. Rationing is fundamentally unavoidable, and therefore, we are not avoiding it.

In any advanced society, where a centralized agency of one species or another creates a pool of money from which most of the society's healthcare bills are to be paid, whether that pool of money is controlled by the government, or by private insurance companies, or by some combination of these, then even if that centralized agency is very large, very powerful, and very coercive, and even if that agency is able to borrow (say) trillions and trillions of dollars, there will always be limits on how much money can be placed into the pool. On the other hand, the amount of money that could conceivably be spent to purchase every bit of all the available, potentially useful healthcare for every individual in the population who might benefit from it is essentially limitless.

This limited supply, and limitless demand, means that somebody, somewhere, will not receive all the available healthcare that would be potentially useful to them. So rationing is occurring. Q.E.D.

Point #2: We're Americans, and Americans don't ration. So the unavoidable rationing must be, and is being, done covertly.

An endearing trait of Americans, endearing to us Americans at least, is our limitless optimism, our undying belief that anything good that we can imagine can, and will, and must actually be accomplished. This refusal to recognize limits is responsible for much of the creativity, inventiveness, and productivity that has come from our American culture. And it has led to much good in the world, resulting, for instance, in most of the remarkable advances in healthcare we've seen over the past half-century.

The American culture of no limits, however, can be carried to counterproductive extremes. And that is what has happened with regard to healthcare.

Our "no limits" attitude about healthcare is typically American. It goes like this:

In America we have, and will continue to have, the best healthcare in the world – the best doctors, the best hospitals, and the best technology. Since one cannot place a price on a human life, anything that can be done for a sick person must be done, as long as there is some small hope of even a tiny benefit. Every disease is potentially curable, and as a matter of policy we will strive to learn how to cure every disease that exists (and when we run out of diseases to cure, we'll invent new ones). Indeed, death itself is merely a manifestation of insufficient technology.

In summary, where healthcare is concerned, there are, and can be, no limits.

We can see the problem right away. While we have inherent spending limitations that unavoidably require healthcare rationing, we find that there can be no limits, and therefore, no rationing. Indeed, there can be no discussion of rationing, except to bitterly condemn the very idea. Any political leader or policymaker who would seriously suggest the idea of healthcare rationing would run squarely into this deeply ingrained culture of no limits, and would immediately become toast.

So, these two basic imperatives shaping our healthcare system – the unavoidable need to ration that will always accompany publicly-funded healthcare, and the culture of no limits – are, in their essence, completely incompatible with one another. Given our deep-seated need to simultaneously cling to both of these incompatible imperatives, our only option is to do the unavoidable rationing in a way that allows us to deny that rationing is occurring; in a way that allows us to ration while declaring that there are no limits. We can ration secretly. We can ration deceptively. We can ration covertly.

And (QED) that is what we are doing.

Point #3: Covert healthcare rationing is inherently and extravagantly destructive, not only to patients and their doctors, and not only to the healthcare system, but also to our national budget, and to our basic American social contract.

While there are plenty of problems with the American healthcare system, the truly intractable ones are intractable largely because of our need to ration covertly. As long as the need to ration healthcare covertly exists, these problems will persist.

By its very nature covert healthcare rationing is a deeply ironic construction. The whole purpose of rationing is to reduce spending on healthcare, and to control costs. But covert rationing (ironically) always increases expenditures. If we could ration healthcare openly, then it would be at least possible that we could arrange, or at least try to arrange, the rationing in such a way as to optimize the efficiency, effectiveness and equity within our healthcare system.

But rationing covertly fundamentally means rationing in whatever way you can get away with. So, in order to hide the rationing, it is imperative to obfuscate, misdirect, complicate, juke, jive, shimmy and shake and do whatever else you must to convince everyone – often including yourself – that whatever it is you're doing, it's not rationing. That is, you've got to create an environment of complexity and opacity in which you can get away with it.

As a direct result of this simple truth, simplicity, transparency and efficiency are lethal to a system based on covert rationing, and thus, are systematically rooted out. Covert rationing absolutely requires opaque processes and procedures, superfluous complexity, bizarre incentives, Byzantine regulations which are arbitrarily enforced or ignored in various times and places, astoundingly wasteful transactions, and the diversion of healthcare dollars to a complex host of non-healthcare ends, such as commissions, study groups and panels, various czars of this and that, ever-expanding layers of government bureaucracies, and the establishment of other massive bureaucracies within the healthcare system whose purpose is to defend against or manipulate those aggressive government bureaucracies. Covert rationing, by its very nature, demands and creates waste within our healthcare system, and therefore costs us far more money than it can ever save us.

So, while the fiscal mess in which we find our healthcare system is destined to screw all of us, by attempting to fix it with covert rationing we're converting a simple screwing into a gang rape.

It will be instructive to have a look at how this has all worked out.

A RECENT HISTORY OF AMERICAN HEALTHCARE (CONTINUED)

It did not take long after the institution of Medicare and Medicaid in 1965 for astute economists and politicians to realize that, perhaps, we had just stepped off a financial cliff.

Smart people became alarmed about healthcare spending as early as 1970, when we were spending a "mere" 7% of our GDP on healthcare (a little more than a third of the proportion we're spending now). And indeed, in 1972 Richard Nixon, demonstrating in yet another way that not all Progressives are Democrats, planned to propose in his second term a universal healthcare system. (So perhaps if those Progressives who today are so desperate for one hadn't made such a big deal about Watergate, they would have had their heart's desire 40 years ago.)

After Nixon was deposed, Gerald Ford got distracted trying to "Whip Inflation Now;" Jimmy Carter busied himself actually whipping inflation to heights not seen since the Weimar Republic; Ronald Regan dedicated himself to spending the Soviet Union into oblivion; and George Bush 41 beat up Sadam Hussein and raised taxes while trying not to move his lips. You know, stuff happened.

And the next thing you know it was 1992 and healthcare spending had nearly doubled as a proportion of the GDP since the time of Nixon.

Subsequently, the Clintons took up healthcare reform as their signature issue. Bill turned the effort over to Hillary because (as he explained it) she was smarter than he was, but some say possibly also as a reward for her amazing loyalty in the face of, well, you know.

In any case, at the beginning of the Clintons' effort to reform healthcare, they had the goodwill and support of most Americans, of doctors, the media, and most importantly, the American health insurance industry. Hillary appeared to start off well, making a successful appearance before Congress, and, with great fanfare, convening numerous expert panels and other groups to gather their ideas, suggestions, and recommendations on healthcare reform, as if she intended to take them into account. Optimism was high.

But Hillary is a true Progressive, and so she already knew how to reform healthcare. Having made a great show of democratizing the process, she then retreated behind closed doors with a few hand-selected advisors, and soon emerged with a 1300 page bill of her own devising – Hillarycare.

Many were horrified by what was in that bill, which in fact gave the government full control of our healthcare system. Not the least among the newly-horrified were executives of the health insurance industry, who to that moment had been major supporters. They realized that if any law passed that was remotely like Hillarycare, their industry would soon become infeasible if not illegal. And so, acting with the alacrity of people who are in imminent mortal danger, the insurers quickly introduced the American people to Harry and Louise, a typical middle class couple who were depicted, in print ads and on TV, discovering numerous appalling provisions of the Clinton plan.

The rest was history.

The collapse of the Clintons' reform plan caused a sudden deflation in Americans' expectations, but the fiscal crisis remained. In fact, the one thing the Hillarycare effort had indeed accomplished was to create a general awareness among the public that the healthcare system was in dire financial straits, and that business as usual was not an option. And nobody (except for the doctors, wallowing as usual in wishful thinking) believed things could simply go back to the way they were before.

Into the breach stepped the very health insurance industry that had just torpedoed Hillarycare. And they had a plan.

"Citizens!" they said, "We have just dodged a bullet. Thanks to us, the frightening socialist reforms of the Clintons have been soundly defeated. But where does this leave us? We stand now between Scylla and Charybdis, between the specter of nationalized healthcare on one hand, and continued, wasteful, traditional fee-for-service medicine on the other. And we cannot countenance either.

"But wait! Here is a third way, a painless way, based on the sound principles of managed care, open markets, and free enterprise. Let us in the health insurance industry, successful businessmen all, wielding the tools of efficiency and sound business practices, step in and save the day. We will apply our proven tools and methods of efficiency to American healthcare, through our new vehicle for medical excellence – our for-profit HMOs. And we will demonstrate to the world the wonders that modern, free-market management principles can bring to American healthcare."

And not having any other viable choice that any of us could see, we Americans gave the go-ahead.

THE BRIEF BUT REMARKABLE ERA OF FOR-PROFIT HMOS

By this time, HMOs had been around, here and there, for 20 years. They were inventions of pipe-smoking, elbow-patched academics and other well-meaning naïfs, who envisioned user-friendly, non-profit organizations which, by inculcating their clientele to the benefits of good health habits, disease-prevention lifestyles, and regular check-ups would – you know – maintain the health of its members. Until the collapse of the Clinton health reforms, HMOs were widely regarded with some bemusement, as the typical sort of ineffectual but benign social engineering experiment you generally get from cloistered academics, or as an eccentric aunt puttering about the attic of the healthcare homestead.

The for-profit HMOs which the health insurance industry introduced to America after the fall of Hillarycare were a different species altogether. If you asked the CEO of one of the old-fashioned HMOs what the mission was, she would say something like, "Why, it's to maintain the good health of our clients, of course." Not so for the new-style HMOs. Their mission (quite explicitly, since this is the message they used to sell all of us on the idea of turning American healthcare over to them) was to apply the modern management techniques of American business to make American healthcare efficient at last. And how does one assure that such modern business techniques will be fully and enthusiastically applied? By doing what every business must do to be successful – by focusing like a laser beam on profitability.

So if you asked a 1990s, new-style HMO executive what was his mission, he would reply, "Why, it's to take this wasteful, inefficient puppy and turn it around into a profit-generating machine. Of course, as a spin-off you will get more efficient healthcare and the like. But the mission – and indeed the measure of our success, the evidence that we're making healthcare more efficient – is our profitability."

And with the mantra, "Profits = Efficiency" emblazoned on their standards, and with "Deus Lo Volt!" on their lips, the new-style HMOs went forth in the crusade to save American healthcare.

However, just as the real Crusaders became distracted on their way to the Holy Land by the opportunity to sack and pillage Constantinople, so did the HMOs become distracted by an unprecedented opportunity to sack every city, town and village in the land. Because it was the prospect of profits which would at last make American healthcare efficient, HMO executives argued, it only made sense for all the non-profit hospitals in America to be turned over to them. This way, the HMOs could incorporate those old, creaky, inefficient institutions into their new, machine-like, ultra-efficient, healthcare paradigm. When the city fathers and state commissioners of America seemed interested, the CEO would add, "We'll even pay you for them."

During the next six or seven years, virtually every non-profit healthcare organization in America – hospitals that had been owned and operated for decades by cities, counties, states, or religious organizations – were acquired by for-profit institutions. The way these transfers worked was: a) the hospital's board of trustees (many of whom later wound up with well-paying jobs with the acquiring HMO) would approve the transfer; b) the state insurance commissioner or state attorney general would determine the intrinsic value of the hospital; c) the HMO would reimburse the appropriate entity with the assessed amount of money, often by establishing a charitable foundation.

For reasons I cannot fathom, the state officials seemed congenitally unable to estimate, even within an order of magnitude or two, the true intrinsic value of the transferred asset. Only the hospital's value as a charity was considered, and not its potential as a business. They failed to consider the market value of trademarks, name recognition, decades of community goodwill, provider contracts, or subscriber lists. There were no competitive bidding processes; no formal valuations. So the new HMOs acquired thousands of major, publicly-held community assets, all across America, for pennies on the dollar.

If state officials were inefficient in this process, the markets were not. And the HMOs found that each time they acquired a formerly non-profit institution, the market would immediately reward them with a nice boost in their market valuations. HMOs suddenly became hot investment vehicles, and investors jumped in with their dollars. HMO executives were very, very happy.

This asset-acquisition phase of the for-profit HMOs was largely responsible for the great financial success these organizations enjoyed in the 1990s. And the hugely important story of the massive transfer of public assets to private companies went largely unreported.

Once they had gobbled up all the public hospitals, the for-profit HMOs immediately entered into a prolonged period of negotiated mergers with one another, thus consolidating the industry into a few massive players. This interval also produced large boosts in their market valuations, and it sustained the facade of corporate success for a few more years.

And that pretty much covers the glory years of the modern HMO. For a decade or so these companies were extremely successful, and performed very nicely for their shareholders. But their success, such as it was, had relatively little to do with their ability to make American healthcare more efficient. Rather, like those holy warriors who fought in the Fourth Crusade, their profits came mainly from sacking Constantinople, the city of their supposed allies and co-religionists.

To be sure, HMOs did work as hard as they could at improving healthcare efficiency during this period of time. They did this mainly by instituting efficiencies of scale. When you are managing several hospitals, or several scores of hospitals, you can streamline and consolidate your processes and procedures in some very big ways – with more pointed negotiations with vendors, for instance, or by computerizing and standardizing billing and ordering, or limiting drug formularies. You can also conduct fancy efficiency studies to show that, really, you could probably get away with an 8:1 nursing ratio instead of a 4:1 ratio. (By "get away with," apparently, the efficiency experts meant that while the "downside" of such cutbacks might be suspected or even perceived by people on the ground, it was unlikely that it could ever be accurately measured – or therefore, proven – by a few local troublemakers.)

So the efficiencies of mega-corporate bigness were broadly applied, and as a result, during the latter half of the 1990s we saw less healthcare inflation than during any 5-year period over the previous 30 years. But the thing about applying this kind of cost-cutting measure – the kind that is applied on a global basis to the whole system – is that it is a one-time event. That is, the savings are realized right away, and as a result you successfully establish a new and lower spending baseline. But because (as we saw in the last chapter) the rate of growth in healthcare spending is not caused by the inefficiencies you've just eliminated, the increase in healthcare spending will thereafter simply resume and continue apace (albeit from a lower baseline).

This is just what happened. By the turn of the century, healthcare inflation was headed back up into the double digits.

And so, if they had not realized it before, by the early 2000s it finally occurred to the HMO executives that, at long last, if they were going to remain profitable they were going to have to figure out how to cut healthcare costs by doing what they'd always told everyone they were so good at doing, but which they had never yet accomplished – actually managing the medical care of sick people.

This is when the panic began setting in.

Their panic was not inappropriate. For the HMOs had not been sitting on their hands when it came to making actual patient care less expensive. In fact, they had already tried everything they knew how to try – and it had not worked.

The business model of the HMO, simply put, is to gather the health insurance premiums from its subscribers, use that money to efficiently manage their healthcare, and keep whatever is left.

Therefore, to the HMO executive (the steely-eyed business executive we had all deputized to control our healthcare costs), the biggest risk to the business is: sick people.

Sick people are a huge problem. They are not subject to the usual "efficiencies" you can apply to most businesses. Simply streamlining business processes (admission and discharge procedures, consolidating laboratories, computerizing records and the like) does not work with sick people. You could implement these sorts of efficiencies all day long, and sick people will still be sick, and each one of them could blow through tens of thousands of your dollars each and every day.

Sick people, unlike the widgets which businesses typically process and manipulate to make their money, are not all alike. Each of them has a different constellation of medical problems, different needs, and different responses to testing and therapy. A medical service that makes Patient A recover in two days puts Patient B in the ICU for three weeks. Patients who recover enough to go home, but then stop taking their medications (or cannot afford to take them), or immediately resume an all-pizza-diet, will bounce right back in your hospital, and recommence consuming even more of your resources.

There can only be one answer to this problem. What you need to do is something you learned on your very first day of MBA school (where basically all you did was get your seat assignment, and eye-up the rest of the class to decide which ones you think you can work with and which ones you'll need to sabotage in order to smooth out the curve). Namely, eliminate unnecessary expenditures. Which means: you need to avoid the sick.

Find ways to keep the sick (or potentially sick) from enrolling in your HMO. For sick people who manage to make it through the obstacle course you are going to set up for them, you will need to find ways to make things so unpleasant for them that they'll go elsewhere. For the really sick who won't (or more likely, can't) leave, you'll need to find ways to just toss them out.

And so, naturally, this is what HMOs did.

They made their best insurance products available to employers only, on the theory that people who have jobs are less likely to have serious, chronic illnesses or severe disabilities, or addictions. The inferior, "individual" insurance products (when HMOs could not avoid them altogether) were pre-loaded with onerous pre-existing condition clauses, so that only healthy young people were likely to be eligible. When HMOs held "open enrollment" drives for Medicare patients, they were invariably located on the second or third floor of buildings without elevators, often in affluent suburbs or at country clubs, and in any case in places that were at least two bus transfers away from "undesirable" neighborhoods. Such methods came to be known as "skimming" or cherry-picking, and were aimed at avoiding the sickest 10% of the population that accounts for 75% of all healthcare spending.

Sometimes, despite increasingly sophisticated cherry-picking techniques, a sick person would still get through the door. Or more likely, a formerly healthy subscriber, by virtue of a newly-acquired illness, would transform – werewolf-like – into a voracious, healthcare-consuming monster. Techniques were developed for these, as well. In fact, the academic managed care literature (and yes, there is such a thing) paid particular attention to this issue – that is, how to frustrate undesirable patients sufficiently to entice them to go elsewhere. One interesting article titled "Demarketing of healthcare services," appeared in the *Journal of Healthcare Marketing* in 1994. It said, among other things:

> *Decreasing accessibility to services . . . can be accomplished by "managing" the information distributed to patients regarding services available and how to access them. For example, an organization might excessively promote less-costly preventive procedures . . . and repress information about other elective and/or expensive services. In addition, providers can strategically locate and number specific services to make them easy (e.g., primary care) or difficult (e.g., specialists) to utilize. Furthermore, lag periods . . . also serve as containment strategies. Lags may be affected by the need for referrals, limited number of contracted specialists, restricted or inconvenient appointment availability, and increased office-visit waiting periods.*

I would like you to notice a couple of things about this excerpt. First, of course, it nicely demonstrates that driving patients away was not an unintended consequence of HMO inefficiencies. The inefficiencies were manufactured specifically to achieve that end. But second, please observe that this is probably the most straightforward statement about covert healthcare rationing you're ever likely to see from the people who are actually doing it. It graphically demonstrates that much of the inefficiency in our healthcare system is not accidental. It is carefully engineered for a very specific purpose. It is, in fact, an investment, aimed at improving the bottom line.

Here's another example. In the late 1990s, the famous Jim Clark, the first Internet genius, the man who had founded both Silicon Graphics and Netscape, decided to launch a new venture which he called WebMD. While today WebMD is muddling along as a reasonably successful information portal, it was originally conceived by Clark as a powerhouse that would revolutionize healthcare in America. He wanted WebMd to become a platform for seamlessly interconnecting all the players in the healthcare system – doctors, patients and insurers – to improve communication, streamline transactions, reduce medical errors, and otherwise create efficiencies that would benefit American healthcare (and at the same time build shareholder value for WebMD). When he finally had built up the infrastructure for doing all this, at enormous cost, he went to the health insurers with his first can't-miss proposition, the very can't-miss proposition that had enticed his investors to put up the money for WebMd in the first place. Namely, he offered (in exchange for a tiny transaction fee) to process the HMOs' medical claims for 70 cents per transaction (as compared to the $7.00 per transaction it was currently costing them), and furthermore, to complete the transactions in a matter of minutes instead of a matter of months. Much to Clark's amazement, there were no takers. None. And his dream died on the spot.

Astute readers will see the problem right away. HMOs, of course, have no interest whatsoever in streamlining their transactions. Quite the opposite. HMOs only make money if they do not have to pay out claims. And if they do have to pay claims, the longer they can hold on to the money before they actually pay it out, the longer they can keep it invested. And so, claims processing procedures have been carefully engineered into the most inefficient, Byzantine, and frustrating endeavors the devious human mind can conceive of. Unless a doctor's practice hires a cadre of "claims specialists," who spend all their time in an elaborate dance with the "claims specialists" employed by the HMOs, they would never collect any money at all. As it is, it is so expensive to chase smaller claims that many doctors simply don't send in bills for them – which means the HMOs get to keep that money. Which means that doctors are reluctant to offer the medical services for which only a small bill is generated.

Are you starting to see how covert rationing works?

THE END GAME FOR HMOS

By the middle of the last decade, the health insurance industry realized it had run out its string. It saw no pathway forward to continued profitability.

The insurers had tried every sneaky and underhanded idea they could think of for reducing costs – cherry-picking the healthy patients, treating chronically ill patients like pariahs so they would go away, making access to specialty care as inconvenient as possible, forcing doctors to sign "gag clauses" to prevent them from telling their patients about certain treatment options (more on this later), browbeating primary care physicians into zombie-like compliance with handed-down care directives, refusing to cover expensive-but-effective medical services, and canceling the policies of tens of thousands of patients after they got sick, based on trumped-up technicalities. Indeed, they had tried everything short of dispatching teams of Ninjas in the dark of night to slaughter their most expensive subscribers in their beds. And still, their costs – essentially, the money they could not avoid spending on people who needed healthcare services – increased relentlessly.

All these efforts were to little avail. The cost of providing healthcare continued to skyrocket, entirely unabated. Finally, when all else failed, the insurers began instituting huge and unsustainable annual increases in premiums, to the point of driving their customers out of the market.

This latter move, of course, was an open acknowledgment that the industry had entered its death spiral. In fact, it was an SOS, a cry for help. It was the health insurance industry wailing, "No mas!"

THE HEALTH INSURANCE INDUSTRY AND OBAMACARE

By 2009, when President Obama began his push for healthcare reform, the insurance companies knew they had no prospect of long-term profitability. Their business model was no longer viable, and, while telling soothing stories to avoid shareholder panic, they were urgently casting about for an exit strategy.

A drowning man will cling to any piece of flotsam that comes his way. What the insurance industry found floating by was Obamacare.

In return for its support in the healthcare reform battle, President Obama offered the insurance industry the graceful exit strategy it so desperately needed. Under Obamacare, for at least a few years the insurers hope to get One Last Windfall – namely, profits from the influx of previously-uninsured Americans whose premiums will be paid, or at least subsidized, by taxpayers. Here, the insurers are relying on the likelihood that the inflow of new premiums will, for a year or two at least, greatly outweigh the outflow of money they will have to spend caring for these new subscribers. Obviously, they will use every trick in their well-worn book to stave off expenditures for these new subscribers for as long as they can, but if they actually knew how to avoid paying healthcare costs indefinitely, they wouldn't have sought a government bail-out. In any case, an inflow of new subscribers will be a very temporary source of profit for insurers. Hence, at best it is One Last Windfall.

What happens to the insurers after they exhaust this last windfall is still up in the air. Obamacare may, of course, eventually transition to a single-payer system, an outcome which many Conservatives desperately fear, and many Progressives fervently desire. Should this happen, there may very well be some final compensatory buy-out (or a buy-off) for the insurance companies – a truly-last windfall.

But more likely, the insurance companies under Obamacare will continue to exist essentially as public utilities. That is, they will exist as companies chartered by the government, which administer healthcare under the direction of the government, with the products they may offer, the prices they may charge, the profits they may keep, and the losses they may incur, determined solely by the government. It's not glorious, but it's a living.

And it's a far better exit strategy than anything the insurance companies could devise for themselves.

So, when the time came, the insurance industry did whatever it needed to do to make sure President Obama's reforms became law. Their assistance consisted of four simple steps:

1) Do not actively oppose Obamacare. In stark contrast to its behavior during the Clintons' effort to reform healthcare, this time the insurance industry never employed its vast public relations resources to stifle healthcare reform. While they resurrected the original Harry and Louise, this time, like the insurance industry itself, they were older, wiser, sadder, and fully in support of the proposed reforms.

2) Submit quietly to demonization. A key strategy of proponents of Obamacare was to remind Americans repeatedly that the for-profit health insurance industry is fundamentally evil. This strategy was based on the time-honored precept that it is easier to get the unwashed masses to cooperate through hatred than through reason, and so, to gain their cooperation, one must give them something to hate. Obviously, this strategy meant that the health insurance industry had to accept its role as the bad guys in the reform debates without complaint, and without engaging in any serious self-defense. They did so.

3) *Offer subdued public support to Obamacare.* The AHIP (America's Health Insurance Plans) issued public statements every so often that cautiously supported President Obama's healthcare reforms. But its support had to remain subdued and tepid, since Satan can't be seen leading the hymns. It was just enough public support to signal opponents of Obamacare not to expect much help this time from this quarter.

4) *Whenever necessary, rise up and demonstrate to the world just how evil you really are.* At the end of the day, this was the most important role the insurance industry played in advancing Obamacare. It was certainly their most active role.

It was not a difficult role to fill. Since 1994 the health insurers had engaged in the sorts of truly evil, inhumane, and reprehensible practices that are naturally engendered by covert healthcare rationing, and that harmed or killed many of their subscribers. The only difficult part was choosing which reprehensible behaviors to feature, and when to do it.

In at least two key moments during the fight over healthcare reform – June, 2009 and February, 2010 – when the proponents of reform felt their momentum lagging, the insurance industry intervened with gratuitous evil behaviors whose chief function was to remind Americans just how unremittingly wicked and inhumane they really are. In the second case, at least arguably, the insurance industry turned the reform effort from apparent defeat to almost certain victory. Indeed, it is not too much of an exaggeration to assert that, in the end, the health insurance industry saved Obamacare.

JUNE, 2009: SAY HELLO TO MY LITTLE FRIEND

The debate over Obamacare entered a new phase in May and June of 2009. It was during those months that the opposition to healthcare reform found its voice, and it began to seem as if perhaps the Obama steamroller could really be slowed, if not stopped. People were even beginning to say that many Democrats in Congress, after getting an earful from their constituents when they held their summer town hall meetings, would abandon any idea of supporting President Obama's healthcare reforms.

Supporters of Obamacare decided it was time to invoke the demons. So in mid-June, the House Subcommittee on Oversight and Investigations called three health insurers to testify on the practice of rescission, and to face not only indignant Congresspersons, but also some of the people who had been personally harmed by their practices.

"Rescission" is when an insurance company voids subscriber's health insurance when they get sick (after happily accepting premiums from that subscriber, often for many years). Under some circumstances, rescission might be justifiable. It is legal and proper to cancel a policy if the subscriber is found to have purposely lied on the insurance application about a prior illness that is material to the current illness.

But health insurance companies for years have actively and aggressively practiced rescission on subscribers whose insurance applications contained inadvertent and non-material inaccuracies. Furthermore, the health insurance industry does not merely engage in occasional unfair rescission practices; it has industrialized the process (which, after all, is what they've always told us they would do to reduce costs). It employs health insurance detectives whose job is to comb the prior medical records of subscribers who are newly diagnosed with certain, expensive medical conditions, looking for even trivial discrepancies on insurance applications, which they can inflate to "fraudulent" omissions, thus voiding the policy. These health insurance detectives are paid by commission, according to how much money their efforts can save the company. Many of them find it a very lucrative career.

So, at the cost of perpetrating a bit of inhumanity, rescission can save insurance companies a lot of money.

Consider some of the individuals who testified in Congress along with the insurance companies on that day:

- A nurse in Texas had her insurance canceled after she was diagnosed with breast cancer because she had failed to reveal that, years before, she had consulted a dermatologist about acne.

- A man (whose surviving sister had to testify) had his insurance canceled before he could begin expensive cancer therapy, because he had not revealed (and indeed he had not known) that a prior CT scan had showed gallstones and an aneurysm – conditions unrelated to his cancer.

- A woman had her insurance canceled – and due to the rescission could not find replacement insurance – because she failed to reveal that, at one time, she had been on medication for irregular menstruation.

During the hearing, the three health insurance executives were caused to listen, on camera, to these and other mind-bending stories describing some of the inexcusable pain, suffering and death their unfair rescission practices had caused, and then were forced to listen to withering commentary by stunned Republicans and Democrats on the Subcommittee, whose own investigation had found that the three companies on the docket had retrospectively canceled the policies of 20,000 sick subscribers over the past 5 years.

After these heart-rending testimonies and the blistering attacks from extremely angry congresspersons, the executives were challenged by Chairman Stupak (D-Michigan) to now commit to discontinuing the practice of rescission unless intentional fraud could be shown.

All three replied, in turn, "No."

Such a reply, in such a setting, almost defies belief. The only possible explanation, in fact, is that the insurance industry was stepping up to the plate, and embracing its assigned role as the Evil One in the great healthcare debate.

Even the most stone-hearted insurance executive can see that canceling the health insurance of a newly-diagnosed cancer patient, because she'd forgotten she had required acne medicine before the prom 20 years ago, is just a bit unfair. But how did these three executives react? They did not attempt to deny such reprehensible behavior, or to explain it, or to defend it. They were simply defiant about it.

One is put in mind of Tony "Scarface" Montana, bereft of friends, family, allies and bodyguards (albeit because of his own actions), hopelessly surrounded by an army of heavily-armed assassins, screaming, "Say hello to my little friend!" then launching defiantly into a wild, bloody and spectacular suicide.

One cannot for a moment believe that Richard A. Collins, chief executive of UnitedHealth's Golden Rule Insurance Co., Don Hamm, chief executive of Assurant Health, and Brian Sassi, president of consumer business for WellPoint Inc., would have been stupid enough to publicly defy Congress over such an indefensible practice, if doing so was against their own long-term interests. Appearances to the contrary notwithstanding, they were not auditioning for a remake of Scarface.

This is not how an industry behaves which wants to court the goodwill of Congress at a critical juncture in its life cycle. This is not the strategy of an industry that wants Congress to defy its own party's President and defeat healthcare reform, or that is begging Congress to give them another chance to figure out how to bring healthcare costs into check. This is not the behavior of any industry that wants to elicit any sort of favorable action from Congress. Indeed, these executives would have seemed more sympathetic and deserving if they had proposed instead to place live puppies on a spit and roast them over an open fire during half-time at the Super Bowl.

There is only one explanation for their astounding public defiance on this matter. Which is, it must have suited their long-term interests.

Recall that at the time of this remarkable hearing, there was growing skepticism about President Obama's healthcare reform efforts, not only on the part of Republicans, but also on the part of a critical minority of Democrats in Congress. And for the first time since the election, there was some question about whether his reform plan would succeed in gaining sufficient support.

In this light the stark, defiant, public "no" uttered by the three insurance executives makes sense. "Look at us," they were saying, "See how evil we are! We are utterly devoid of human decency, ethical constraints, or a sense of fair play. If we behave this defiantly when we are in the position of mere supplicants to your eminences, just think how we will behave if you fail to rein us in with new reforms! Abandon all hope, those of you who rely on us for your healthcare, and behold the congressional dogs that placed us in this position of power over your very lives!"

Given the headwinds the healthcare reform effort was to face during the next nine months, it is difficult to say with any certainty how much good the insurance industry did in June, 2009, when it took such an extraordinary step to remind Americans just how incredibly evil it is. But when the time came to help boost the President's reform efforts, nobody can deny that the insurance industry stepped up and did its duty.

February, 2010: Raising Obamacare from the Dead

Things looked especially bleak for healthcare reform in early February of 2010. The incredible, Constitution-defying, machinations Congress had employed in its desperate attempt to pass healthcare reform had disgusted a majority of Americans, and momentum was clearly shifting to the opponents of Obamacare. And when Republican Scott Brown incredibly won the Senate seat in Massachusetts, robbing the Democrats of their crucial, filibuster-blocking 60th vote, many thought healthcare reform was dead.

But then out of nowhere, in early February, Wellpoint's California subsidiary, Anthem Blue Cross, announced it was raising its already-astronomical health insurance premiums by as much as 39%, a move that promised to greatly increase the number of Californians who are uninsured.

The demoralized Democrats in the administration greedily capitalized on this new opportunity.

Secretary of HHS Kathleen Sebelius immediately fired off a very public letter to the company, demanding that they justify this unconscionable rate increase. And Wellpoint, lustily assuming its assigned role as villain, was delighted to reply, equally publicly.

We're in a recession, Wellpoint brazenly asserted, and in a recession, like it or not, people exercise their prerogative to drop their health insurance. The only people who don't drop their health insurance are the sick people, or those who are likely to become sick, which means that our cost per subscriber goes way up. So naturally, we have to increase premiums. By a lot. It's just business. That's just the nature of our current, unreformed healthcare system. So choke on it.

Wellpoint was also kind enough to mention (for anyone dense enough to have missed the point) that the need for higher insurance premiums would be nicely mitigated if everybody was mandated by the government to purchase health insurance.

Wellpoint's announced premium increase immediately triggered great volumes of delighted outrage by thankful Democrats, who desperately needed a large dose of "evil insurance company" at just that time. Wellpoint's action reignited the proponents of healthcare reform, who were inspired to remind all Americans that this is what would happen to everyone if healthcare reform failed, and the greedy insurance companies had their way.

Stunned Republicans, seeing their impending victory over Obamacare evaporating before their eyes, could only issue a few lame and uncomfortable attempts to diminish the significance of Wellpoint's unfortunate action. But to little avail. The momentum had shifted. At least arguably, it was Wellpoint's decision to announce an unconscionable rate increase at this extremely critical juncture that put healthcare reform back on the road to adoption.

From a pure business standpoint, there was no good reason for Wellpoint to stir the soup at that moment. Wellpoint at the time was the most financially sound private health insurance company. While its California subsidiary did lose money in 2009, overall the company performed quite well, and reported a very nice profit growth for the year. And with several of its competitors in trouble, Wellpoint stood to do comparatively well for the foreseeable future.

Furthermore, it has since been learned that Wellpoint's math was bad. An independent actuary working for the California Department of Insurance reported on May 5, 2010 that the company had made "numerous errors" in calculating its rate increases, and further, that Wellpoint could cut its rate hikes substantially, and still meet its required 70% medical-loss ratio threshold. So, uh, oops.

It stands to reason that if Wellpoint really wanted healthcare reform to go away, they would have first checked their math before announcing seismic rate increases, and then, if such astounding rate increases were really needed, they would have waited a few months – while Obamacare died – before announcing their rate hike.

The last thing they would have done is to throw the reformers a critical lifeline just as they were going under for the last time.

In any case Wellpoint's action, especially at that moment, seems entirely gratuitous. Wellpoint could only have chosen to do its demon dance, at such an inopportune moment, in order to revive Obamacare during its darkest hour.

And that's precisely what happened.

WHAT THIS MEANS

What this means to those of us who would like for Obamacare to go away ought to be quite obvious. Simply nullifying or repealing Obamacare will not do. The insurance industry simply will not tolerate it. If we decide we need to get rid of Obamacare, to shed ourselves of the specter of government-controlled healthcare (and far worse, government-controlled covert rationing), we'll need to have another solution in hand.

CHAPTER 3 - THE COWING OF THE MEDICAL PROFESSION

"Did you really think that we want those laws to be observed? We want them broken. You'd better get it straight that it's not a bunch of boy scouts you're up against . . . The only power any government has is the power to crack down on criminals. Well, when there aren't enough criminals, one makes them. One declares so many things to be a crime that it becomes impossible for men to live without breaking laws. Who wants a nation of law-abiding citizens? What's there in that for anyone? But just pass the kind of laws that can neither be observed nor enforced nor objectively interpreted and you create a nation of law-breakers."

- Floyd Ferris, bureaucrat, *Atlas Shrugged*

The doctor who tells his patient to open wide and say moo is, in fact, projecting.

For the once proud, once ethical medical profession has been officially broken and domesticated. This, of course, is incredibly sad for the profession.

But it is life-threatening for patients.

And while it began a long time ago, the gradual destruction of the medical profession became a headlong rush in the 1990s, and ended with a final, formal capitulation in 2002. To be sure, doctors did not go voluntarily, but were coerced – by both the avaricious insurance companies and the ruthless government – to sacrifice their professional autonomy for the sake of their personal comfort and safety. The coercion was intense, but still, their resistance was remarkably feeble. In the end they did not fight as they might have to protect either their profession or their patients' welfare. When the time came they chose not to defend their professional integrity with their lives, their fortunes or their sacred honor.

It is a sorry tale, but it must be told.

After the collapse of the Clinton healthcare reform plan in 1993, both the triumphant HMOs and the beaten-back government plotted their moves. For the insurers, the pathway seemed open and clear. For government policymakers, chastened as they were, the pathway forward seemed no less clear – but it would have to be negotiated in a somewhat less open manner than they had originally hoped.

When these two powerful entities sat down in their respective bunkers to figure out next steps, they each came to the same conclusion: At the end of the day, the key to controlling the healthcare system was to control the behavior of physicians.

This became apparent the moment the accounting experts from the HMOs and various government agencies studied the matter in order to determine where all their money was going. What they saw horrified them.

They saw, 1.5 million times per day, a single doctor sitting down with a single patient, and – just between the two of them – deciding which extraordinarily expensive healthcare resources they would like to consume for the possible benefit of that individual patient. And, once reaching a decision, the doctor then would calmly scribble something on a prescription pad, or write a line in a hospital chart, and instantaneously all the resources of the massive, mindless healthcare system would heave into action, bending to the doctor's will. And, seeing all this, the HMO executives and the government policymakers, separately but with equal fervor, each sat up and cried, "My God! They're spending MY money!"

Something had to be done to get these doctors – the engines of all healthcare spending – under control. The strategies the insurance industry and the government used to control the behavior of doctors were quite different from one another – but both were effective. And as a result of these efforts, as we enter the era of Obamacare, the Central Authority will find the medical profession to be quite compliant and docile to its needs. To be sure there will be a bit of whining from physicians, and expressions of dissatisfaction and similarly ineffectual complaints, but these are easily dealt with. Doctors will not pose any real obstacle to Obamacare. They have been fully domesticated.

WHAT THE HMOS DID

HMO executives, being businessmen, set out to control doctors the only way they knew how – by attacking them in their wallets. Promise them riches beyond belief (or at least the wherewithal to make a decent living) if their behavior pleases you, but make sure they know that destitution awaits if they should displease you.

It did not take long for these smart business experts to figure out that to control the physicians' wallets, you need simply take control of the flow of their patients.

Doctors in the early 1990s were used to getting their patients by the hard work of establishing their professional reputation, and relying on referrals from appreciative colleagues and by word of mouth. When the HMOs suddenly moved in, before physicians ever realized what was happening, that model disappeared virtually overnight.

Under the HMOs, insurance products no longer covered patients for whichever doctor they chose to see. Instead, in exchange for reduced premiums, their health insurance covered them only if they received their care from doctors who had been admitted to the HMO's "physician panel." Doctors all over the land quickly learned that patients they had cared for, sacrificed for, and worried over for years, and who (they thought) regarded them as part of their family, dropped them like a hot potato the moment they had the opportunity to choose a health insurance plan which was marginally cheaper, but which did not include them on its panel of physicians.

And it quickly dawned on doctors that, if they were going to maintain themselves in anything like the style to which they had become accustomed, they needed to get on every panel of every HMO that served their area. It was the only way to allow all their patients to continue to have access to them.

But once doctors were "captive," (i.e., completely dependent upon their position on HMO panels for their livelihood), the game was all over except the shouting. Physicians were cooked virtually before they knew what had happened to them.

At first, the HMOs were happy to have all physicians on their panels. This is because at first, the HMOs' major priority was signing up just as many patients as they could – so including as many doctors as possible on their physician panels was an important aspect of recruiting subscribers.

But once this initial sign-up phase was over, the HMO executives no longer had use for all those doctors on their panels. Some were expendable. They let their doctors know it by terminating a few of them from time to time, apparently arbitrarily and without explanation – leaving the surviving doctors to guess the reason for it.

But since doctors are generally pretty smart, they were good at guessing the heart's desire of the HMO executives.

It should be obvious that HMO executives would be anxious to get rid of doctors who spent a lot of their money, and retain the ones who did not. To distinguish between the two, HMOs set up "performance standards." These standards, following the usual fiction, were billed as "quality" measures, but in general they actually seemed aimed at determining how much money various doctors were spending. Often, something like 10% of the physician's annual reimbursement was held back as a "withhold," payable to the doctors only if they met the published performance standards. Doctors who failed to meet performance standards not only did not get the rest of the money they had earned, but worse, were in danger of being cut loose from the HMO's panel altogether, thus jeopardizing their livelihood.

This system quickly got physicians into the right frame of mind, and focused them quite nicely on whose interests they actually needed to keep at the forefront when they were making clinical decisions for their patients. It also prepared them to put up with more of the HMOs' new management techniques.

Once each quarter, some men in dark suits would come to visit. They were "practice consultants," and they were there to help. The practice consultants would use data the HMO had accumulated to assist the doctor in re-titrating his or her decision-making processes, in order to guarantee they were practicing medicine to everyone's best advantage.

For instance, the practice consultants might say, "Dr. Smith, we notice that the patients in your practice cost our HMO an average of $342 each last quarter. This is unfortunately higher than the target we set for you of $315. We are distressed to have to mention that this puts you in some jeopardy regarding your "withhold," and possibly of further action as well. But we are here to help. Let's see how we can do that. Ah! Here's something. Notice that you sent four patients last quarter to Cardiologist Jones, and Cardiologist Jones spent an average of $4300 doing whatever it is he did to evaluate and treat those patients. And you sent three patients to Cardiologist Wilson. And she only spent $2100 per patient. That is quite a difference, isn't it, Dr. Smith? Hmm. Well, Dr. Smith, you know we would never tell you how to practice medicine – you're the doctor! – but we thought you might find this cost differential interesting, as you decide where to refer your next patient."

And while Cardiologist Jones and Cardiologist Wilson have entirely different areas of expertise, which Dr. Smith had formerly taken into account when deciding where to refer his patients, his new-found wisdom now dictates that it might be best if Cardiologist Wilson would become his new go-to cardiologist for all cardiac-related problems his patients might have. And Cardiologist Jones, when he notices a marked decrease in his referrals during the following quarter (since the men in suits visited lots of primary care offices in the area), will probably never know that he (as well as many patients) has become the victim of trickle-down covert rationing.

Another common methodology to improve the quality of care, in a manner that would save the HMO money, was to institute Pay for Performance programs. P for P initiatives provided primary care doctors with a checklist of 10 or 12 items that they would need to accomplish during each patient visit, if they would like to be paid. The checklist consisted mainly of things that everyone would have to agree are useful – things like checking and discussing blood pressure and cholesterol levels, and reviewing their dietary and exercise habits, smoking habits, etc. There would be nothing on the list that anyone could possibly object to. However, the lists were so constructed that it was impossible to complete them in less than 10 minutes or so. And that, too, would have been fine, except that in order to meet the patient load the HMOs required, doctors needed to see a patient every 12.5 minutes. And here you can begin to see the true brilliance of P for P.

P for P saw to it that the routine health maintenance stuff got done each and every visit. But P for P also saw to it that there would be little or no time for "ad libbing," that is, for the patient to bring up new, potentially-expensive medical issues, or, if the patient managed to blurt something out, for the doctor to adequately assess it. At best, the patient would have to reschedule another visit, for perhaps a month or two later. By that time the problem might be resolved, or might have run its course. Or perhaps something else might happen to make the new medical issue, well, moot.

Severely limiting the doctor's face time with patients, then carefully scripting, down to the minute, what is to take place during that limited time, creates an opportunity for real cost savings. This is the kind of benefit you get when you apply modern management techniques to a trade whose processes really hadn't changed much since the Middle Ages.

Through these and other creative applications of business principles, in a matter of a couple of years the HMOs owned doctors, lock, stock and barrel. And to make it official, in the middle years of the 1990s (once doctors realized that being retained on HMO physician panels was a matter of life or death), HMO executives invented the "gag clause," which they added to the doctors' contracts when it came time for renewal. Gag clauses said something like this:

> "The physician agrees not to take any action or make any communication or representation to patients or patients' families, potential patients or potential patients' families, employers, unions, the media, or the public that would tend to undermine, disparage, or otherwise criticize the healthcare coverage provided by [insert name of HMO here]. The physician further agrees to keep all proprietary information such as payment rates, reimbursement procedures, utilization-review procedures, or other processes and procedures related to billing, collection, or review, strictly confidential."

Agreeing to keep such potentially vital information from their patients – information which might materially affect a patient's decisions regarding his or her own healthcare – was of course a direct violation of medical ethics. Medical ethics, however, had long since gone by the boards. The moment they had acceded to "performance standards" that enticed them to withhold medical services – and also acceded to sundry other coercions which HMOs had dreamt up to make sure physicians answered to their needs instead of their patients' – doctors had already become deeply complicit in bedside healthcare rationing, essentially, rationing by omission. The gag clauses just put it in writing. So, apparently believing they had no good options, and already having lost the professional integrity which they ought to have held dear, doctors signed contracts by the thousands with gag clauses in them.

After a few years the gag clauses were noticed by "patient advocates" and other species of troublemakers, and strong objections were raised to them. The objections were based on the notion that it's not nice for HMOs to gag physicians from telling their patients things that they ought to know. So, gag clauses were finally removed from HMO contracts.

But the damage had been done; the essential point had been made. When HMOs had asked doctors for a declaration of fealty that superseded all pre-existing professional obligations, doctors gave it, and with barely a protest. Whether or not gag clauses continued to appear in the contracts was immaterial. Once a dog learns to heel you can get rid of the leash, and the dog still heals just fine.

WHAT THE GOVERNMENT DID

The defeat of the Clintons' healthcare reform plan certainly set the government policymakers back. The Progressives' plans for a government takeover of the healthcare system, all in one grand campaign, had been foiled.

But Progressives always take the long view, and they were undismayed. They quickly regrouped, and began stealthily instituting as much of the defunct Clinton plan as they could, piece by piece, through various laws, budgets, executive fiats and riders on Congressional bills.

Like the health insurance companies, Progressives in the government also recognized that it was imperative for them to gain control of the behavior of doctors. Hillary probably had said it best: "The problem with our healthcare system is too many greedy doctors using too much expensive technology." So the name of the game was controlling the greedy doctors, the decision-makers on the ground.

The methodology they employed to do so was fundamentally different from the methods used by HMOs. HMOs naturally concentrated on controlling physicians by the power of economics, through simple threats to their livelihood. But as Ayn Rand taught us so many years ago, the power of the government over its citizens derives from regulatory (ultimately, prosecutorial) intimidation.

There is no need for the government to go all Robespierre, however. Actual bloodshed can be minimized. The Central Authority can usually get the effect it needs by sending in the regulators – always backed by the threat of legal violence, of course – to harass a few people, ideally for what appear to be entirely arbitrary reasons. This action always proves wonderfully intimidating to the rest, and is an effective way to focus people's attention on that which you would like them to focus.

I will be devoting much of the rest of this book to the abuse of government power with regard to healthcare, and don't want to get too distracted by that topic here. So I will simply describe a single foray the government made in the time frame we're talking about – the late 1990s – aimed at teaching doctors what is expected of them, and letting them know who they really work for. By doing so, I hope to make a bit more understandable why the medical profession made a complete and disastrous capitulation in 2002.

THE E&M GUIDELINES

During the second Clinton administration, a new set of tortuous documentation requirements were imposed on American physicians by our government. The E&M guidelines, for "evaluation and management," apply to the documentation that physicians are obligated to provide in support of their Medicare billing. The E&M guidelines, first instituted in 1995 and revised in 1997, were part of the Clintons' great healthcare fraud reduction initiative. Ostensibly, the new, very strict documentation requirements would reduce the opportunity for fraudulent billing.

However, the E&M guidelines were, from the very beginning, a Regulatory Speed Trap of the first order. Regulatory Speed Traps work like this:

1) Over a long period of time, regulators will promulgate a confusing array of disparate, vague, poorly worded, obscure and mutually incompatible rules, regulations and guidelines.

2) Individuals or companies which need to provide their products or services despite such hard-to-interpret regulations, will necessarily render their own interpretations (usually with the assistance of attorneys, consultants, and the regulators themselves), and will act according to those interpretations.

3) By their apparent concurrence with, or at least by their failure to object to, such interpretations of the rules, the regulators over time allow de facto standards of behavior to become established.

4) When it becomes to their advantage, the regulators will reinterpret the ambiguous regulations in such a way that the formerly tolerated de facto standards suddenly become grievous violations.

5) Regulators aggressively, but selectively and arbitrarily, prosecute newly felonious providers of those products or services.

The E&M guidelines are so convoluted as to be unworkable in any objective way. Through their utter opacity and complexity, only partially reflected by the 48 pages of dense prose that comprise them, the E&M rules (for "rules" is what they are) in fact greatly magnify the doctor's opportunity for making inadvertent documentation errors, and thus of producing a "fraudulent" bill.

Under the E&M rules, writing what used to be a simple progress note in a patient's chart requires the physician to assemble a complicated set of "elements" from Column A and Column B, as from a Chinese menu, for each of four subject areas of the patient "encounter" – the history, the physical exam, the assessment, and the plan. Then somehow, one must translate the result (which reads like – and often is – a computer-generated form letter) into a billing code.

Despite the morass of confusion caused by the E&M guidelines, any failure to follow them to the complete satisfaction of the Central Authority is a priori evidence of Medicare fraud or abuse. And therefore, the E&M guidelines assure that with each and every patient encounter, the thing that will be foremost in the physician's mind is not the needs of the patient, but how to fill out the complex documentation in such a way as to avoid the appearance of committing a crime.

In practical terms, this means filling out the documentation so as to blend in with the masses, so that one's records will be passed over by the sharp eyes of the greedy forensic accountants (who are paid by commission for detecting instances of substandard documentation, now construed as "fraud or abuse"), or even worse, by the sophisticated software now being deployed to detect ever-more nuanced gradations of "outliers."

Even if this documentation mess resulted in a straightforward means of determining proper billing codes (which it does not), it results in a medical progress note that is virtually undecipherable. This means that when another doctor (or even the same doctor on a different day) tries to read the progress notes to figure out what's been going on with the patient (which used to be the point of medical progress notes, before they became primarily a vehicle for auditors), they cannot. Compliance with the E&M guidelines often actively confounds patient care.

The E&M guidelines were recognized immediately by doctors as a complete abomination. Indeed, the great hue and cry from angry physicians caused the Secretary of HHS to appoint a special commission to review the E&M guidelines in 2001. The special commission reviewed the evidence and concluded that indeed, the E&M guidelines were entirely counterproductive to patient care. In June, 2002 the commission voted (20-1) to recommend abandoning them altogether.

But HHS declined to follow the recommendations of its own commission, instead leaving the E&M guidelines in place "temporarily," and vaguely promising to revise them "soon" in order to make them less dangerous to patient care – knowing full well that the saurian lassitude of the bureaucracy would easily outlast the fleeting indignation of the medical community. And, as the bureaucrats predicted, there has not been any substantial noise from doctors about revising these guidelines for several years now. A whole new generation of doctors has been weaned on them, and does not know any better. The E&M guidelines have become as permanent as the IRS.

(This simple example ought to teach us how difficult it will be to roll-back any of our new healthcare reforms in the future, even ones that are officially deemed to be harmful.)

Not only has HHS failed to take (or, alternately, succeeded in not taking) the steps it promised to take to revise the E&M guidelines, they also have vigorously pressed forward with audits and prosecutions for the federal crime of healthcare fraud, based on physicians' inadequate compliance with them.

In a well-publicized test case, instituted by the government shortly after the E&M guidelines were first implemented – apparently to let doctors know they were deadly serious about this – criminal charges were brought against a Montana family doctor, alleging medical coding violations. But the government's own expert concluded that the prosecutors were holding the doctor to standards that were not yet in force at the time the bills were submitted, and that the government was applying its new rules retroactively. The expert was so disturbed by his findings that he even offered to switch sides and testify for the defendant. Unfazed, the government simply switched tactics, dropping criminal charges and instead initiating a civil suit against the doctor for $37 million – which is way more money than the average family doctor has on hand. The defendant, breaking from the usual pattern, fought the government instead of settling. And after a long, long time, she was finally cleared – but not before she had spent over $300,000 out-of-pocket in legal fees.* Nonetheless the Feds had made their point to the physician community, loud and clear: We intend to vigorously prosecute physicians for violation of these guidelines, whatever you may think of them, and whether we're acting fairly or unfairly.

---

*Paul Rosenzweig, Senior Legal Research Fellow, The Heritage Foundation, testimony on "Sentencing and Enforcement of White Collar Crimes," Subcommittee on Crime and Drugs, Committee on the Judiciary, U.S. Senate, June 19, 2002.

Every doctor in America suddenly realized just how serious the Feds were about enforcing these ridiculous, clinically counterproductive coding guidelines.

Frightened by the prospect of prosecution for Medicare fraud, many doctors adopted the tact of systematically "downcoding" their Medicare bills, figuring that they are unlikely to be brought up on fraud charges for under billing. And normally one might think that the Feds would consider this a victory, since it would result in their keeping money they should be paying out. But the Feds' purpose here was only secondarily to save money. Their primary purpose was intimidation – showing those doctors who's the boss. So Medicare let doctors know that systematic downcoding may also be considered a fraudulent act, since it shows contempt for the law, and doctors suspected of doing so will be audited.

Because of the clear and present danger the E&M guidelines pose to every doctor, a multi-million dollar industry has sprung up to help physicians better comply with these coding guidelines. Physicians across the country are spending the time and money allotted for their continuing medical education learning to become better accountants, rather than better physicians.

Which brings me to a very interesting point about the E&M guidelines: It is not actually possible to follow the E&M guidelines accurately.

It turns out that coding correctly is impossible. This was proven in a formal study conducted a few years after these guidelines were instituted. A group of government-sanctioned coders took a sample of typical doctor-patient visits, coded them according to the E&M guidelines – and they all got different answers. If government-approved coders, using the government's own guidelines, cannot figure out how to arrive at what prosecutors will always insist is the singular correct answer, then what hope do mere doctors have? (The results of this study were published in the *Annals of Emergency Medicine* in September, 2002.)

Obviously, then, since there is no "right" way to comply with the coding rules, all a doctor needs in order to become guilty of abusive billing, if not outright fraud, is for the fickle finger of the Feds to point his way, and initiate an audit. Violations are virtually guaranteed to be found during any audit. So what we've got here is a well-documented, openly acknowledged, published-in-peer-reviewed-literature Regulatory Speed Trap.

Here's what happens to doctors who are suspected of committing coding abuse (which is to say, to any doctors who are visited by Federal auditors):

1) A small sample of their patients' charts is audited.

2) The coding error rate (which is determined by the auditor) will be calculated for that sample, then that error rate is applied by extrapolation to every Medicare bill the doctor has submitted for the past 6 years (the statute of limitations).

3) For each violation in coding the doctor is estimated to have committed during those six years, the doctor must pay: a) triple the amount of restitution, plus b) $11,000.00 per coding violation.

It is not unusual for audited doctors to be hit with hundreds if not thousands of coding violations over a 6-year period, and the fines will almost always amount to well over 7 figures, if not 8. However, if it's just abuse the doctor has allegedly committed and not fraud, often the Feds may offer a settlement deal in the low 7 figures.

And here's what happens if the coding violations are judged by the auditor to be fraudulent (which involves the determination of intent, and therefore, unfortunately, often appears a somewhat arbitrary designation):

1- 3) As above.
4) Jail

And, as we have seen, if you somehow escape being convicted on criminal charges, the government still has the prerogative to come back at you with civil charges, where the burden of proof is lower.

Any doctor who has come anywhere near such a process wishes fervently for the good old days, when it was only the HMOs making your life miserable. Yes, HMO executives can be nasty sons of guns. But they can only decide not to pay you what you are owed, or perhaps throw you off a panel. They cannot decide to wipe out your life savings, take your professional license, or put you in jail.

The Central Authority knows that the E&M guidelines are harmful to patient care. Its own commission came to that very conclusion in 2002. The Central Authority knows that failing to comply perfectly with the E&M guidelines in each and every case does not really indicate fraud and/or abuse, but is the necessary outcome when you institute a complex set of rules that not even the government's own approved coders can interpret.

That the Central Authority continues to impose the E&M guidelines on physicians, despite the harm this is acknowledged to cause, tells us something very important about the underlying motives. When you are in the business of covertly rationing healthcare, controlling the behavior of physicians – getting them under your thrall – is Job One. And as George Orwell observed for us, when you want to control the behavior of some people, a critical step is to control the mode, the rules, and even the very language of communication.

That physicians continue to comply with such oppressions, despite the harm it does to them and to their patients, and (with notable exceptions) without serious complaint, tells us something important about them, too.

WHAT THE DOCTORS DID

Despite the intense, unrelenting attacks against them by the health insurers and the government, it remains striking how completely physicians capitulated to the pressure and abandoned their professional responsibilities, and how quickly they did it. And in doing so, physicians threw away two thousand years of tradition, jurisprudence and ethics.

Medicine was one of the three original professions, the other two being the clergy and attorneys. Today, anyone working in any area of endeavor, as long as they have sufficient expertise that that somebody is willing to pay them to do it, calls themselves a professional. So we have professional hairdressers, chefs, sanitation workers, hit-men, and athletes. And by this definition, I suppose doctors can still call themselves by that name as well.

But by the original definition of the word, they gave up that privilege in 2002.

Originally, the term "professional" was defined not merely by somebody's knowledge or expertise, but rather, by the special quality of the fiduciary relationship they had with their clients – a relationship marked by an absolute duty to place the needs of the client ahead of the professional's own personal interests, or the interests of any third party.

In the case of physicians, this relationship is called the doctor-patient relationship.

To really understand what the doctor-patient relationship is supposed to be like, it is quite sad that today it might be necessary to have a look at a different profession, one whose members are often despised by physicians, but one that has managed to hang on to its professional integrity to this day – namely, the lawyers.

Say you are arrested for robbing a bank. Say the arrest was not unexpected, since you actually did rob a bank. Say that while you didn't actually mean to do it, you shot a teller in the process, and the teller subsequently died. And finally, say you were caught red-handed.

Given this series of unfortunate circumstances, what rights can you expect?

It turns out that under the law, you have many rights. Despite the overwhelming evidence against you (the surveillance tapes, the eyewitnesses, the being-caught-at-the-scene-with-the-smoking-gun-in-your-hand, etc.), you have the right to a fair trial; you have a right to be considered innocent until a jury of your peers declares you guilty; and you will have the right of appeal (assuming you won't like the verdict). But more importantly than anything else, you have a right to counsel, to an advocate, a knowledgeable professional who is obligated to defend you to the limits of her abilities, and to fully protect all of your interests under the law.

Society recognizes that the legal system is a morass of rules and regulations that ordinary citizens cannot hope to navigate on their own. Society acknowledges the need for any citizen caught up in the complex legal system to have a personal advocate who will hold that citizen's interests above all others. Even when the accused party is as obviously guilty and as deserving of punishment as you clearly are, most of us would shudder to think of the abuses that would occur if people (even the likes of you) had to face a hostile legal system without the guidance of their personal attorney.

When you are sick, you are no more capable of navigating the complex healthcare system than is the accused felon of navigating the complex legal system, and you are no less in peril if you run afoul of that system. And your need of a personal advocate, a professional whose job is to protect your interests against the conflicting aims of a hostile healthcare system, is no less acute.

When you are sick, you should be entitled to at least the same protections as when you rob a bank. And this is what the doctor-patient relationship is actually for.

In recent years the "doctor-patient relationship" has been taken in hand by certain "experts," who (in the way of teaching doctors to work more "effectively"), have reduced the whole thing to a series of tricks from the interpersonal-relationship trade. These may include looking your patients in the eye; displaying sympathetic expressions (practicing with the use of mirrors may be necessary); nodding as they speak (with all the sincerity of a Dr. Welby bobble-head); freely showing them your emotions (even if you have to manufacture them); remembering their birthdays and children's' names (yet another benefit of computerized medical records), and similar strategies for convincing patients that they have your full attention, and that nothing can be more important to you at this moment than their welfare. Such techniques are designed to get your patient's thinking to the right place – which is to say, to get them to understand without too much fuss or muss why the efficient course of evaluation and treatment you have selected for them (with the kind assistance of various government expert panels) is the correct one.

I think it's the same training they give annuity salespersons.

Obviously, none of that has anything to do with the real doctor-patient relationship. The real doctor-patient relationship is a sacred covenant, one which is formed when a patient goes to a doctor for help, and the doctor agrees to give that help. Under that covenant, the patient agrees to take the physician into his confidence, and to reveal to her even the most secret and intimate information related to his health. The physician, in turn, agrees to honor that trust, and to become the patient's advocate in all matters related to his health, placing his personal best interest above all other considerations. This strong relationship of mutual trust is what patients have always expected, what most doctors have striven for, and what everyone else (medical ethicists, professional societies, and those who enforce the law of the land) have traditionally agreed – and even demanded – must be the standard.

And for over 2000 years, the precepts of medical ethics were aimed squarely at guaranteeing the integrity of that relationship. Fundamentally, these ethical precepts held physicians to the high standards of behavior embodied in the classic doctor-patient relationship, and further, gained physicians admittance to the small society of "professionals."

Unfortunately, by the late 1990s, perceptive physicians noticed a big problem. Namely, thanks to the various perfidies being visited upon them by HMOs and the government, doctors could no longer act in accordance with their fundamental ethical precepts. They were being pressured to place the vital interests of the insurers and the government ahead of the vital interests of their patients. They were coerced into violating their sacred duties under the doctor-patient relationship. And, as we have seen, doctors gave in to that pressure.

Soon, influential thought leaders in medicine and medical ethics expressed alarm at what was going on. Clearly, they said, something needed to be done about it. And they decided to act.

But the action which the medical thought leaders finally took was not to fight back against the pressures being placed on physicians to violate their most fundamental ethical principles. Instead, the medical thought leaders launched an effort to change the precepts of medical ethics, to make medical ethics comport with the actual behaviors which modern doctors were being coerced to adopt.

Changing millennia-old ethical precepts proved to be surprisingly easy. This is because it is surprisingly easy today to find respected ethicists who will sanction just about any nefarious activity you can think of, as long as that activity furthers some higher cause which is to their liking. These ethicists are called utilitarians.

The solution to the physicians' ethical dilemma was initially proposed as early as 1998, in an article by Hall and Berenson in the *Annals of Internal Medicine*, which stated: "It is untenable for the medical profession to continue asserting an idealistic ethic that is contradicted so openly in clinical practice. . ..We propose that devotion to the best medical interests of each individual patient be replaced with an ethic of devotion to the best medical interests of the group. . ."

This influential article, among other things, led to the formation of a commission to formally study the issue (the issue, again, being that if it becomes difficult to follow ethical precepts, then one ought to go ahead and change them).

This effort was led by the American College of Physicians, the main professional organization of experts in internal medicine, and this organization was quickly joined by virtually every other major physician organization in the world. Physician-leaders completed their ethical overhaul of the medical profession impressively quickly, and published it in 2002. They called it "Medical Professionalism in the New Millennium: A Physician Charter. "(*Annals of Internal Medicine*, February 5, 2002). With its publication a two-thousand-year tradition of medical ethics was ended. It is the suicide note of the medical profession.

The innovation of the Millennialists was to proclaim a new ethical precept: the precept of Social Justice. The precept of Social Justice charges physicians with effecting "the fair distribution of healthcare resources." That is, it renders it ethical for doctors to decide which patients ought to get those limited resources, and which ought not to get them; it specifically and directly justifies covert bedside rationing by physicians.

The reason this new ethical precept was deemed necessary is explicitly because doctors cannot any longer adhere to the old ones. ("It is untenable. . .to continue asserting an idealistic ethic," according to Hall and Berenson. "Indeed, the medical profession must contend with complicated political, legal, and market forces," according to the Millennialists themselves.)

Ostensibly, the precept of Social Justice gives doctors who are too introspective (admittedly, not a big problem with many of us) an out when they find themselves having to place the interests of payers ahead of the interests of their patients by, say, failing to mention certain medical options that might be available. "Sure, I'm violating classic ethical principles," they can now tell themselves, "but I've got to do that to honor this new one."

The bottom line is that, having been coerced by the insurers and the government (both of which control the doctors' professional viability, and one of which also controls their status regarding incarceration vs freedom) to place the payers' needs ahead of the needs of patients, doctors found themselves in utter violation of their fundamental ethical precepts. The proper response of physicians (and their professional organizations such as the ACP) would have been to reassert those ethical obligations, to push back against the payers, and enlist the cooperation of their patients (who, after all, have a particularly vital interest in the matter) in doing so. Instead, they have taken a path of lesser resistance, re-defining medical ethics to comport with their new, coerced behavior.

WHAT DOES THIS "NEW ETHICS" DO TO THE DOCTOR-PATIENT RELATIONSHIP?

The addition of the precept of Social Justice to the ethical obligations of the physician renders the classic doctor-patient relationship inoperative.

The New Ethics breaks the covenant from the outset. It renders "ethical" the divided loyalty of the physician. Today, when patients go to a doctor for medical advice, they do not know – and cannot know – whether that advice is being given to advance primarily the patient's own well-being, or the well-being of the society that desires a "fair distribution of healthcare resources."

With the formal adoption of this New Ethics, patients essentially have been cut loose, and set adrift to fend for themselves in an increasingly hostile healthcare system, without being able to rely on the kind of personal advocate they've been conditioned to expect, the same kind of advocate an accused murderer is still granted without question or hesitation. What's worse, nobody has told patients that they have been abandoned in this way. They think their doctor is still working for them.

Less obvious, but no less profound, are the consequences this New Ethics has on the profession of medicine. Abandoning their primary obligation to the individual patient means that physicians have committed the "original sin." They have abdicated their traditional, ethical, and legal roles as patient advocates; they have broken a sacred pact. They have fully compromised themselves as professionals; indeed they have become professionals in name only, and not in fact. And as a result, to their utter frustration, they find themselves standing naked before their enemies, the very insurers and regulators who forced them to abdicate their sacred obligation in the first place.

And it is in this utterly subservient position that we find our doctors – our protectors, our advocates – when Obamacare comes to town.

CHAPTER 4 - THE FOUR WAYS TO CONTROL HEALTHCARE SPENDING

"Unfortunately even the pope could not achieve significant reductions in the cost of American health care over the next few years."
- Uwe Reinhardt

In the first three chapters of this book, I have attempted to show how and why our nation's healthcare expenditures have become entirely untenable, and why the heroic measures we have taken so far to contain those expenditures have been not only an abject failure, but also quite counterproductive. Indeed, the cost-containment measures at which we have been flailing away for twenty years (primarily employing the multifarious techniques of covert rationing) have left more than merely our treasury in a "spent" state.

Our health insurance industry has worn itself down to a still-blustering but empty shell. And our physicians have allowed themselves to be reduced to an abject community of supplicants. In neither the insurers nor organized medicine are we likely to find the ideas, the energy, or in any manner the wherewithal that will be necessary to lead us toward a real solution to the mess we have made of our healthcare system. At best, they will be followers.

It is true that our political leaders are certainly not spent. Our Progressive leaders, using their typical end-justifies-the-means approach to the Constitution, have made Obamacare the law of the land. And our Conservative leaders are invigorated with the idea of repealing that law after the next election.

But amidst all the accusations and counter-accusations, vituperations, abuse, and scurrility that passes for debate between these two factions, neither faction has clearly articulated its plan for controlling our healthcare expenditures.

Any Progressive healthcare system – including Obamacare – will of course have an inherent, built-in methodology for reducing expenditures. Namely, government-approved experts will determine that some healthcare services will not be provided to anyone, and that other services will not be provided to some. But our Progressive leaders do not like to talk explicitly about that methodology in public. So instead, they talk about fairness, reducing the number of uninsured, and stifling the greedy doctors and biomedical companies.

With a few notable exceptions, Conservatives seem to be in an even sorrier state, since they seem to be relying on the health insurance industry and a vague notion of "free markets" to take care of everything once they get rid of Obamacare. They seem not to realize that we have already tried this strategy, and it has failed abysmally. This kind of talk most likely frightens health insurance executives more than anyone else.

Worse, the less-than-useful debate that has taken place between the two parties – with neither party forthrightly addressing the kinds of actions that will really be necessary to rescue our healthcare finances (and thus our society) – has created a general sense among the public that the problem is so confused and chaotic, so rifled by conflicts of interest, and so very complex, as to be fundamentally unsolvable. If that were the case, it would mean that our society is doomed, and in the relatively near future.

I myself have suggested, just a chapter or two ago, that this outcome does not seem particularly unlikely at this moment.

However, there are, in fact, solutions to our healthcare spending crisis, and so descending into chaos is not the only possible outcome. In fact, I will assert in this chapter that there are actually four (but only four) entirely different ways to meaningfully reduce our healthcare expenditures.

By understanding these four methods of solving the problem, it is entirely possible – as we listen to all the debating, fighting, and reciprocal castigations, aspersions, distortions and lies being exchanged by and amongst the various interest groups – to understand which method is actually being espoused by which parties.

We have, obviously, already settled upon one of these methods, at least for now. Obamacare is a nice example of Method Two – the Progressive plan. We have settled on it above the others, I believe, because it is easiest (if you do not dig too deeply) for its proponents to make Method Two sound a lot less difficult, a lot less painful, and a lot more fair than the other methods. Indeed, while the people "selling" Method One or Method Three (nobody is trying to sell Method Four) usually make it sound like they're asking us to pick the least bad of all the bad choices, proponents of Method Two are true proselytizers. They honestly believe that their option will represent a pinnacle of human achievement (and thus, that people who disagree with them are tools of the devil).

As I have already stated, I believe the Progressive viewpoint is dangerously incorrect. Before giving a detailed picture of why I think this is the case, it is only fair for me to briefly review all the alternatives that will remain to us if we should decide to turn away from the Progressive style of healthcare reform.

And so, without further ado -

METHOD ONE: MAKE ALL HEALTHCARE SPENDING THE RESPONSIBILITY OF THE INDIVIDUAL.

That Method One, when baldly stated as I have just done, seems so outlandishly inappropriate and hard-hearted today is a tribute to just how far down the Progressive path all of us have already traveled. But it is, in fact, a legitimate method for getting control of our national healthcare expenditures.

Further, the necessity of paying ourselves for products and services we consume ourselves, as we have seen, is a fundamental law of economics. And, as our society is about to learn, while we can get away with violating this law for a couple of generations, we cannot get away with it forever.

Also consider the fact that, just a few decades ago, this is exactly how we all paid for healthcare. Indeed, this is the method by which all of mankind has paid for its healthcare for all but a few brief decades out of the millions of years we have graced (or plagued, if you must) the planet. It has always been thus: If you want or need healthcare (and if it exists), simply pay for it yourself.

Those few brave souls who remain proponents of this method – who often count themselves as Libertarians – offer two general arguments to support their position; an ethical one and a practical one.

It is fundamentally unethical to insist that your own individual healthcare services must be provided by others – claiming, as you do so, that healthcare is somehow intrinsically different from any other product or service which you may wish to acquire (such as food, clothing, housing, and iPads). Proponents of Method One quaintly cling to the now-outmoded idea that there is no such thing as a right that creates an obligation upon another person. So to them, insisting that healthcare is a right that must be provided by others is, a priori, unethical. Furthermore, they point out, much of a person's health (and therefore, a person's healthcare needs) is determined by lifestyle choices, so it is only right and proper for the individual to bear responsibility for those choices. But more importantly, demanding any "right" that creates a burden on one's fellow citizens will inevitably lead to tyranny by some Central Authority. Therefore, this demand is unethical.

Method One also holds that, by returning to the individual the responsibility of paying for healthcare, we would be achieving a great good – namely, we would be returning healthcare back into the realm of actual market forces. When that happens, the laws of supply and demand will kick in once more, and will determine which services are actually needed, and what the rightful price for those services ought to be.

So from a practical standpoint, Method One will truly recruit the efficiencies of the marketplace into the workings of the healthcare system. (In contrast, placing dictatorial powers into the hands of insurance executives, which is what the HMO movement of the 1990s actually did, accomplished no such thing.) And the cost of healthcare services will at last come back down to a level which individuals can actually afford. As an added bonus, since everyone will know that paying for future illnesses will be their problem, people will suddenly become more likely to begin making lifestyle choices that will lower their odds of having to do so.

But whether or not individuals can afford medical services, at least the spending on those services will no longer be the burden of society – and the fiscal doom we now face will be cured.

Opponents of Method One point out that, inevitably, there will be individuals – and likely many, many individuals – who simply will not be able to afford to pay for healthcare services which are needed, and which are readily available for the right price, and will therefore suffer preventable pain, disability, and death. Without some kind of public support for healthcare, heart-rending tragedies will abound, our civilization will become coarsened, anger will build, and insurrection will become a constant threat. Such a result, of course, would be suboptimal.

METHOD TWO: MAKE ALL HEALTHCARE SPENDING THE RESPONSIBILITY OF A CENTRAL AUTHORITY.

Proponents of Method Two hold (because of ethical reasoning that is as obvious to them as the opposite ethical reasoning is to proponents of Method One), that healthcare is a fundamental right; that whether one receives a healthcare service – a service that can relieve pain or prevent disability or death – ought not to depend on one's ability to pay, but instead, that such services, so fundamental to human life, ought to be equally available to everyone. And the only way to achieve this goal is to collectivize and centralize healthcare decisions and healthcare spending.

This is what I have called the Progressive plan.

For proponents of Method Two, healthcare services are indeed fundamentally different from all other human needs – food, clothing, etc. – since the kind and the amount of healthcare services one needs are most often not a matter of individual choice, but are very often foisted upon one by fate. Burdening individuals with the need to pay for such arbitrary and uncontrollable costs is not only unethical, but destabilizing to our society.

Requiring individuals to pay for their own healthcare is destabilizing because, if a person's lifetime of work and saving can be wiped out in an instant by an unexpected illness, people will be much less willing to work hard, take risks, and otherwise engage in the economic activities that drive our society. "Healthcare security," which can only be provided by collective efforts, is thus necessary to a robust and sustainable civilization.

The methods by which healthcare costs can be controlled under a centralized system are straightforward. Obamacare, for instance, does so by explicitly empowering a (nearly) all-powerful Independent Payment Advisory Board with all macro-level healthcare spending decisions. Furthermore, "guidelines" promulgated by various other government-approved expert panels will control spending at a more granular level, by determining which specific services doctors will be permitted to offer to which patients, and under what circumstances. Doctors will be strictly held, under the threat of criminal prosecution, to these guidelines. Finally, recognizing implicitly that many healthcare needs are indeed determined by individual lifestyle choices rather than purely by chance, public health experts will advance enforceable policies that will determine what individual Americans will be permitted to do and not do, purchase or not purchase, eat or not eat. (The public health experts are off to a very good start in this effort!) If everyone within the healthcare system (and in our society) will simply follow the multitudinous directives laid out by the legions of sanctified experts, everybody will have their healthcare, costs will at last be contained, and all will be well.

Proponents of Method Two obviously do not sell their plan to the public by saying such things. Rather, they emphasize that the benevolent, caring, non-conflicted, government-approved experts will make sure that all the inefficiency and greed are squeezed out of the system, and that by doing so, everyone will get what they need, and costs will be controlled.

I will spend Part II of this book showing why Method Two is a bad choice. Here I will only state the bottom line: Implementing Method Two requires an all-powerful Central Authority, which will inevitably lead to tyranny (or anarchy), and will necessarily destroy the Great American Experiment.

Method Three: Provide Strictly Limited Public Support for Some Healthcare Services, with Individuals Responsible for the Remainder.

Method Three attempts to combine the benefits of Methods One and Two, while avoiding the major disadvantages of each.

Method Three recognizes that paying for all of one's own healthcare is beyond the means of many individuals, and that therefore a modern, civil society ought to provide at least some healthcare to at least some of its citizens. At the same time, Method Three recognizes that the public funding of all healthcare is beyond the means of society, leads to tyranny, and that (both for these practical reasons and for ethical reasons) individuals ought to be responsible for paying for as much of their own healthcare as they can, within reasonable limits.

The key to controlling costs is that the dollars which society will spend on healthcare for individuals must be strictly defined and strictly limited, and cannot be open-ended. Economic principles dictate that public healthcare spending must be limited to pay-as-you-go, and cannot accumulate inter-generational debt. Any other healthcare expenditures beyond those which society is able to provide in an economically responsible way must be paid for by individuals. Therefore, most individuals should not and cannot rely entirely on public funding for their healthcare.

At the same time, Method Three seeks to assure that individuals will have ready access to, and the means to pay for, basic healthcare services, and that the chances of being financially ruined by a catastrophic illness are very low.

Numerous configurations are possible under Method Three, and indeed, the creativity it allows (in distinction to Methods One and Two) is one of its attractions. Possible configurations might include something like the plan

Congressman Ryan proposed in 2011, which would place a strict limit on Medicare expenditures by providing seniors with a fixed amount of money – on a means-tested sliding scale – with which to purchase their health insurance of choice.

But a more radical (and I humbly submit) a more complete Method Three configuration would be that which I proposed in my 2007 book, *Fixing American Healthcare*. That book describes my plan at great length, but in outline here it is:

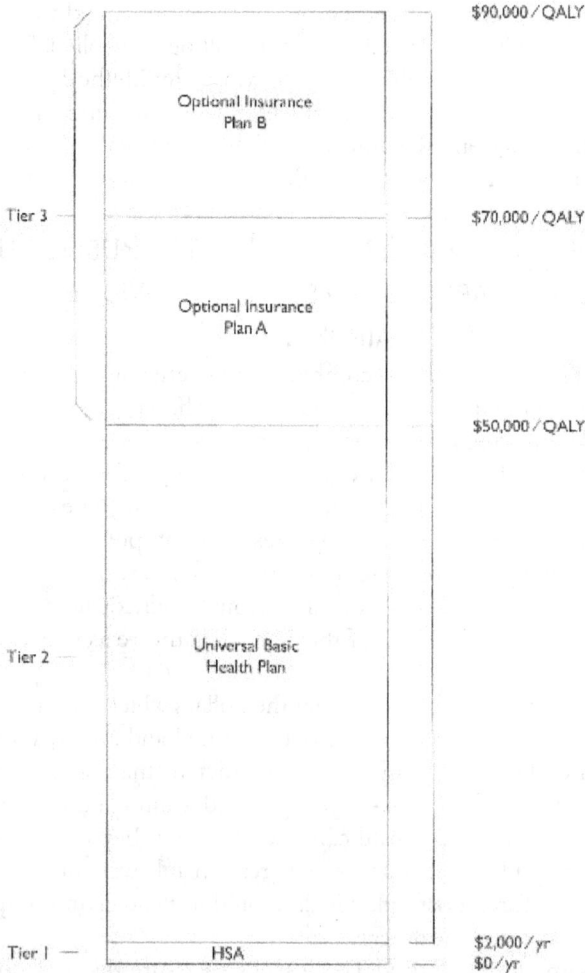

My model calls for a 3-tiered healthcare plan. (See the figure.) Tier 1 consists of a modified Health Savings Account. Each individual has his or her own HSA, into which they can deposit some amount of money each year (say, $2000) tax-free. For people in lower income levels, HSAs will be funded by the government on a sliding scale. Funds in the HSA can also grow tax-free, are the property of the individual, and cannot be taken away. Unspent funds that have accumulated above $10,000 can be transferred to an IRA at age 70.

The HSA is there for a very specific purpose: All individuals are responsible for paying for all their own healthcare expenses, up to $2000 per year. The HSA is aimed at providing funds for these annual personal expenditures.

Tier 2 is a Universal Basic Health Plan (UBHP), which will cover every person who resides in the United States legally. The UBHP kicks in after the individual has maxed out his or her $2000 annual personal healthcare expenditures. The UBHP I described in my book would operate under a system of completely open, completely transparent healthcare rationing. That is, it would cover all healthcare services that achieve a target level of cost-effectiveness, and would not cover anything else. The methodologies used to determine what is covered and what is not must be objective, measurable, and fully transparent to the public. My book describes such a rationing methodology in great detail*. However, the kind of open rationing system I described in my book is admittedly very complex, would likely be difficult to operate, and would certainly be difficult to explain to the public. There are simpler ways to administer Tier 2, and these simpler ways should be entertained.

_____

*My earlier book employed a novel method of calculating Quality Adjusted Life Year (QALY) values for various medical services, in order to rank the cost-effectiveness of those services. That section of my book was extremely boring and tedious and full of math, and I am led to understand that several individuals who actually tried reading that section died in situ. I am only mentioning it here because the term QALY shows up in the figure. For the purpose of the present discussion you can think of the QALY values in this figure as indicating "some defined amount of money that can be spent on your healthcare."

_____

The key point, however, is that the UBHP must indicate, very openly and plainly and for everyone to see, which medical services are covered, and which are not. It will not pretend to cover all beneficial healthcare services, or that uncovered services are necessarily worthless. It is a basic health plan, and not a comprehensive one. Its mission will be to cover all the proven healthcare services it can afford to cover without unreasonably jeopardizing the security of future generations of Americans.

Tier 3 is optional for individual Americans. It consists of insurance products which will be designed to cover healthcare services that a person wants or needs, but which are not covered (for whatever reason) under the UBHP. Accumulated funds in HSAs may be used to help pay premiums for Tier 3 coverage. Among other things, Tier 3 insurance products would resurrect our moribund health insurance industry. It would give them the opportunity to develop an array of products that do what insurance is actually supposed to do – to provide financial protection against the unlikely chance of something prohibitively expensive occurring.

If you don't like my plan, that's fine. I'm merely offering it as an example of the kinds of schemes that are possible under Method Three. The main points I want to emphasize are: a) This plan strictly limits the amount of public funding that will be spent on healthcare (and therefore solves our healthcare fiscal crisis). b) At the same time, it provides for both basic and advanced healthcare for every American (The advanced healthcare is provided with limits, to be sure, but those limits are completely transparent, and can be mitigated by electing to participate in Tier 3.) c) Since everyone will be paying out of pocket (from their HSAs) for basic healthcare services, those basic services will become subject to normal market forces for the first time in a half-century, and as a result their cost will inevitably drop.

How Will We Choose?

At this moment it appears that we have chosen Method Two. This is perfectly understandable. Progressives, in promoting their solution, have been able to make it seem far more desirable to the average American than have any proponents of Methods One or Three. Their message is: We will make sure that fair-minded, dedicated government agents (who care nothing for the evil of profits) will squeeze all the waste and inefficiency out of the system, and distribute just the right amount of healthcare at just the right time, and everyone will get exactly what they need. Even better, the rich people (i.e., the profit mongers) will bear most of the freight by paying high taxes.

That's a far more pleasant message than the ones that have been tried by those who favor Method One or Three, both of which require different – but significant – degrees of personal responsibility on the part of every American. Therefore, these other two methods, on the surface at least, sound a lot riskier, more difficult, and a lot more complicated than the easy, Let-Uncle-Sam-Do-It Method Two. In fact, given the way these choices have been sold to the public, it's hard to imagine we would choose anything except Method Two at this critical juncture.

Still, one can always hold out hope that we might reconsider. The main point of this book is to induce such a reconsideration by showing what Method Two will really be like for all of us.

And, if we do reconsider, I suppose it is obvious by now that I am partial to Method Three.

Method One is simply a non-starter. For all practical purposes, and for good or for bad, we moved irreversibly beyond a purely self-pay healthcare system over 60 years ago. So if there is to be a real battle, it will be between Method Two and Method Three.

The key difference between these two methods, both practically and philosophically, is whether individuals are to be expected – indeed, whether they are to be permitted – to pay for at least some of their own healthcare with their own money. Progressives, for reasons I will describe later, are absolutely adamant about the answer to this question – by no means will individuals be expected (or permitted) to pay for any of their own healthcare. It is absolutely imperative, if we are to achieve the perfect healthcare system that Method Two promises, that all healthcare decisions and all healthcare spending be centralized. There can be no compromise on this.

Indeed, the moment a compromise is made, true Progressives understand, we will inevitably wind up under a Method Three healthcare system. So Progressives are in no mood to compromise.

I will be delving into this crucial question – whether some amount of personal responsibility should be expected, or even allowed – later on in some detail, as I believe it is the most pivotal as-yet-unanswered question we will have to face going forward. For, while we have ostensibly chosen Obamacare, we have not all agreed on what that ultimately means for each of us. And once we do understand what it means, I believe we may be in the mood to reconsider our decision.

For now, I will make a simple assertion which I would like you to begin thinking about.

Here it is: If I am correct that Progressives will fight very hard – possibly to the death – to prevent individuals from spending their own money on healthcare, that fact carries with it an unavoidable implication. The only logical reason Progressives would fight so extremely hard to prevent such a thing is that their actual prime objective must be something other than merely fixing the healthcare system and controlling healthcare expenditures. Rather, their actual prime objective must be to employ our healthcare system's fiscal crisis as the most immediate and expeditious, and indeed the most ideal, vehicle for achieving their overall Program.

If you will allow even the remote possibility that this is the case, then we had better take a look at what the Progressive Program actually is. In the next chapter, that is what we will do.

WAIT! WHAT ABOUT METHOD FOUR?

Oh, yeah. I forgot to talk about Method Four.

There's really very little reason to talk about the fourth and final method for controlling our healthcare expenditures. This is because nobody likes it. There are no proponents for it, so nobody discusses it.

Still, Method Four, at this moment, seems to be the most likely outcome for us. Indeed, at this moment it appears to be our default method of choice.

Method Four is formulated as follows: Our skyrocketing healthcare expenditures are the chief driver of our national debt. Our national debt burden, unless we get control of it by controlling healthcare expenditures, will inevitably destroy our civil society. At the same time, our modern, sophisticated and very expensive healthcare system utterly requires a complex, modern, highly organized, high-tech society in order to function.

Therefore, our skyrocketing healthcare expenditures ultimately provides its own cure. Once society collapses, "healthcare services" will revert back to the roots-and-poultices methodologies that served mankind so well for millions of years. Healthcare will become very cheap again. And healthcare, as well as other modern gewgaws like cable TV, Internet, iPhones and automobiles, will no longer be considered by so many to be fundamental human rights, but will become a mere afterthought (if thought of at all), in a more primitive kind of society where life is nasty, brutish and short.

If we neglect to settle on any one of Methods One, Two or Three, or if we pick one and execute it poorly, we will, Chutes-and-Ladders-like, be deposited right back to Method Four where we all started.

Method Four is therefore only important in the way of helping us to keep things in perspective. For, whatever the outcome turns out to be, our current fiscal crisis in healthcare will ultimately be viewed by posterity, should any record of it remain for posterity, as a temporary matter of not much immediate concern.

CHAPTER 5 - A PRACTICAL THEORY OF THE PROGRESSIVE PROGRAM

"Unfortunately, in the last 30, 40 years, [liberal] has been turned up on its head, and it's been made to seem as though it is a word that describes big government, totally contrary to what its meaning was in the 19th and early 20th century. I prefer the word 'progressive,' which has a real American meaning, going back to the progressive era at the beginning of the 20th century. I consider myself a modern progressive."
- Hillary Clinton, 2007

My goal in Part I of this book has been to describe the sorry state of the American healthcare system pre-Obamacare. Before moving on to Part II – which will attempt to show why "fixing" the problem by instituting Progressive healthcare reforms is precisely the wrong thing to do – it occurs to me that I ought to explain exactly what I mean by "Progressive."

What I have done so far in this regard has largely consisted of offering unflattering innuendoes, casting negative aspersions, remarking snidely, and quoting from Ayn Rand (who I think was brilliant in characterizing the diagnosis, but whose prescription – unfettered and godless self-interest – I find disturbing). This has not exactly constituted an exercise in probity and precision. In this final chapter of Part I it is my intention to remedy this shortcoming.

To really understand where our healthcare system is headed, and for that matter where our society is headed, we need to understand Progressives and the Progressive Program.

I have personally found this understanding hard to come by. This is because Progressives, and especially American Progressives, have always been a bit enigmatic about their real goals. In my view their behavior tends to be persistently, almost defiantly counterproductive to the rights Americans traditionally hold dear, and which the Progressives themselves insist they revere – in particular, our inalienable rights to life, liberty and the pursuit of happiness.

Even a superficial analysis of the words and deeds of Progressives should reveal that, their protests to the contrary notwithstanding, they never really bought into the "inalienable" thing. It is quite apparent, to anyone who cares to look, that for Progressives such "natural rights" can and must be abridged whenever it is necessary to achieve some higher goal.

Since the behavior of American Progressives is so often inconsistent with the values they (most of them, at least) insist they love as well as any American, I concluded long ago that they must either be prevaricators or self-deluded when it comes to telling us what they are really up to. Either way, if we want to know what they really think, and what their agenda really is, we'll have to figure it out for ourselves.

And perhaps we'd better do just that, since it is looking a lot like the Progressives are going to be running things around here for a while.

I am not a political scientist. But I am a scientist. And for a scientist, one useful way to learn about any kind of system is first to make as many observations as you can about that system, then devise a theory to fully explain those observations, and then apply that theory to attempt to predict future behaviors of the system. As you observe how your theory is working, you can then go back as needed and readjust it to comport with your new observations. Repeat until done.

When you get to the point where subsequent, otherwise-difficult-to-explain behaviors have become predictable, your theory is reasonably likely to be in the ball park.

And so, I am going to present a theory of Progressivism. It is a theory that I have found useful in explaining many of the otherwise confounding and enigmatic behaviors which Progressives habitually display. I am not claiming that this theory is absolutely correct, merely that it is useful in practice. Since it is a theory whose value you can assess objectively with your own observations, its practical value should not depend on my own character, morals, intelligence, or psychological status, all of which have been impugned by readers of my blog in the way of proving that my theory cannot possibly have any merit.

You may not like this theory. A lot of people don't. But the thing about the scientific application of theories is that if you are going to make any, well, progress, you cannot simply write off or ignore theories whose implications you do not happen to like. Whichever theory is currently the best at explaining the known facts necessarily takes precedence, until such time as you can devise a new or adjusted theory that explains those facts even better.

I would welcome hearing about such a theory. In the meantime, here's mine.

A HOPELESSLY ABBREVIATED HISTORY OF PROGRESSIVISM

When I started my study of Progressives, I honestly did not know where to begin. So, like Descartes before me, I decided to proceed from the simplest and most irreducible of truths. Namely, that Progressives are really, really smart. We know this because all the best professors in all the best Ivy League schools are Progressives.

From this simple truth we can deduce that, whatever it is that Progressives are actually up to, it must have its roots in the writings of The Philosopher.

And sure enough, it was not at all difficult to discover the roots of Progressivism within the teachings of Aristotle. Aristotle tells us that man is innately a political animal, an animal with an inherent propensity to gather into increasingly complex communities. The essence of man, according to Aristotle, is society.

The formation of complex societies is what defines mankind; it is what differentiates man from the rest of the animal kingdom. Hence, because man is defined by society, society is inherently on a higher plane of importance than the individual. Individuals are entirely beholden to and dependent upon and subservient to the society to which they belong. Indeed, they are defined as individuals by their place and status within that society. Without society, a man is just an ape with better thumbs.

And so the precedence of the collective over the individual is not something we can simply choose to accept or reject; it is the very essence of mankind. It is nature. It is just the way it is.

Aristotle, as we can see, is a great friend to the Progressives.

The general idea that mankind is essentially a creature of society, and that the worth of the individual is defined by his/her worth to their society, is thus a very old idea, and in fact has been the normal way of looking at the relationship between individuals and society throughout most of history.

This really started to change just a few hundred years ago, when humanists began to cautiously explore the radical notion that individuals (rather than the collective) constitute the fundamental unit of humanity. The new humanist heresy – which declared the innate and irreducible worth of the individual and began to celebrate individual "autonomy" – came to be called "liberalism." Classical liberalism stressed individual freedom of thought and action, the right of private property, individual responsibility, free markets, and the limited power of the state. Classical liberalism reached its zenith a mere two and a half centuries after its painful birth, with the Declaration of Independence and the Constitution of the United States. The formation of a new nation whose government was explicitly established on the grounds of classical liberalism is what I've been calling the Great American Experiment.

The Great American Experiment, so far at least, appears to be a once-in-a-species event. So if we're about to abandon it, I would caution that perhaps we should first really think about it for a while.

In any case, even in America the collective countercurrent never really went away. And it never will, if only due to its extraordinarily deep roots in the history of men. And so, after only a century or so of relatively unfettered capitalism (the natural economic system of classic liberalism), during which the industrial revolution had been whipped to new heights, leading to unimagined progress and economic growth but also, alarmingly, to the creation of a large new underclass of hopelessly poor and horribly oppressed urban dwellers, collectivist thinkers were stirred to new action.

In some countries the "action" consisted of violent revolutions and all the bad stuff that typically follows such things. In the United States, the collectivist movement followed a much more prudent, much more practical, much more gradualist approach.

Taking its cue from the industrial revolution, which by radically transforming the modern world had graphically introduced the idea of "progress," and fascinated by the ideas of Darwin (which suggested not only that a system could be steadily and unrelentingly directed toward some state of "perfection," but also that the very nature of things seemed to dictate that it should be so), the new collectivist movement at the turn of the 20th century adopted the name "Progressive." To Progressives, classical liberalism has always been an aberration. Despite what America's founding documents might say, society takes precedence over the individual. It takes this precedence by way of the very essence of mankind, as was taught by The Philosopher, and so it cannot be otherwise.

(Within a couple of decades, "Progressives" had gotten such a bad reputation that they brazenly began referring to themselves as "liberals," usurping the terminology from a philosophy that was nearly its opposite, as if to convince the public that they actually held to those foundational American precepts of individual liberty, limited government, etc. But true to form, by 2007 they had pretty much trashed the name "liberal" as well, at which time Hillary Clinton famously declined to call herself a liberal any longer, and insisted instead that she was a "Teddy Roosevelt Progressive." It is therefore in deference to Ms. Clinton's explicit instructions that I am using that original terminology in this book.)

The Progressives, following unrelentingly their steady, Darwin-inspired evolutionary-not-revolutionary approach, have made astounding strides. Today they are on the verge of rendering their Program irreversible. And taking over the healthcare system will likely lead them to the final victory for which they have striven, so patiently and for so long.

THE PROGRESSIVE PROGRAM

Progressivism is a political movement whose premise is that the society of men can be perfected, and therefore it is the highest duty of any "good" society to constantly strive toward that achievable state of perfection. And so the Progressive Program – the thing that makes Progressives progressive – is to develop the perfect society. This program is not optional; it is dictated by the nature of mankind. It is therefore "right," and objecting to it is therefore "wrong."

The perfect society has three fundamental requirements. First, it must meet all the basic needs of the individuals within that society (such as food, clothing, shelter, sanitation, and health), without which individuals will always be tempted to engage in the counterproductive behavior of striving for things. Second, the social and economic benefits of society must be fairly distributed among all people. Therefore, there must be social justice – there must be no big winners or big losers. Big winners are an especial problem, because the presence of big winners just encourages greed and self-aggrandizement on the part of others, and will discourage citizens from dedicating themselves to the good of the whole. Third, once perfection is finally achieved, the social order must be of such a nature that it can persist, theoretically forever, without fundamental change. Indeed, the very notion of perfection implies that any change, of any type, is bad, since it will necessarily constitute a movement away from perfection. (This means, of course, that once the Progressives reach their goal, they will need to change their name. Of necessity they will become Conservatives.)

The perfect society therefore requires that people be granted "rights" to things – food, clothing, shelter, healthcare, etc. These rights obviously do not come from any Creator – so where do they come from? They can only come from a Central Authority – from the sovereign entity within a society that has the ultimate authority (backed by the legal use of violence or the threat thereof) to distribute the fruits of the society in such a manner that all those rights can be realized.

Progressives love to grant new rights to everyone, because each time they do, the Central Authority accrues that much more power over the behavior and the property of individuals.

The perfect society demands social or redistributive justice in all areas of social and economic endeavor, even in areas that have not yet been defined as a formal "right." Once again, only a strong Central Authority can determine what is fair or not fair, and can have the power to affect the appropriate redistributions it determines are necessary to achieve such fairness. The aforementioned creation of "rights," of course, will guarantee that such a powerful Central Authority will be established, so that social justice can progress steadily forward.

The perfect society requires complete stability. This would include (at a minimum) a stable population size, the preservation of natural resources and the earth's environment (indeed, when one hears the word "sustainability," one is usually listening to Progressive gospel), the careful management of the economy, and the careful control – if not suppression – of unplanned innovations.

This latter refers both to material (or scientific) innovations, and innovations of thought, either of which will always threaten hard-won societal stability.

Achieving the perfect society being the paramount work of mankind, any method which may help in achieving this perfection is to be embraced; none discounted out of hand. The only considerations one must make in choosing methods of action are: Is this method practicable? And: Is this method more likely to be successful, or counterproductive?

These two questions fully define Progressive ethics.

And finally, the Central Authority exists purely to grant essential rights to the people, to determine what is fair and then act to effect that fairness, and to establish the executive structures needed to achieve and maintain societal stability and sustainability. Therefore, by definition, as long as its actions are directed in these ways, it is an inherently ethical entity and must be regarded as such; and further, resistance to it is (equally inherently) unethical.

That's it. That's my theory of the Progressive Program. If you object to it, then, despite whatever personal shortcomings, sins, and wants you may perceive in your humble author, you are obligated (by all that is righteous and good) to postulate your own theory of Progressivism that explains, at least as well as my theory does, all of the following phenomena:

RULE BY EXPERTS

Despite its lip service to the contrary, Progressivism is not egalitarian. It simply cannot be.

For, while Progressivism is not by definition a system of rule by the elite, in practical terms it can only end up this way. Progressive leaders (themselves being quite elite) are never slow to perceive this truth.

It works like this: The duty of mankind is to strive for the perfect society. The chief tool by which mankind is to achieve this program is man's intellect and logic. It is axiomatic that only a minority of people will have the intellect and logic necessary to direct the Program of mankind.

Therefore, Progressivism ultimately relies on an elite corps of individuals — formally called "experts" — to guide our progress toward the perfect society. The perfect society will not just happen, it must be engineered by those who are expert enough to know what to do, and who are gifted enough to lead.

Those leading experts, the rare individuals without whom we will never achieve our state of perfection, are to be carefully nurtured and valued by society. Because their work is so critical to the essential Program, the elite must be removed from worry over the mundane necessities of life. That is, providing the leadership class with certain luxuries and privileges, and even freedom from having to follow all the rules that apply to the masses, is therefore not hypocrisy, but is an essential good. It redounds to the benefit of the Program, and therefore, to everyone.

This is why Progressive leaders habitually accept special privileges and perquisites that would make the King of Siam blush, and they do so with an air of matter-of-factness and entitlement that is impressive to behold.

THE DUTY OF WE THE PEOPLE

Just as it is the sacred duty of those who have been blessed with the intellectual tools to lead us toward the Promised Land, it is no less the sacred duty of the rest of us — we in the unwashed masses — to do whatever it is that the experts determine is best. The determinations and directives which the experts hand down may apply to all people, or they may be specifically directed toward you or me (which indeed would be a very great honor for us, would it not?) Either way, it is our duty to comply with all central directives, for the greater good of the whole.

This explains why Progressives express such indignant wrath over the Tea Party. Tea Party enthusiasts insist that their own individual autonomy must remain paramount, and utterly deny that they have any duty to comply with the Progressive Program. This attitude, of course, makes members of the Tea Party stupid, crazy or evil. And, because the current Progressive-in-Chief happens to be an African American who is acting within the prescribed range of behaviors for African Americans, it also makes them racist. (More on this latter point shortly.)

PROGRESSIVES VS. PROGRESSIVES

Progressives (capital P), as I use the term, are the thought leaders of Progressivism. They are the experts, the leadership class. They are the political leaders, the academics, the authors, the bureaucrats, and the pundits and spokespersons who set the agenda, make the decisions, form and transmit the message, and pass the judgments that make the Progressive engine run. They are the ones who know the way to the perfect society, and are driving us to it.

On the other hand, progressives (the "small-p-progressive," the rank and file, one-of-us progressives who spend their lives toiling away within the general population), who form the large majority of American progressives, are basically just nice people. For the most part progressives honestly believe that their political philosophy is the right philosophy, the fairest philosophy, and innately the kindest and most humane political philosophy there can be. They are not trying to drive society toward perfection as much as they are merely aiming for more fairness in the distribution of the good things that come from being in a society in the first place.

Small-p-progressives do indeed tend to look at non-Progressives, and especially Conservatives, as being driven chiefly by vice – usually selfishness and greed – and so are subject to being induced to states of great indignation and anger (by Progressives) against specific non-Progressives, and can often be mobilized to action against same.

So, within the great unwashed masses, progressives are seen by Progressives as the ones who bathe at least weekly.

THE FUNDAMENTAL FLAW OF PROGRESSIVISM

The fundamental flaw of Progressivism is the same as the fundamental flaw of all collectivist political systems. Namely, Progressivism ultimately relies on all members of society to subsume their own individual needs to the needs of the collective. That is, the Progressive Program requires a fundamental change in human nature. And alas! This change will never be forthcoming.

All ideal political and economic systems – including capitalism – eventually founder on the shoals of human nature if certain adjustments are not made. However, collectivist systems are especially vulnerable to human nature. Unlike capitalism (which incorporates, utilizes and makes the best of the individual's innate self-centered nature), collectivist systems require the complete suppression of man's natural impulses (again, unless you are lucky enough to be amongst the leadership class). So collectivist systems are rapidly and deeply challenged by human nature. It is their fundamental flaw.

This fundamental flaw will almost always lead to great frustration on the part of the leadership of any collectivist system, dooms their attempts at societal perfection, and finally results in tyranny or anarchy. This is why, while collectivist systems often sound quite attractive to the inexperienced youth or their unaware elders, collectivism always tends to end badly.

So, despite their frequent hymns of praise to the worthiness of the common man, Progressives invariably develop an underlying contempt toward the unwashed masses. It is not difficult to spot this contempt if you are alert to it.

MANAGING THE UNWASHED MASSES

Instead of surrendering to the inevitabilities of human nature, Progressives will instead try to "manage" the unwashed masses.

Now, for your typical American progressive, getting people to go along with the Progressive Program will be a simple matter of education. The Progressive Program is so obviously Right, and anything else so obviously Wrong, that anyone can see it with a minimum of instruction. These progressives believe this because it is how they themselves were won over.

But the Progressives – the elite class of leaders, who have probably been to Harvard – understand that education (i.e., indoctrinating the public to the great benefits of the Progressive agenda), only goes so far. It does indeed get you a substantial number of believers (probably 20 – 25% of the population), but it still leaves you with a very large proportion of the people who will only go along to the extent that they themselves benefit.

And so Progressives attempt to control the unwashed masses by means of pacification (i.e., attempting to meet all their basic needs, so as to eliminate their impulse to strive). This helps quite a bit – in fact, it is one of the main strategies of the Progressives for controlling the people.

Unfortunately, even this does not work in a substantial number of people. Some people, no matter what kind of indoctrination you provide for them, or what benefits and entitlements you may offer them, will simply refuse to place the needs of the collective above their own.

In other collectivist systems we have seen around the world, the utter frustration that develops on the part of political leaders because of this innate human recalcitrance seems nearly inevitably to lead to coercion, intimidation, peer-pressure, and, ultimately, violence*. When the expediency of violence is finally reached, you inevitably end up with the tyranny or anarchy I mentioned earlier.

---

* According to R.J. Rummel in his book *Death by Government*, during the 20th century the world's governments killed four times as many of their own people, on purpose, as were killed in all wars combined.

In the United States, while the frustration of our Progressive leaders with us folks is often palpable, and while their growing contempt for us occasionally breaks through the surface, so far whole scale violence has been avoided. I think this is at least partially because of a unique invention of American Progressives – Diversity.

THE IMPORTANCE OF DIVERSITY

"Diversity" was once merely a pleasant feature of some population or group, a nice-to-have, a quality that implied a certain open-mindedness, an acceptance of different kinds of people, or thoughts, or music preferences. In recent years, however, Diversity has been transformed into the Uber-Virtue, the highest virtue of all, the virtue from which all the other subsidiary (formerly cardinal) virtues must necessarily spring. Today, when planning any new endeavor, no matter of what type or for what purpose, your chief and overarching consideration must be – can only be – to achieve Diversity.

How did it get to be this way?

It all comes from the Progressive Program, which, again, is to create the perfect society. The Progressive elite know just how to do this, of course, but individuals within every population throughout human history have insisted upon acting in their own self-interest, which is counterproductive to the collective goal. In many places which have made similar efforts to perfect human societies, such individual recalcitrance has been dealt with by means of concentration camps and pogroms and the like.

"Diversity" is a much kinder and very much gentler approach to curing the problem of individualism. With such a critically important function, Diversity has naturally assumed a primary place in our society.

Specifically, the doctrine of Diversity defines the range of permissible behaviors and thoughts – Right Actions and Right Thoughts – for a given group of people within a society. Diversity informs you of how to be a legitimate and accepted member of your group.

The numerous celebrations of Diversity we see all around us invariably turn out to be strategies to reinforce those allowable ranges of thought and behavior. In this way, members of a particular group can be individually celebrated as embodying the characteristics assigned to the group. Conversely, those who begin behaving and thinking outside the allowable range can be quickly identified and dealt with, either through correction (which brings them back into the group), or through vilification (which completely marginalizes and devalues them within society). So, for instance, Al Sharpton and Jesse Jackson are celebrated individuals, whose accomplishments nicely reflect their assigned group identities. In contrast, Clarence Thomas and Thomas Sowell are not celebrated by Progressives, and indeed are castigated as abominations, because their individual accomplishments do not reflect their assigned group identities.

This concept, I believe, also helps us to understand what Progressives mean by "racism." Racism is when you criticize a person, for any reason, who is acting entirely within the expected range of behaviors of their assigned group. On the other hand, it is not racism – and indeed, it is strongly encouraged – to criticize a person who is acting outside of his/her allowable range of behaviors. So criticizing Louis Farrakahn for calling Jews devils is racist. Saying anything nasty about Thomas Sowell, for any reason whatsoever, is perfectly acceptable.

Similarly, the concept of Diversity helps us to understand why it is laudable for Progressive commentators to say extraordinarily vile things about Ms. Palin and Ms. Bachman (and their children); but it is the height of sexism (sexism being a mortal sin) for Conservative commentators to say equally vile things about Sandra Fluck (the Georgetown law student who voluntarily testified before a Congressional subcommittee in early 2012 to ask for free contraceptives). I was raised in an era when it was unacceptable to say such horrible things about any woman, and believe Mahar, Letterman and Limbaugh all ought to be ashamed of themselves. But by the lights of Progressivism, since those Conservative women are acting well outside the bounds of acceptable behavior for their group (i.e., Women), making defamatory statements about them (and theirs) is no less than they deserve. Ms. Fluck, needless to say, was acting in precisely the prescribed manner, and so any negative statements (vile or not) about her are entirely verboten.

I want to emphasize the beauty of this formulation. It allows Progressives to make passionate and heart-felt – but highly selective – charges of racism, sexism, homophobia, etc. against their adversaries, while engaging in precisely the same behavior themselves, and all without being in the least bit hypocritical. Hypocrisy is when one espouses certain principles, but then acts in a way that violates those principles. But the actions of Progressives in making charges of racism, etc., are entirely consistent with their Diversity dogma, right down the line, and hence do not constitute hypocrisy.

To a great extent the potential worth of an individual in society is pre-determined by the group to which the individual belongs. People belonging to White Male, for instance, appear to have lesser intrinsic value to the ultimate goal of societal perfection than people belonging to Hispanic Female, even if they are particularly exemplary members of the White Male group.

Therefore, while individuals within Progressive societies can achieve a certain level of importance, individual importance is merely of tertiary concern, rather than primary or even secondary concern. Individuals can become officially "important" only if their importance reflects the essence of their assigned group; and the importance of the assigned group (the secondary concern), in turn, is proportional to its ability to advance the Progressive Program in general (which, of course, is the primary concern).

In summary, Diversity is critical to Progressivism because group identity is the best available mechanism by which the Progressive leadership can attempt to control and direct individual behaviors without resorting to violence. It is, in fact, a brilliant invention.

I know it is easy to become confused about this, since classically "diversity" means something other than "conformity." You may find it helpful to remember a general rule about Progressives: If you want to know what Progressives are really up to, listen to what they say and then look to see if their deeds are actually working toward the opposite thing. Frequently you will find that they are.

PROGRESSIVISM AND RELIGION

Progressives have a natural aversion to organized religion. This is for three reasons. First, most major religions find a higher authority than the enlightened leadership the Progressives propose to create for us. Second, most religions are too concerned with some sort of afterlife, and insufficiently concerned with creating paradise right here on earth. And third, the major religions stress individual conscience and individual salvation over collective priorities.

Apparently realizing that abolishing religion is far too difficult a task, Progressives have adopted the long-term strategy of infiltrating and co-opting religious establishments, and by means of introducing new ideas – such as "group salvation," and the concept of social justice as a religious imperative – rendering religion, this "opiate of the masses," less incompatible with the Progressive Program.

Progressives do find certain religions more acceptable than others at various times. Such partiality certainly does not appear to depend in any way on the precepts or beliefs of any particular religion, but rather, on whether temporarily showing sympathy for it might in some manner advance their Program.

GOOD AND EVIL IN PROGRESSIVISM

In a similar vein, Progressive intellectuals are known for asserting that there are no absolutes, and so there is no such thing as inherent good or inherent evil, or inherent right or wrong. So, for instance, being against gay marriage because you believe it is "wrong" on religious grounds simply does not signify.

This general attitude toward good and evil is easily explained by the simple fact that true Progressives deny any authority, any arbiter of values, that is above their own enlightened leadership. Saying that something is intrinsically "good" or intrinsically "evil" clearly implies such a higher authority, and so, such statements must be delegitimized.

In general, this kind of moral relativism in Progressive thought holds up quite nicely, except in one area. That is the area of Progressivism itself. Because the Progressive Program is the innate agenda for mankind, there indeed exists a standard by which one can (and must) determine good and evil.

"Good" is anything which advances the Progressive Program; and "evil" is anything which threatens it.

Anyone who doubts the existence of good and evil within the Progressive Program need only observe the scores of behaviors and figures of speech which are condemned as unrelentingly evil by Progressives, with all the wild-eyed fervor of a Jonathan Edwards.

Accordingly, individuals who hinder the Progressive Program are a danger to mankind's very essence. They are evil, and must be rehabilitated or eliminated.

PROGRESSIVISM AND ENVIRONMENTALISM

Radical environmentalism and the Progressive Program are not perfectly compatible with one another. But they are close.

Radical environmentalists believe that humanity is a plague upon Planet Earth. Everything man has done since the day he first learned to cultivate crops (and thus for the first time became a different kind of animal) has been bad. And anything which delays, halts or reverses the sins mankind has perpetrated upon sacred Gaia, since that day he first departed from Nature, is a good thing. So the radical environmentalists tend to favor strong central governments which (with the help of their Progressive allies) they can influence to control the destructive behaviors of individuals.

Progressives are certainly on board with controlling man's effect on the environment, but (in most cases) they are not in favor of returning mankind to a hunter/gatherer condition (since most Progressives do not view this condition as the embodiment of a perfect society). Rather, they view the environmental movement – in particular, the Global Warming Theory – as a good way to get the populace to grant sweeping new powers to the Central Authority, which they can then use to carry out their Progressive Program. So Progressives have completely embraced the Global Warming Theory, chiefly as a means to their own political ends. Accordingly they have awarded it the status of Progressive Dogma, pronouncing man-made global warming to be "settled science." They suppress any efforts to study it further, and declare anyone who dares question it to be the moral equivalent of a Holocaust denier.

This is really too bad. I suspect that global warming is occurring, and I will even concede that human behavior may be playing a role. So I am saddened that this scientific question has been declared off limits, and has been absorbed into the Progressive Program in such a way that we are not allowed to find out what's really going on. It leaves people like me (who think the Progressive Program is deadly) little choice but to oppose the environmentalist and global warming agenda.

PROGRESSIVISM AND THE INTRINSIC VALUE OF HUMAN LIFE

Progressivism values the individual primarily (and often, solely) as a function of their value to society. Unfortunately, this means that - especially under times of duress - Progressivism tends not to impart any real, intrinsic value to human life itself. Under a Progressive system, the lack of an intrinsic value to human life is manifested most often by a willingness, sometimes an enthusiasm, to assign arbitrary values to various categories of human life. In Chapters 12 and 13, I will elaborate on some aspects of this feature of Progressivism.

While I find this tendency very troubling from a religious point of view, I concede that religious points of view generally carry no weight with true Progressives. So I will simply note that, looking at the matter in a purely hard-nosed, objective and practical way, when the value of human life is determined arbitrarily, that value is necessarily changeable given the exigencies of the day. And during times of stress (say, severe fiscal stress), terrible abuses become almost inevitable.

The changeability of the value of human life is most easily observable, in recent years, by the apparent "slippage" we have seen in what ought to constitute a legal abortion. We began by saying that abortions ought to be conducted only during the first trimester. But Progressives are now indignant at efforts to stop late-term abortion, and near-infanticide (killing babies who are born alive after a botched abortion). Some respected Progressive ethicists are even proposing that laws to be changed to allow frank infanticide, that is, to allow parents to kill their recently born children if they decide they would rather not have them. (I will elaborate in this proposal in Chapter 13.) Whether you're religious or not, this kind of slippage in what constitutes "human life" might seem troublesome to you.

Historically, of course, the most visible example of the Progressive attitude toward the sanctity of human life was their enthusiastic support of eugenics in the early decades of the 20th century. Since World War II, of course, openly espousing eugenics has become unfashionable, and we have successfully developed a collective amnesia regarding just how mainstream the idea of eugenics was prior to the War. It was, in fact, quite mainstream. For decades, eugenics was openly celebrated by Progressive leaders, and in fact was openly practiced - mainly by conducting involuntary sterilizations in women who were deemed to be of substandard stock, and by letting babies born with congenital defects die without care.

The enthusiasm Progressives displayed for eugenics is easy to understand when you consider that, one way or another, a perfect society will require far more perfect citizens than we have today. Indeed, the seething contempt with which Progressives regard the current genetic pool that comprises the unwashed masses is often difficult for them to suppress. The idea of "culling the herd" in order to improve the quality of the populace is an idea that comes to them naturally. Theodore Roosevelt, Woodrow Wilson, Bertrand Russell, H. G. Wells, and Margaret Sanger (the founder of Planned Parenthood) are only the most well-known Progressives who publicly extolled the idea of eugenics.

Now that Progressives are in charge of our healthcare system, and will be the ones determining who gets what, when, and how, this history – and this tendency – is something we ought to keep in mind.

PROGRESSIVISM AND POLITICS

Under the Progressive Program, just as Aristotle says, mankind is essentially a political animal. In fact, the Progressive Program (in general) can only be achieved by political action. This means that politics – and to be clearer, political control – is the fundamental work of Progressives. Without politics, without political control, there is nothing. To lose political power is oblivion.

Not all Progressives, of course, run for elective office. Many more of them go into "public service," wherein they spend their entire careers becoming deeply imbedded into the multitudinous governmental bureaucracies, in all three branches, and at all levels.

For Progressives, politics is everything, the essence of human behavior. And it is worth any cost, any desperate measure, to maintain political control. Indeed, to fail to lie, cheat and steal in order to keep political control would be unethical. This is why they think any proposal that would limit their ability to commit what most Americans would consider election fraud is immoral, and must be indignantly put down.

This attitude toward politics is in stark contrast to the attitude of non-Progressives, and especially of Conservatives, for whom government (and therefore politics) is merely a necessary evil, with which one must occasionally contend when it cannot be avoided. For most Conservatives politics is an afterthought.

What this means of course is that Progressivism has progressed continuously, for over a century, despite the fact that a majority of Americans still appear not to subscribe to their Program. Even in those intervals where Conservatives roust themselves into action, and take temporary control of the Presidency or a house or two of Congress, the deeply-imbedded Progressives are still there, busily gumming up the system at every level, until such time as their leaders again are in the ascendancy.

PROGRESSIVISM AND THE GREAT AMERICAN EXPERIMENT

Unlike any other nation in the history of mankind, the United States was not founded because of geography, race, religion or ethnicity. It was founded on an idea. It was founded on the still-radical idea that individual autonomy – the individual's God-given right to life, liberty, and the pursuit of happiness – is the chief Fact of humankind, and that the only legitimate role of government is to create an environment in which individuals can enjoy those rights to the fullest extent possible.

One can see immediately that the Great American Experiment – which awards primacy to individual autonomy – is fundamentally incompatible with Progressivism. But because a majority of Americans still like the ideas expressed in the Declaration of Independence, the Progressives need to play their cards close to their chests. They need to proceed carefully – but relentlessly.

By slowly re-interpreting the Constitution, and slowly addicting a critical mass of Americans to an array of government programs, Progressives are certain they will ultimately prevail. They have been at it for over 100 years, and have come a long way.

I personally cannot tell whether or not we have already passed the Event Horizon, the point beyond which restoring the Great American Experiment will become impossible. But we are at least very close.

In fact, one plausible theory for President Obama's headlong pursuit of healthcare reform (and other policies which tend to anger the majority of Americans), is that he sees America as being at the very cusp of that Event Horizon. One, last, great push – Obamacare – will sufficiently expand government control, and government dependency, to render the Progressive Program irreversible, whatever might happen in the next election or two.

In any case, whether the President's gamble pays off or not, the Progressive assault on the Great American Experiment has at least placed it in mortal jeopardy, and mankind's one (and possibly only) shot at creating a society in which individual rights are paramount is in grave danger of oblivion.

PROGRESSIVISM VS. SOCIALISM, COMMUNISM, AND FASCISM

To this point I have avoided directly comparing or contrasting Progressivism to the more commonly discussed economic and political systems of Socialism, Communism, or Fascism. And actually, I would have preferred to leave it this way. As I have said, I am not a political scientist, and so I am not as interested in relating Progressivism to these other -isms, as much as I am in simply characterizing the behavior of the people who will actually be running my life, and the lives of my family and loved ones.

But I know from experience that if I do not directly address this topic, readers with a certain frame of mind will be dissatisfied with my theory of Progressivism, no matter how well it predicts the behavior of Progressives.

So I will do my best, very briefly, to place Progressivism into its proper place relative to these other major political/economic systems.

Progressivism falls into the larger category of collectivist systems. That is, it is a political system in which individual rights and individual freedom of action are subservient to the needs of the collective, and whose chief goal is to run things for the optimal benefit of the collective whole.

Also within the category of collectivist systems are Communism, Socialism, and (some authorities maintain) Fascism.

Communism (the kind that has actually existed in various countries, not the impossible kind which Marx described) is a system in which all property is owned by the state, which in theory acts as a proxy for the "people". The job of the state is to arrange things so as to achieve a reasonably high and reasonably equal level of "good" for everyone.

Socialism is a much broader and much less restrictive form of collectivism, since, while the state may own all or much of the property, socialism is also fine with a certain species of private ownership. Under socialism, individuals or private organizations may own even large amounts of property, but their control over that property – what they are permitted to do with it, or how they may dispose of it – is largely controlled (or "regulated") by the state. The state also reserves the right to decide when somebody owns too much property, and has the authority to "redistribute" some or all of it, to further the goals of collective fairness (i.e., social justice).

Under Fascism, individual freedoms are also subservient to the collective goals, and the state has the right to confiscate private property any time it deems it desirable to do so. This (and the fact that Nazis referred to themselves as socialists) causes many authorities to classify Fascism as a collectivist system. But Fascism differs greatly from Communism and "real" Socialism in that the overarching goal of the latter two systems is to achieve a reasonably high and reasonably equal level of good for everyone, whereas the overarching goal of Fascism is to establish a certain faction of the population (an ethnic group, or the party) as a master race, and anyone else who is suffered to continue living as subservient peoples. So Fascism is collectivist only in the narrow sense that by the "collective" you are referring only to the favored group.

Given these constructs, Progressivism is a species of Socialism. As I have just defined Progressivism, it is in fact a fairly uniquely American form of Socialism. It is a harder-edged, more muscular form of Socialism than, say, European Socialism.

European Socialism has been the most successful form of collectivism to date. In particular, unlike other collectivist systems we have seen around the world, it has not led to violent suppression of the people by the Central Authorities. I believe this is largely because of the history of Europe – centuries of monarchies and non-mobile societies in which status was related to birthright, culminating in several extraordinarily destructive wars that deeply and directly affected virtually every member of society. This history rendered the idea of socialism (subsuming individual freedom – which had never amounted to all that much anyway – for the promise of stability and security) quite attractive to most Europeans. When Western European countries adopted Socialism, their leaders could afford to be open an honest about what they were attempting to do. And Socialism was broadly embraced by the people, to a large extent, with open arms and a sense of relief. Even today, with the European debt crisis (which is the other end-result of collectivism) threatening to wreck the entire system, most Europeans still love their brand of Socialism, and the relative (though temporary) security it has brought them.

In contrast, American Progressives have the difficult task of having to upend – as surreptitiously as possible – a foundational philosophy that is the polar opposite of collectivism; a system founded on the inalienable rights of the individual, in which the chief job of the government is to provide national security and a reasonably level playing field on which individuals can compete – and otherwise stay out of the way. It is a system that most Americans still like, and do not want to end. So the Progressives' task has been monumentally difficult. They have had to carry out their Program without being able to say openly what their Program is really all about. Even now, when they are on the verge of success, their success relies largely on the fact that most Americans don't realize what is about to be taken away from them.

Having to operate in the milieu of the Great American Experiment has made American Progressives – the ones who are really running things, not the large majority of progressives – hard-edged and realistic. They are not immersed in the usual bright-eyed idealism that characterizes most Socialists who first ascend to political victory. American Progressives don't expect things to go smoothly. They have had, of necessity, to be cagy about what they were doing. They had to prevaricate. And they realize that most Americans are only slowly awakening to the realities of Progressivism. Progressive leaders know they will have to use coercion, cajoling, bribery, threats, selective prosecution, intimidation, and lots and lots of smooth talk to maintain their newly-won positions. American Progressives know what they are up against, and promise to be relatively ruthless, relatively merciless, in consolidating their authority. They have worked long and hard for this opportunity and will be ready for it, and they will be very formidable indeed.

I realize that this synthesis of Progressivism will be highly objectionable to many progressives, who honestly believe that their political philosophy is simply the fairest one there can be. To these, some of whom I have counted among my closest friends, I beg only three things. First, please take an objective look at the history of collectivist systems in the world during the last hundred years. Second, try to articulate, with an equally objective view, exactly how my synthesis is mistaken, and specifically, how it fails to explain the actual behavior we see from American Progressives. And third, ask yourself whether you are really prepared to assist in scuttling the Great American Experiment.

In any case, if there is going to be a fight to slow the march of Progressivism, it will have to be on the battleground they themselves have chosen, and on which their forces already have been fully arrayed. That battleground is our healthcare system.

Part 2 - What We Can Expect from Obamacare

CHAPTER 6 - SOME IMPLICATIONS OF A RIGHT TO HEALTHCARE

"It will be of little avail to the people, that the laws are made by men of their own choice, if the laws be so voluminous that they cannot be read, or so incoherent that they cannot be understood."
- James Madison, *The Federalist* #62

———

Apoplexy is a frequent condition among Conservatives today. This is because triggers abound.

And, among these fine Americans, one of the more common and more malignant triggers of apoplectic vocalizations is the assertion that healthcare is a right.

To a Conservative, a right is an attribute that accrues to every person naturally, by virtue of the fact that they are members of the human race. Such natural rights, which invariably are rights to take some action, are considered to descend from the Creator (as the Declaration of Independence asserts), or at the very least from the inherent nature of the Universe, and thus are not subject to addition or subtraction by any human authority – such as by governments. And because natural rights are granted equally to every human, it is an inherent truth that there can be no such thing as a right that imposes obligations or limitations on the natural rights of others. Indeed, the very notion that a right can exist that imposes such obligations on another person is an utter abomination.

Progressives see rights differently. To them, a right is not a right to act, granted by nature, but rather, it is a right to receive something (invariably the product of another's actions), granted by a man-made Central Authority.

And hence, apoplexy.

Franklin Roosevelt started it. In his 1944 State of the Union message, he said:

> *"This Republic had its beginning, and grew to its present strength, under the protection of certain inalienable political rights – among them the right of free speech, free press, free worship, trial by jury, freedom from unreasonable searches and seizures. They were our rights to life and liberty.*
>
> *As our nation has grown in size and stature, however – as our industrial economy expanded – these political rights proved inadequate to assure us equality in the pursuit of happiness.*
>
> *We have come to a clear realization of the fact that true individual freedom cannot exist without economic security and independence. Necessitous men are not free men. People who are hungry and out of a job are the stuff of which dictatorships are made.*
>
> *In our day these economic truths have become accepted as self-evident. We have accepted, so to speak, a Second Bill of Rights under which a new basis*

of security and prosperity can be established for all, regardless of station, race, or creed."

Roosevelt then proposed, in his Second Bill of Rights, that each American is entitled by rights to:

- A living wage
- Freedom from unfair competition
- Housing
- Education
- Social security
- Healthcare

All this, of course, just goes to show how bad an idea the Bill of Rights was from the very beginning. If I had been around in 1789, I would have counseled Mr. Madison thusly: "Jim, don't do it. You have crafted a perfectly good Constitution already. It carefully enumerates the very few powers which We the People have granted to the Federal government, and it explicitly states that any such power not explicitly granted herein is specifically NOT available to the Feds. If you go amending the thing, before it ever gets going, with a list of specific things the government cannot do to us, you will undermine that overarching prohibition. Your list of restrictions on the government's power will necessarily be incomplete, and eventually proponents of big government will notice, "It doesn't say we can't do such and such." And furthermore, even your enumerated prohibitions will be quibbled with, twisted, and reinterpreted over time, in a very lawyerly fashion. And the next thing you know (say, in a quarter millennium or so), you'll have a huge, powerful Federal government doing all kinds of nasty things to We the People (though no doubt only with the best of intentions), and referencing your fine Constitution as their authority for doing so."

The Bill of Rights, as President Obama has noted, is a negative list. It enumerated specific items, which were particularly important to Americans at the end of British rule, which the government was not permitted to do to the people.

Franklin Roosevelt turned the whole concept of the Bill of Rights on its head – his was a list of items the government was required to "provide" for the people. His formulation was masterful, and it is a formula that has been carried forward by Progressives to this day. He claimed to derive the authority for his new Bill of Rights from the Declaration of Independence itself, saying that the "pursuit of happiness" requires everyone to have (i.e., to be given) this whole list of stuff (thus neatly eliminating the need to "pursue" the happiness in the first place). He added that failing to provide these rights will lead to dictatorship, ignoring the very reason for the original Bill of Rights – that any government with the power over individuals necessary to provide all these "rights" will itself have to be an extremely authoritarian one.

In any case, Roosevelt's Second Bill of Rights has been the Progressive's Shining City on a Hill for nearly 70 years. And it graphically illustrates how differently the Progressives view "rights." (Conservatives will note that it is entirely possible to address the problem Roosevelt invoked – an unreasonable inequality of opportunity – without creating any new "rights" that will forever increase the power of the government over the people.)

American Progressives generally do not explicitly deny the existence of "natural rights" altogether. (Doing so would cause them embarrassment when they assert their own inalienable "truths," such as the superiority of Diversity over all other human virtues). But at their core Progressives do not (and cannot) actually subscribe to natural, God-given rights that accrue equally to every person. This is because in the Progressive Program, rights are attributes granted by a Central Authority, aimed at achieving the social justice which is necessary to a perfect society. Therefore, almost by definition, Progressive rights are differential rights. That is, they are rights that, for the sake of social justice, must be at least somewhat different among various defined groups, and accordingly, not only must such rights be actively manufactured, but also they must be appropriately assigned and carefully distributed.

Natural rights granted by some sort of Creator obviously cannot handle such a job. Only a Central Authority can do this.

"Rights" granted under the Progressive Program will necessarily create involuntary obligations upon at least some individuals, at the very least confiscating the products of their efforts, and therefore from the Conservative point of view will always fundamentally violate the essence of what is truly a "right." A Progressive may or may not be willing to allow that a few natural rights may exist; but they won't let such rights hinder them. This is because rights granted by the Central Authority, deriving from political power*, take precedence; and any "natural rights" can simply be suspended whenever necessary.

---

* As Ron Bloom (President Obama's former Manufacturing Czar) explained, "We kind of agree with Mao that political power comes largely from the barrel of a gun."

Nothing pleases Progressives more than an opportunity to grant a new right. Every time they do so, the Central Authority gathers yet more power over the actions and the property of individuals, and therefore becomes more capable of moving us all toward societal perfection.

In Part I of this book, I tried to describe the American healthcare landscape as we enter the era of Obamacare. Here in Part II, I hope to show what we should all expect from Obamacare. And the first thing we need to know in this regard is that the passage of Obamacare, for its proponents at least, finally establishes healthcare as an American right, and thus achieves a goal which has been an explicit part – and likely the most critical part – of the Progressive agenda since at least 1944.

This accomplishment – establishing healthcare as a right – carries with it certain implications.

WHAT IS HEALTHCARE, ANYWAY?

When healthcare is a right, then for the very first time, that which constitutes "healthcare" will have to be explicitly defined. This is because if a medical service is deemed to be "healthcare," then people have a right to it. Conversely, if a medical service is deemed not to be "healthcare," then not only don't people have a right to it, but they also should not have access to it. (If people were allowed access to medical services that the Central Authority deems not to be "healthcare," people might get the idea that the Central Authority is holding back on them. And that would be a dangerous idea indeed.)

So you can see how important it will be to define, specifically, what healthcare is – and what it is not. Since the Central Authority will be administering the right to healthcare, naturally the experts appointed by the Central Authority will be the ones who will be doing this job.

It will be a job as difficult as it is important. For instance, most people would agree that medical services that aim to prevent disease, restore health, optimize functional capacity in the face of illness, or control symptoms, ought to be included under the umbrella of "healthcare."

But nitroglycerin and stenting can both relieve angina. One is very cheap and marginally satisfactory; while the other is very expensive and usually much more effective. Should both constitute healthcare, or only one? An expensive new drug prolongs survival with a certain type of cancer by an average of six months. Is that healthcare?

Is a treatment that does not actually cure or ameliorate a disease, but, that, say, slows the normal aging process, to constitute healthcare? If not, we should put a stop at once to the large volume of research currently being done on the aging process.

What about other treatments that enhance the life of individuals in the absence of serious disease or disability, such as face-lift surgery, hair transplantation, Lasik surgery, oral contraceptives when used for the express purpose of preventing pregnancy, or Viagra? Should those be healthcare?

And then there are conditions famously subject to "disease creep" – such as autism spectrum disorder, or ADHD, or even obesity – conditions for which the diagnosis has been increasingly expansive, so as to roll in more and more people who, in earlier times, would have been considered variants of normal. Should treatment of those conditions be considered healthcare?

Since the availability or non-availability of treatment will likely hinge on the answer to this question, there will be a lot of pressure, in both directions, on the Deciders. If it were not for the fact that the people who will be doing this job will be entirely objective and totally non-conflicted government-appointed experts, the process of deciding what is and what is not "healthcare" would be quite worrisome.

ALL RATIONING WILL HAVE TO BE COVERT

Since healthcare is a right, useful healthcare obviously cannot be withheld. Therefore, all the healthcare rationing that is done under Obamacare will have to be covert.

Under Obamacare many of the methods of covert rationing which were traditionally used by health insurance companies (e.g., cherry-picking, driving sick subscribers away, rescission, etc.), will not be available. This means that other covert rationing techniques will have to be developed.

Thankfully, physicians will be a big help here, since their New Ethics makes it OK for them to ration healthcare at the bedside. So it will be important for Obamacare's administrators to continue establishing incentives for doctors to withhold medical care.

But to really cut down on healthcare expenditures, a lot of creativity will be needed. Fortunately for the Obamacare administrators, while they do not have all the options that were available to the HMOs, they do have the wind of the sovereign authority in their sails. They will be able to try new things that the HMOs could only dream of.

Here is a brief survey of what some of those "new methods" will be. I will be discussing the more remarkable ones in detail in the following chapters.

CENTRALIZED DECISION-MAKING

The big driver of medical expenses, as we have seen, arises from individual doctors making independent spending decisions along with their individual patients. And even though the Central Authority can coerce doctors all day long to withhold expensive medical services, the HMOs graphically demonstrated that you simply can't coerce doctors enough to make a real dent in skyrocketing healthcare expenditures.

Fortunately for the Central Authority, a right to healthcare naturally leads to a situation in which all those spending decisions must be centralized. After all, a thing so noble as a right to healthcare – with the comprehensive fairness that is demanded by such a right – cannot possibly be achieved by hundreds of thousands of individual doctors acting independently. Comprehensive fairness absolutely requires central direction.

As a bonus, of course, centralized control of the healthcare system also gives you the opportunity to cut costs.

Centralized decision-making is a hallmark of Obamacare. The most notable features of centralization in Obamacare include:

1) The Independent Payment Advisory Board. The innocent-sounding IPAB (for how much damage can any mere "advisory" board do?) actually represents a truly astounding attempt to create a nearly all-powerful, unelected, immutable (in the sense that no governmental body can terminate it) board which will determine the ceiling for all of America's healthcare expenditures.

2) GOD panels. Numerous expert panels will be created – which observers less sophisticated than myself have referred to as "death panels," but which I choose to call by the much less insulting and much more justifiable name of GOD panels ("Government Operatives Deliberating") – for the purpose of publishing the clinical "guidelines" that will tell doctors which specific patients can get which medical services, and when and how they can get them.

3) Stifling preventive medicine. While preventive medical services might actually prevent a disease here or there, the Central Authority has figured out that preventive services of all kinds, without exception, will always cost far more money than they can ever save. So Obamacare has instituted new processes to limit preventive services, and (as you will already have noticed if you are paying attention) to indoctrinate us in the great unwashed that expensive preventive services actually do more harm than good.

4) Herd medicine. A natural by-product of a system in which medicine is practiced strictly according to centrally determined guidelines is that all patients with a particular disease process will be treated the same way. The treatment guidelines generally will reflect clinical studies that report on the average response of patients given treatment A as compared to the average response of those given treatment B. Thus, treatment guidelines will necessarily be directed toward the average patient. If you are interested in improving the average outcome for the entire herd of patients, this might be a good thing to do. But for patients themselves, (who are still stuck on the idea of optimizing therapy for each individual, and 50% of whom will necessarily fall on the wrong side of "average"), this could be very bad news.

5) Slow medical progress. As we have seen, it is runaway medical progress (along with the greedy doctors) that has created this whole mess in the first place. Therefore, making it as difficult as possible for innovators to get their new products to market is a critical feature of the Central Authority's strategy.

GROUP MEDICINE

Group medicine, which is analogous to Diversity, is different from herd medicine. Group medicine means that different groups of patients (grouped according to one or more characteristics) need to be treated differently from other groups of patients, even if they have the same medical disorders.

Within each designated group, of course, herd medicine will apply.

An example of group medicine is life-cycle medicine, in which your relative priority to receive medical services is related to your position within the life-cycle. One system that has been suggested by a prominent advisor to President Obama would award persons under the age of 5 and above the age of 75 a very low healthcare priority, those between 5 and 14 and between 55 and 75 an intermediate priority, and those between 15 and 54 the highest priority. Such a system would assure that fewer healthcare expenditures are used to help individuals who are not actively contributing very much to the collective.

Another example would be caring for people who are deemed to be at or near the end of their life. While thoughtful and compassionate end-of-life care can be a great boon, when it is implemented primarily as a cost-saving measure it is open to many abuses.

And then there is the variety of group medicine in which individuals are grouped according to their inherent worthiness, as judged by some feature other than age. Presently, the group known as "the obese" is serving as a test case. If our leaders can set a precedent of implementing medical discrimination against fat people, it will be relatively easy to expand the concept greatly.

CONTROLLING INDIVIDUAL BEHAVIORS

Successfully demonizing the obese will set a precedent that goes beyond merely establishing group medicine. Fat people are fat, we are told, because of the choices they make (such as the choice to be slothful and gluttonous), and because of these choices they are consuming far more than their fair share of healthcare. This "fact" is already beginning to lead to regulations that propose to control food choices.

If the Central Authority succeeds in making this case – and they probably will, since who cares about fat people? – they can use the same argument to regulate any other human behavior that they decide might influence a person's odds of having to consume a bit of healthcare. Some of these behaviors (in addition to what you eat) might conceivably include your hobbies, listening to advertisements for unhealthful products, the number of miles you drive, or owning a firearm.

LIMITING INDIVIDUAL PREROGATIVES

I have said earlier that the key battle, the one most likely to determine the outcome of whether Americans will retain at least some semblance of individual freedom, or whether the Progressive takeover of our healthcare system – and of our society – will be complete, will be in regard to whether individuals will retain the ability to purchase at least some of their healthcare with their own money (and also, necessarily, whether providers will be allowed to sell it to them).

The very fact that healthcare is now a right means that it must be provided for you; you should not have to provide it for yourself. And this is how Progressives state their case. But what they really mean is that you should not be permitted to provide it for yourself.

I understand how outlandish this sounds. I also understand that almost nobody seems to be talking about it – so how can it be the case?

Well, I will show you. And since, as I maintain, this question occupies the key position in the battle over healthcare and in the battle over individual freedom, I will get right to it, and show you in the next chapter.

SUMMARY

Every new "right" granted to citizens by a Central Authority, while it may or may not succeed in providing the promised thing to the citizens, will always expand the power of the Central Authority over the liberty of individuals. In the case of a right to healthcare, as we have seen, it is simply not possible to provide "the promised thing" in its entirety to everybody. And worse, in the case of healthcare, the very essence of individual liberty is direly threatened.

Chapter 7 - Limiting Individual Prerogatives in a Progressive Healthcare System

"..[R]ightful liberty is unobstructed action according to our will within limits drawn around us by the equal rights of others. I do not add 'within the limits of the law,' because law is often but the tyrant's will, and always so when it violates the right of an individual."
- Thomas Jefferson

Of all the seemingly outlandish things I am going to assert in this book – all of which I will fervently desire the reader to, if not swallow whole, then at least take into serious account – the most outlandish of all is probably the one I am addressing in this chapter. Namely, that any Progressive healthcare system will necessarily attempt to curtail the ability of individual Americans to spend their own money on their own healthcare, and thus, will try to limit the most essential freedom of all – the freedom to act to preserve oneself.

To those many readers who at this moment are expressing alarm over my apparent paranoia, I thank you for your concern. But fear not, for if it turns out I am wrong about this (and I sincerely hope that I am), then not only do they have medication for paranoia, but also, I would be permitted to purchase it legally.

Progressives, of course, deny that they have any such thing in mind. And undoubtedly the majority of progressives, and even many actual Progressives, do not. Indeed, I will happily concede it likely that very few Progressives actually start out with this idea.

What I am saying is that limiting this vital individual liberty turns out to be such an essential component of any Progressive healthcare system that the people who run such a system, perhaps despite themselves, will, sooner or later, find themselves acting forcefully to limit it. This is my proposition.

My intention in this chapter is (once again) to present my proposition as a theory. It is a theory that takes into account two things. First, it incorporates the natural and necessary inclinations of the Progressive Program to limit an individual's freedom of action regarding his or her own health. And second, my theory incorporates objective observations we can make today, relating to actions which Progressives have already taken in this regard. I contend that my theory best explains both of these things. And of course, as always, I invite (and in this case, greatly desire to hear of) any alternative theories that explain these observations better than mine does.

But if my theory is correct, then if we Americans are to avoid severe restrictions on our ability to purchase healthcare services with our own money (and, ultimately, on our ability to expend any individual resources for any individual benefit), such a favorable outcome will only result if we remain vigilant and alert to the aims of our Progressive leaders, and fight vigorously against their efforts to suppress our liberties, whenever and wherever we find them. It will not result from our complacency, or from placing our trust in the beneficence, the common sense, or the respect for fundamental American precepts, of our political leaders.

THE INDIVIDUAL IS THE PROPER GUARDIAN OF HIS OWN HEALTH

It really ought to go without saying that a person should be able to expend his or her own resources to purchase any healthcare service he or she desires. This is a primary corollary of classical liberalism, and was recognized as a fundamental human right by the likes of John Locke and Thomas Jefferson.

It is also an idea deeply imbedded in American jurisprudence. The great Supreme Court Justice Joseph Story, in his *Commentaries on the Constitution of the United States* (1833), noted that the individual "is the proper guardian of his own health." This precept was repeated by Louis Brandeis in 1890, and became the foundation of the Supreme Court's assertion of an individual right to privacy. In particular, the writings of Story and Brandeis were specifically relied upon by the Court in its 1965 finding (*Griswold v. Connecticut*) that a right to privacy is not only guaranteed by our Constitution, but is also a right which is "older than our Bill of Rights." I would like to remind my Progressive friends that it was this very precept that laid the basis for deciding *Roe v. Wade* in 1973.

Fundamentally, both classic liberal philosophy and the American judicial system have always recognized a liberty to act to preserve one's own health to be an inherent, inalienable right.

WHY INDIVIDUAL PREROGATIVES MUST BE RESTRAINED

Despite this long history in political philosophy and in jurisprudence in favor of such an inherent liberty, it is nonetheless natural and unavoidable for any Progressive healthcare system to strive to limit it. This is because Progressive healthcare systems are necessarily universal.

They are universal in two senses. First, they attempt to cover all people. Second, they purport to cover all healthcare services.

Under Obamacare, for instance, health insurance – which every American is required to have – must cover (as laid out in Section 1302 of the law): ambulatory patient services, emergency services, hospitalization, maternity and newborn care, mental health and substance use disorder services, including behavioral health treatment, prescription drugs, rehabilitative and habilitative services and devices, laboratory services, preventive and wellness services and chronic disease management, pediatric services, and oral and vision care.

Fundamentally, this "universality of features" reflects a particular philosophy. It is, in fact, the Progressive philosophy. Healthcare being an essential component of any ideal society, it is thus necessary to assure that everybody receives everything that is officially deemed to be healthcare. In Section 1302, the Central Authority is telling us, everything will be taken care of for all of us, from soup to nuts. So there is no need to worry our pretty little heads.

But, as always when the Central Authority assumes all responsibility for providing some aspect of security (in this case, healthcare security), it also assumes all control.

Complete central control is necessary not only to assure the societal perfection promised by the Progressive Program. Central control is also the method by which Progressives propose to manage America's healthcare spending. Which is to say, controlling all healthcare expenditures is essential for the purpose of covert rationing.

Allowing individuals to spend their own money fundamentally undermines a Progressive healthcare system. It implies that the Central Authority is actually not supplying all useful healthcare services (when, by definition, it is), and thus implies that the government is holding back, and indeed, may be engaging in some kind of rationing. Such an implication cannot be permitted.

To say it another way, when individuals are allowed to purchase "extra" healthcare, that's a graphic admission to the unwashed masses that there is extra healthcare to be had. The real problem is that this behavior raises expectations for everybody, and these higher expectations make it that much more difficult for the Central Authority to ration covertly.

The critical importance of controlling expectations in a Progressive healthcare system is nicely illustrated by some of the problems being experienced by the British and the Canadian healthcare systems. Both of these systems, naturally, initially outlawed private healthcare spending. But unfortunately, the very visible medical progress that continued unabated in the American healthcare system – new drugs, new techniques and new technology – were noticed by Canadian and British citizens, and created new demands upon their respective healthcare systems. Essentially, seeing what was possible, a critical mass of the population demanded some of these medical advances, even if they had to pay for them themselves. Ultimately the authorities were forced to relent, at least to a degree, on their desired restrictions on individual freedom.

Some have argued that such "loosening" of individual restrictions in Great Britain and in Canada proves that any restrictions on individuals simply will not stand – so we Americans don't really have anything to worry about. For, if such restrictions cannot be maintained in those countries, how will they ever be maintained here? Perhaps. But I would suggest instead that the need to loosen individual restrictions in Canada and Great Britain graphically illustrates the critical necessity, in any universal healthcare system, of managing expectations. It in fact proves that a failure to manage the expectations of the people leads to a loss of control.

Had it not been for the very visible example of advances in American healthcare, citizens of Canada and Great Britain quite possibly never would have agitated for "more." As it is, thanks to the unfortunate example of the high-cost healthcare their citizens saw in the United States, British and Canadian officials were simply unable to manage the expectations of their own citizenry. (Which means that healthcare officials in those countries were likely among the happiest people, anywhere, when Obamacare became the law in America.)

Once we have a universal healthcare system in America, it will therefore become critically important for the Central Authority to manage the healthcare expectations of American citizens. Fortunately, American healthcare bureaucrats won't have any annoying, external healthcare systems to worry about, busily spinning out advances in medical technology and thus continually raising expectations. Their job likely will be somewhat easier than it was for their counterparts in Canada and England.

For American bureaucrats, managing public expectations will largely become a matter of restraining individual American citizens from going outside the system, and buying extra healthcare with their own money. And for this reason, restricting individual prerogatives in the United States will be critical, even more critical than it was in our cousin nations. And we should not be surprised if our bureaucrats employ some very devious and even draconian maneuvers to do so.

IT'S ALL ABOUT FAIRNESS

The official rationale which the Central Authority will always invoke for taking such restrictive actions will be to achieve "fairness." Allowing the rich to go outside the system would create an unfair, two-tiered healthcare system, etc. The goal of fairness, as is being taught to every schoolchild, is unquestionably and obviously a righteous one, and indeed, its achievement is a chief responsibility of the Central Authority*. Equally obvious is the fact that its hindrance is always threatened by the greed of a certain kind of person. Therefore, the Central Authority is fully justified in constraining the individual liberties of those enemies of righteousness who would stifle fairness.

---

*As I write this, President Obama is campaigning very hard for a special new tax on the very rich. While this is nothing new in itself, what is new is the rationale that is being advanced for this new tax, i.e., "fairness." The President and his spokespersons have all acknowledged that this new proposed tax would do next to nothing to reduce our deficit, or to create new revenue for the government. Rather, the purpose they articulate for taking the property earned by these very successful people is, quite explicitly, redistributive justice, or "fairness." This argument, possibly for the first time, explicitly creates "fairness" as a principle goal of taxation, and makes achieving such fairness a chief responsibility of the Central Authority (which is convenient, since the Central Authority also gets to define what "fairness" is). This explicit new principle is readily extendable to government actions outside the tax code – such as healthcare.

And so, restricting the right of individuals to use their own resources to benefit their own health is something that will always be conducted only for the best of reasons – to achieve the fairest and the most ethical healthcare system possible.

But whatever the reasons Progressives might offer for their actions, and whatever the dictates of classical liberal philosophy or American jurisprudence to the contrary, their attempt to restrict individual prerogatives will become deadly serious, because doing so is essential to their real aims.

HILLARY STARTED IT

The natural propensity of Progressives to limit individual prerogatives was manifest as early as 1993, with the Clinton Health Security Act, more affectionately known as Hillarycare.

The question of how much individual freedom Hillarycare would permit came to a head in early 1994, just as the debate over this bill was reaching a crescendo, and played a significant role in defeating the legislation. What brought the question to a head was the publication of an article by Betsy McCaughey, entitled *No Exit*, in (of all places) *The New Republic*.

Ms. McCaughey, who quickly became for Progressives a sort of practice version of Sarah Palin, was at the time a frequent denizen of Conservative think tanks and an occasional editorialist. But what made her an acknowledged expert on Hillarycare was the fact that she was one of the few people who actually had read the legislation.

No Exit revealed that many of the claims being made by proponents of Hillarycare (for instance, that patients could keep their present insurance; that specialty care would be readily available; and that there would be no rationing) were actually false. Despite the fact that the White House quickly released an official response to Mcaughey's article insisting that many of her conclusions were untrue, her accusations stuck. And according to many observers McCaughey's article was at least as influential as the Harry and Louise commercials in turning the tide against Hillarycare. Indeed, the importance of her article was formally recognized when it won her the National Magazine Award for excellence in the public interest.

One of McCaughey's chief assertions – and likely its most striking one – was that Hillarycare would make it illegal for patients to pay doctors directly, and that doctors could be paid only through the government-sanctioned insurance plans. And of all her claims this one in particular made proponents of Hillarycare angry, because the legislation explicitly stipulated that this was not to be the case. Here is the actual language from the bill: "Nothing in this Act shall be construed as prohibiting…an individual from purchasing any health care services."

Because one of the main assertions in her highly effective article so obviously ignored this explicit statement to the contrary, for the past 20 years McCaughey has been widely painted in the general media as being totally incompetent at best, and more often as a congenital liar and/or a shill for various components of the healthcare industry. And in 2009, when she performed a similar analysis of the Obamacare legislation (coming to many of the same conclusions), she was for the most part either ignored or ridiculed.

It turns out, however, at least in retrospect, that McCaughey's analysis of Hillarycare was largely correct.

HILLARYCARE IS THE MODEL FOR OBAMACARE

Before demonstrating how McCaughey was right, I ought to say why spending any time with Hillarycare at this point is still worthwhile. Hillarycare is still relevant for two reasons. First, while Hillarycare itself never became law, many of the provisions of Hillarycare eventually did – and so, we are living under them today. And second, Hillarycare embodies the fundamental aims of any Progressive healthcare system, so understanding the aims of Hillarycare will help us to understand the aims of Obamacare (and whatever Progressive reforms might succeed Obamacare).

When House Speaker Nancy Pelosi famously pronounced that we would have to pass the Obamacare legislation in order to find out what was in it, she did not misspeak. She was not uttering a typical Nancy-ism (such as her contention that paying people not to work is a great stimulus to job creation), nor was she channeling Yogi Berra. She was, in fact, speaking the plain truth, and imparting a nugget of deep wisdom to us in the general public.

I have spent substantial time reading large portions of the 2400-page Obamacare legislation. And having done so, here's what I can tell you about it.

The Obamacare legislation was specifically designed to be obscure; in fact, it is fundamentally indeterminate in its meaning. It was designed in such a way that the unelected regulators who would later translate it into actual rules, regulations and guidelines (under which healthcare providers can then be prosecuted), would ultimately determine what the bill really said. And until those regulators finish their work, what Obamacare actually says is a matter of debate. So Nancy was right.

This fact explains why none of our legislators bothered to read it before voting on it – except for a few pesky Republicans, who were only trying to make trouble. What's the point in reading a long, boring document whose actual meaning will only be determined later?

This fact also raises another question. Where did this extraordinary document – whose true meaning was elusive even to the President and the legislators who were promoting it – come from? Who actually put the words to the page, and crafted this remarkable legislation?

We may never know the names of the people who actually held the pens which scratched out the actual words, any more than we will ever know the real names of the individuals who wrote the gospels of Matthew and Luke. But, just as New Testament scholars have been able to trace these two gospels to a now-lost common prior source – the so-called "Q document" – it is not difficult for anyone with a smattering of interest in the art of legislative exegesis to trace the source document for Obamacare.

The Q Document for President Obama's Patient Protection and Affordable Care Act was Hillarycare.

In preparing to write this book, I decided to go back in time, and re-examine Hillary's original proposal for fundamentally transforming the American healthcare system. What I found surprised me.

While Hillary's Health Security Act was widely castigated by contemporaries as being a vast monstrosity of bureaucratic legerdemain, filled with complexity and labyrinthine passages that attempted to hide its true meaning, I found Hillarycare, in comparison to Obamacare, to be a model of legislative brevity and clarity. In fact, I now believe that its very straightforwardness is one of the things that killed it. (And, it seems obvious to me, so did whoever wrote the Obamacare legislation, an individual or individuals who so clearly and so painstakingly avoided making the same mistake.)

For instance, Hillarycare is only 1368 pages in length. How could they be so concise? Even more remarkably, Hillarycare spelled out pretty plainly what it actually meant to do.

For instance, in the Obamacare bill, in order for a reader to assemble the information necessary to determine that the Independent Medicare Advisory Board is actually to be called the Independent Payment Advisory Board (IPAB), and that its "advisory opinions" which are to be submitted to Congress for "consideration" are actually formal dictates which must be followed to the letter, and that it can inflict its cost-cutting mandates to all of healthcare and not just to government programs, one must jump around to numerous distant sections in the 2700-page document, cutting and pasting the relevant sections, jigsaw-like, into a coherent whole. In the Hillarycare bill, in stark contrast, the analogous National Health Board (which, like the IPAB, was to have been an appointed-not-elected Supreme Court of healthcare, beyond which there was to be no appeal, no revision, and no repeal) is presented in an entirely straightforward way, and pretty much all in one place.

Having now immersed myself in the relatively refreshing model of clarity and precision that was Hillarycare, I find it quite likely that the people who actually wrote the Obamacare bill (and may God keep these invaluable artists of legislative lyricism safe, as we will be needing them), simply began with Hillary's old Health Security Act, disassembled it into various bits, padded each bit with a little more than twice its weight in verbiage, and reassembled the pieces in some nearly random fashion into the exceedingly difficult-to-read document that became Obamacare.

Obamacare's debt to Hillarycare is obvious. Hillarycare required every American to have government-approved health insurance; it reduced private health insurers to government-directed utilities, whose products, rates, and profits were to be controlled by the feds; and it created omniscient and omnipotent panels which were to hand down dictates to "let doctors know" what services they may or may not provide and under what circumstances. This should not be surprising, since any Progressive healthcare system will ultimately have the same goals, and will likely discover similar pathways toward achieving those goals.

HILLARYCARE AND INDIVIDUAL PREROGATIVES

So: if Hillarycare is to a large extent the model for Obamacare, and indeed, if it is a model for Progressive healthcare systems in general, then what did it have to say about the ability of individual Americans to use their own resources for their own healthcare?

Progressives have told us (and have spent nearly 20 years castigating Ms. McCaughey for telling us otherwise) that the answer is obvious – the bill says in plain language that "nothing in the bill should be construed as prohibiting an individual" from purchasing healthcare services. What could be clearer?

I humbly suggest, and ask the reader to suspend disbelief long enough to consider, that when an act of legislation makes an unprovoked, blanket assertion like this, apparently out of the clear blue, sometimes that assertion is being made in order to distract the overly curious from digging through the bill to find out what it really says, or at least, to create plausible deniability. There are lots of examples where legislation begins by saying, "This legislation does not do X," and then immediately goes on to do precisely X.

For instance, the legislation that created Medicare contains the following language: "Nothing in this title shall be construed to authorize any federal officer or employee to exercise any supervision or control over the practice of medicine, or the manner in which medical services are provided, or over the selection, tenure, or compensation of any officer, or employee, or any institution, agency or person providing health care services." (Section 1801, Medicare Act, 1965). This point of law, in light of what Medicare has in fact become, is mind boggling.

Also, in the Obamacare legislation, the introductory language in the section which creates the IPAB (the IPAB being a straightforward and very blunt instrument for rationing healthcare), contains language that prohibits healthcare rationing.

95

Then there's the fact that Hillarycare itself, in its section on fee-for-service medicine, begins by establishing a collective negotiation process for determining what fee-for-service doctors may charge (Section 1322, paragraph (c)(2)). But then it immediately goes on to say (paragraph (c)(5)) that "collective negotiations by providers pursuant to paragraph (2) shall be considered as efforts intended to influence government action." And efforts intended to influence government action is later defined, in the Fraud and Abuse sections of the legislation, as an act of healthcare fraud, and is subject to criminal penalties. To top it all off, the very next section of the bill also prohibits providers from boycotts or even threatening boycotts. So in effect, after asserting that there will be collective bargaining, the bill provides a mechanism for the government to dictate doctors' fees, without input from doctors, and furthermore, these dictated fees are not even presented to doctors in a take-it-or-leave-it fashion, but rather, in a take-it-or-go-to-jail fashion.

All this, of course, is not to say that the language in Hillarycare denying that the bill has any intention of prohibiting individual prerogatives is itself definitive proof that the legislation intends to prohibit individual prerogatives. All I am saying is that such language, so gratuitously offered, may actually not mean anything at all in particular, and certainly should not be treated as being dispositive. If anything, it should make you want to read the rest of the bill with particular care.

And when we read the rest of the Hillarycare legislation we find (Section 1406, Paragraph (d)(1)) that "A provider may not charge or collect from any enrollee a fee in excess of the applicable payment amount...for items and services covered by the comprehensive benefits package." When we deconstruct this language, we find that a "provider" is any individual who provides health professional services (a definition that includes all doctors); an "enrollee" is any American citizen (since all Americans are required to be enrolled in a government-approved health plan); and the "comprehensive benefits package" covers all healthcare services. So: any doctor who treats any patient in America is bound to the fee schedule as determined by the government. Furthermore, the next paragraph (paragraph (d)(2)) prohibits directly billing the patient for any of these services. The plain meaning of these provisions is that doctors and patients cannot contract with one another legally for the delivery of healthcare services.

The Fraud and Abuse sections of Hillarycare also limit the prerogatives of doctors and patients. For instance, under Hillarycare, some activities which would usually be considered compatible with routine medical practice, even when conducted within the government-approved healthcare system, created opportunities for jail time for both doctors and patients. According to Paul Craig Roberts, writing in the *Washington Times* in December, 1993, "Mr. Clinton's plan turns normal patient advocacy into a federal criminal offense. For example, a doctor who wants an earlier date for surgery for a needful patient can be accused of using wrongful influence and accepting a bribe and sentenced, along with the patient, to 15 years in prison."

So, on one hand Hillarycare makes a very direct, blanket assertion that it does not intend to inhibit individual prerogatives. On the other hand the specific provisions of Hillarycare do just that. It certainly appears, then, that the blanket assertion made in Hillarycare that people could buy whatever healthcare they wanted, is just another example of employing such an assertion for the purpose of providing plausible deniability that the legislation in fact (and in less plain language) does just the opposite.

Furthermore, the overall effect of the Hillarycare legislation, when viewed from 10,000 feet, was most striking in the detailed and minute control it assumed over each and every conceivable aspect of American healthcare. And when you consider their work product in its entirety, it becomes difficult to believe that the authors of Hillarycare would really countenance individuals going outside the system to buy whatever healthcare they wanted.

To me, this all indicates that Ms. McCaughey was probably right after all.

But since Hillarycare never became law, we can't really know how its apparent limitations on the freedom of individuals actually would have played out.

Or can we?

AFTER HILLARYCARE

As I have noted in an earlier chapter, the ignominious defeat of Hillarycare in Congress did not stop the Progressives' efforts to overhaul the healthcare system. It simply put them on a somewhat slower track.

For instance, large sections of the onerous Fraud and Abuse portions of Hillarycare were cut-and-pasted into the HIPAA legislation which became law a few years later. We saw, in Chapter 3, just one example of how these new anti-fraud provisions were then employed to change routine medical practice into a maze of regulatory booby-traps, punishable by ruining fines and jail terms. Such methods, which were aimed at wrenching the physician's attention away from what was best for the patient and toward what would best please the Central Authority, were extraordinarily painful for doctors at first, but in the intervening 15 years have come for many physicians – especially the younger ones who never knew anything else – to seem routine and natural. And so, despite the defeat of Hillarycare, the government has succeeded in getting physicians into the correct frame of mind for Progressive healthcare.

Similarly, the downfall of Hillarycare did not deter ongoing efforts by Progressives to limit the freedom of individuals to purchase their own healthcare. These efforts necessarily had to be relatively subtle, and accordingly have been marked by subterfuge and clever legal posing. But their aim cannot be plausibly denied.

LIMITING THE RIGHTS OF MEDICARE PATIENTS

Lest I mislead readers into thinking that I'm blaming only the Clintons for starting all this, I will point out that the first major effort to limit the ability of Medicare patients to purchase healthcare services outside of Medicare was effected by government bureaucrats during the administration of George Bush 41.

In 1991, Medicare administrators published a "carrier bulletin" warning physicians that direct-pay agreements between Medicare patients and doctors (even non-participating doctors) were strictly prohibited, unless the contract was initiated solely by the patient, and even then, the rate of payment for any such direct-pay agreements must be those rates set by Medicare, and further, that any such direct-pay agreements were still subject to all Medicare rules and regulations. Medicare added that if the patient at some later time became dissatisfied with that (patient-initiated) contract, Medicare would severely (and retroactively) sanction the physician. The clear aim of this new policy was to deter any direct-pay agreements, whatsoever, between Medicare patients and doctors, and thus, to limit the patients' ability to spend their own money on their own healthcare.

When a group of physicians and their patients sued Medicare in 1992 to prevent this odious new policy from being implemented (*Stewart et al. v. Sullivan*), the government took the position that the plaintiffs could not prove that Medicare had really promulgated this new policy after all – since they could not "prove" that the carrier bulletin had been initiated by the Secretary of HHS. The judge agreed with the defendants over this legal technicality, and after implying that if Medicare had actually implemented such a policy (which at the time could not be "proven"), it would indeed unreasonably limit individual rights, threw the case out in a summary judgment for lack of "ripeness."

Then, having successfully dodged this challenge on a legal subterfuge, Medicare immediately (and cynically) rendered this very policy official, in its entirety, by formally changing its Medicare Carriers' Manual.

But the Feds were still not satisfied. The new, restrictive policy technically still allowed for private-pay contracts, as long as the patient initiated them. So the Clinton administration engineered an amendment to the Balanced Budget Act of 1997 – Section 4507 – which prohibited any self-pay contracts whatsoever between Medicare patients and their doctors for medical services which are covered under Medicare. Under Section 4507 – which is still the law today – if a doctor provides even one self-pay medical service to a single Medicare patient, that doctor is punished by complete banishment from the Medicare program for at least two years.

The federal government was eventually challenged again in court over Section 4507, but that lawsuit was also thrown out in a summary judgment

(*United Seniors Association et al. v. Shalala*). The rationale the government offered to the court for its actions in this case is instructive: ". . .what you will have is a system whereby the rich can buy what they want and those many beneficiaries who are on fixed income will not be able to afford those services." So again, the interest of collective "fairness" was invoked to justify a law which stifles an individual's fundamental right to purchase medical services he or she determines to be necessary for his/her well-being.

There are several legitimate reasons a Medicare patient might want to self-pay for a medical service that is covered by Medicare. If Medicare "covers" heart valve surgery, for instance, a patient might want to pay for a new, minimally-invasive surgical approach that is inadequately reimbursed by Medicare, rather than the big, open-heart surgery that Medicare reimburses fully. Or, one might want to self-pay for "covered" psychiatric care, or for treatment for a venereal disease, in order to keep embarrassing or harmful medical records out of government-controlled databases – that is, for privacy reasons.

Furthermore, it is important to recognize that just because a healthcare service is "Medicare-covered" does not mean that it will be covered for a given patient. Whether a specific individual is covered is often determined by a "medical necessity" ruling, made by a bureaucrat. Section 4507 essentially precludes a patient's ability to purchase a denied (but "covered") medical service, no matter how badly they want it, or believe they need it.

One can argue, and with some merit, that at this juncture denials of medically necessary services by Medicare have been relatively judicious, and therefore that the "Section 4507 rule" has not had much of an actual impact. In fact, it is likely that most Medicare beneficiaries do not even know that this rule exists.

But while its impact might be relatively small so far, the Section 4507 rule has now been in place for 15 years – it is very well-established. So, once Medicare begins reducing reimbursements to physicians and hospitals to the point where they can no longer afford to offer certain "covered" services to Medicare patients (and Medicare has just recently begun doing so, specifically, for some cardiac imaging studies), patients who need those services will be left out in the cold. Services which are officially covered by Medicare, but which are reimbursed at such a low rate that they cannot actually be provided to them, will become unavailable even to Medicare patients who are willing and able to pay for them.

It is conceivable that some older people who understand the implications of Section 4507, and who want to receive a covered-but-denied medical service, might decide to drop out of Medicare altogether so they could legally purchase that desired service. But this is something Progressives do not like either, because allowing patients to drop out of Medicare threatens to create an unfair, two-tiered healthcare system.

And this is why, also in 1993, the Clinton administration promulgated a rule in its Program Operations Manual System (POMS) to prohibit Medicare-aged Americans from forgoing Medicare. The rule implied that no elderly person could drop out of Medicare unless they also gave up their Social Security benefits, and repaid any Social Security benefits they had already received.

Recently, this POMS rule was challenged in a lawsuit filed by three elderly Americans (one of whom was Dick Armey) who wished to drop out of Medicare in favor of self-purchased health insurance, without having to sacrifice their Social Security benefits.

But in the summer of 2011, Washington DC District Judge Rosemary Collyer ruled for the defendants and upheld the POMS rule. So: elderly Americans do not have the right to drop out of Medicare and purchase their own health insurance, unless they also forgo and repay all Social Security benefits.

Interestingly, in 2009 Judge Collyer had denied a motion by the Obama administration to dismiss the suit, and in her denial pointedly noted that "neither the statute nor the regulation specifies that Plaintiffs must withdraw from Social Security and repay retirement benefits in order to withdraw from Medicare." Her preliminary ruling thereby confirmed the plaintiffs' main contention. So most observers had assumed that the judge's final ruling would also be in favor of the plaintiffs.

It was not. In her final ruling in 2011, Judge Collyer found a new interpretation of the Medicare statute itself that upholds the POMS rule. The Medicare statute, she finally determined, specifies that people who are entitled to Social Security are automatically "entitled" to Medicare, and therefore if one elects to receive the Social Security payments one is owed, one must also accept Medicare. She flatly rejected the notion that when Congress says "entitled" it is implying anything optional, as in, "You can have it if you want it." When you're dealing with Medicare, she said, "'entitled' does not actually mean 'capable of being rejected.'" So, when Congress creates a new entitlement, Congress actually means you must have it – that it's mandatory. Judge Collyer ended her ruling by sympathizing with the plaintiffs (or laughing at them – I cannot tell for sure): "Plaintiffs are trapped in a government program intended for their benefit."

The apparent change in Judge Collyer's reading of the Medicare statute between 2009 and 2011 is disturbing. What made her originally read the plain language of the Medicare statute just like any literate American would, but then two years later read it as if she had to twist it into a presupposed "right" answer? We likely will never know what induced this marked shift.

It is instructive that the Obama administration would go to such lengths to prevent old people from dropping out of Medicare. Medicare is not only in the red, but is a great fiscal threat to our national well-being. One would think they'd welcome the idea that some of our elderly might want to pay for their own health insurance, and thereby save Medicare a lot of money. But instead, the administration fought the idea tooth and nail, to the point of articulating absurdities that even the judge who was sympathetic to their side could not refrain from mocking. One of the Obama administration's arguments, for instance, was that the plaintiffs were lucky to receive such a boon as Medicare, and therefore suffered "no injury" by having to accept it. The judge responded in her ruling: "The Secretary extolls the benefits of Medicare and suggests that Plaintiffs would agree they are not truly injured if they were to learn more about Medicare...The parties use a lot of ink disputing whether Plaintiffs' desire to avoid Medicare is sensible."

So as it now stands, seniors (unless they are rich enough to also walk away from Social Security altogether) must accept Medicare. Admittedly, for most elderly Americans this is not a big deal – of course they're going to accept Medicare. But, as we have seen, current law already makes it nearly impossible for patients on Medicare to self-pay for denied medical services. Once you are on Medicare, you will get the medical services the Central Authority approves for you – and nothing more. In the not-too-distant future, this restriction is likely to become much more apparent to Medicare recipients than it has been to date. When and if the day comes when we would like to buy ourselves some medical care which the Central Authority would rather we did not have, Old Farts like your author will find that we are "entitled" neither to pay for our own healthcare, nor to drop out of the government program that so restricts us.

PREVENTING DOCTORS FROM ADOPTING DIRECT-PAY PRACTICES

Disturbed by the destruction of their professional autonomy, and by their inability to advocate for their individual patients, for the past decade more and more doctors have been dropping out of the "system," and establishing practices under which they are paid directly by their own patients. By eliminating the pressure from insurers and the government to make the patient's best interest a secondary concern, direct-pay practice immediately restores the classic doctor-patient relationship, and therefore restores professional integrity – and so it is a menace to Progressive goals.

Unfortunately, direct-pay practitioners have a serious public relations problem. Part of the problem, to be sure, was caused by these doctors themselves. The first few to set up this new style of practice unabashedly catered to rich patients, and to attract the rich, referred to themselves as "concierge" practitioners. This name (and its elitist connotations) have been forcibly affixed to all direct-pay practitioners, even as this style of practice has evolved into a much more democratic form. Today, more and more doctors are starting direct-pay practices which are easily affordable to anyone who can afford a cell phone or cable TV contract. This evolving variety of direct-pay practice is actually not so radical as Progressives would have you believe. It is the way doctors practiced medicine until very recently. It is, in fact, the way Dr. Welby practiced medicine.

While many direct-pay practices offer patients certain benefits they usually cannot get from primary care doctors who remain in the approved system (such as phone and e-mail access, same-day appointments, appointments lasting as long as necessary instead of the allotted 12.5 minutes, etc.), the fundamental benefit, to both the patient and the doctor, is that it restores the classic doctor-patient relationship. The physician's primary obligation is no longer to the 3rd-party overlord, or to the Progressive ideal of social justice, but to the patient.

And while critics (who abound) attack direct-pay practitioners for their elitism, laziness, and greed, their real issue is that direct-pay practitioners are acting as if their primary duty is to their individual patients, and not to "social justice." It is for this reason that direct-pay practices are a deadly threat.

Having gained nearly complete control over the behavior of primary care practitioners, it is critical for Progressives to shut the door to any alternative forms of primary care. Direct-pay practitioners are a menace because they threaten to raise the expectations of both doctors and patients. Perhaps, doctors might tell themselves, there really is a way to maintain our professional autonomy within the healthcare system. Perhaps, patients might tell themselves, there really is a way for me to have a personal advocate watching out for my interests when I have to interact with the healthcare system.

The issue, as always, is one of "fairness." It is not fair for rich people to be able to buy "extra" access to their doctors, since it will create a condition of inequality. The policy director for the AARP (an organization that is ostensibly interested in the best interests of older Americans) has said that direct-pay practices creates "the prospect of a more explicitly tiered system where people with money have a different kind of insurance relationship than most of the middle class, and where Medicare is no longer as universal as we would like it to be." It is apparent that, to assure fairness, no patient should have email or cell-phone access to their doctors, or same-day appointments – or to a true professional advocate who is dedicated to their own individual interests, instead of the competing interests of the whole.

The attacks on direct-pay practitioners have followed the usual scheme Progressives follow when they discover an idea they need to suppress. First, they were ridiculed. "For a Retainer, Lavish Care by 'Boutique Doctors,'" said a headline in the *New York Times* in 2005. Then, they were demonized and widely attacked for their elitism, for catering to the frivolous desires of the rich, and for their lack of fundamental medical ethics. In this latter effort, it was not difficult to find fellow physicians – generally, from the medical organizations which promulgated the New Medical Ethics (see Chapter 3) – to lead the attacks. There are countless examples. I will give just two.

Anthony DeMaria, then President of the American College of Cardiology, criticized the practice of direct-pay medicine in an article in the *Journal of the American College of Cardiology* in 2005, saying, "Personally, I do not mind if people acquire yachts or personal trainers if they have enough money, nor would I object if they secured a physician at their beck and call. However, unlike yachts, health care is not discretionary, and everyone should be entitled to the same quality." So, direct-pay physicians improve the quality of healthcare only for only some patients (i.e, for their own patients), and so have no place in the healthcare system.

In a 2002 article in the *New England Journal of Medicine*, Troyen A. Brennan M.D., J.D., and M.P.H., really gets to the point. Referring to direct-pay practices as "luxury primary care," he notes that "traditional medical ethics is rather poorly equipped to address issues related to luxury primary care." That is, while "traditional" medical ethics always places the individual patient first, that kind of thinking is now outmoded. "(M)ost ethicists now agree that the financial structure of health care is an important subject for ethical consideration. Access to health care, in particular, is a salient ethical issue." Direct-pay practitioners threaten (by their elitism and the limited size of their practices), to limit access to primary care, and thus are in fundamental violation of medical ethics.

The argument here, for those who missed it (advanced by fellow physicians no less), is that, of the two competing ethical precepts now established by New Medical Ethics (i.e., the physician's obligation to the individual patient vs. the physician's obligation to society), clear primacy is to be given to the physician's obligation to society. Physicians must (like it or not) place the needs of society above the needs of the patient – and participate in covert bedside healthcare rationing. Physicians who take the only path remaining to them that allows them to make the individual patient their primary obligation are to be castigated as ethically deficient.

When ridicule and demonization fail to suppress their opposition, Progressive dogma indicates it's time to resort to force. The first pass in this regard, of course, is always to render the opposition illegal. (Actual violence is reserved for criminals who persist in their misbehavior, despite more polite efforts to get them to behave lawfully.)

Making direct-pay medical practice illegal has not been accomplished yet, but clear efforts have been made in this regard. Noting with alarm the rise of direct-pay primary care, numerous Congresspersons have issued statements of concern, suggesting that perhaps Congress should "look into" the propriety of such activities.

Indeed, the first step by Congress has already been taken. In 2003, as part of the Medicare Prescription Drug, Improvement, and Modernization Act, Congress directed the GAO to study and report on the effect of direct-pay practices on Medicare patients. The GAO did so in 2005, and a fair paraphrase of its report is as follows: "The practice of direct-pay medicine is not currently a threat to Medicare patients, because the direct-pay movement is not large enough yet to have an impact. If it does begin to have an impact on Medicare patients, action will have to be taken." That is, direct-pay medicine was considered OK in 2005 not because it was inherently an ethical and legal form of medical practice, but simply because there were not enough practitioners at that time to bother about. The clear implication is that Congress stands ready to pass laws outlawing – or, at least, severely limiting – direct-pay practices, as soon as those practices begin to "impact" the system.

A follow-up report was done in 2010 which showed a 5-fold increase in the number of direct-pay practices since 2005. It is not yet clear what actions the Feds may take – the numbers are still quite small – but leaders of MedPac (a commission that advises Congress on Medicare) has publicly expressed alarm that this new phenomenon appears to be growing rapidly.

Certain state governments are not waiting for Congress to ban direct-pay practices. The state of Maryland and a few others have taken the creative position that, because many direct-pay practices work on a retainer basis, they meet the definition of a health insurance company. And as a health insurance company, to be considered legal entities, they have to have millions of dollars set aside to pay for unforeseen "claims." (Interestingly, the lawyers in state legislatures who are advancing this argument have never suggested that the same rules be applied to attorneys, who also often work on a retainer model.) According to the *Baltimore Sun*, the state's stance in this regard has already successfully caused several primary care physicians to abandon their plans to become retainer practitioners. This interesting pathway to banishing direct-pay practices is being taken up by other states, as well. In early 2012, for instance, the state of Oregon also began requiring direct-pay physicians to register their practices with the state insurance commission.

As I write this (August, 2012), Massachusetts has just passed a new law that brings physician practices - as a condition of licensure - under the supervision of an 11-member, state-appointed Health Policy Commission. This commission, which appears to be modeled after Obamacare's all-powerful IPAB (discussed in more detail in Chapter 8), has the authority to set rules and limits for both public and private healthcare spending in the state. Among other things, the Health Policy Commission is authorized to control the practice of medicine in Massachusetts, and police how medical practices are organized. For instance, under the new law no medical provider is permitted to make "any material change to its operations or governance structure" without prior approval of the commission. And any physician who is deemed to be engaging in excessive spending can be brought under the direct control of the commission, by means of a "performance improvement plan." Physicians who fail to buckle under will be fined $500,000. (It is not clear how many times or how often this fine can be levied against a physician.) While the stated goal of this new law is to control healthcare spending, one of its likely consequences will be to end direct-pay practices. It is very difficult to see how any direct-pay practice can function - or for that matter, how one can even be established - under such rules. Fundamentally, this new law makes all practicing physicians directly answerable to the government's new panel of experts for the clinical decisions they make, no matter who pays them for their services. As a condition of licensure, physicians become wards of the state, or more accurately, indentured servants.

Since medical licensing is controlled by the various states, theoretically it would take 50 bills like this one to really get rid of direct-pay healthcare. But there are ways for the Central Authority to accomplish this goal much more expeditiously. Now that the federal government directly controls all student loans, for instance, it would be a simple matter to make student loans for medical students contingent on agreeing to become primary care doctors working strictly within the government controlled system, or to offer loan forgiveness for doctors who agree to do so, or to rescind favorable re-payment conditions (retroactively, and decades after the fact, if necessary) for doctors who go to a direct-pay model later in life.

Even without taking such action, the Central Authority may already have poisoned the water for direct-pay practices. Attorneys representing direct-pay practitioners think they have discovered a potentially fatal problem within Obamacare. Under this law, apparently only physicians enrolled in Medicare can order durable medical equipment or home health services for Medicare patients. Worse, the language of Obamacare may award to the Secretary of HHS the authority to expand this limitation to all other medical services they might order. If direct-pay physicians are banned from ordering any medical services for their patients, it is difficult to see how their practices can remain viable.

Direct-pay practices are the last, best hope for patients who want their own individual interests looked after, and for their doctors who want to practice their profession ethically. This is why Progressives are determined to terminate them with extreme prejudice.

WHAT DO CONTRACEPTIVES HAVE TO DO WITH ALL THIS?

In early 2012, President Obama unleashed a firestorm when he ordered HHS to issue a directive requiring all organizations providing health insurance to their employees to cover contraception, "morning after" pills, and sterilization procedures. This directive stunned the American Catholic leadership, whose support for the Obamacare legislation (they tell us) was predicated on assurances that healthcare reform would never require Catholic institutions to violate their fundamental principles. The bishops, and many American Catholics, felt betrayed.

Some felt personally betrayed. Cardinal Timothy Dolan had met in the Oval Office with the President in November 2011 to discuss this very issue, and was assured by Obama's own lips that the administration was committed to protecting the church's principles. This new directive, Cardinal

Dolan said after the President's directive on contraceptives, "seems to be at odds with the very assurances that he gave me." (This is as close as a Cardinal may come, when speaking of the President, to saying, "He lied to me.")

Progressives were delighted with the new rule, which put the principles of religious belief into their proper place. Conservatives, however, along with Catholic leaders and leaders of other religions, expressed outrage at the President's directive, which was a clear assault on religious freedom in America.

The President was ready for them. Supported by his allies in the American media, he portrayed objections to his new directive as a "Republican War on Women." It is instructive to consider the basic premise of this War on Women, to wit: By objecting to the new directive, Republicans are saying that women should not have access to contraceptives.

This twist of logic seems completely absurd, from almost any perspective.

Almost.

If there is one aspect of healthcare services to which American women have plenty of access, regardless of their income levels, it is contraceptive services. That is why we taxpayers fund Title X Family Planning Services, and also why we fund Planned Parenthood. And for any woman who does not wish to avail herself of this taxpayer-funded access to contraception, Walmart sells birth control pills at $10 for a month's supply. There is no lack of ready access to contraception.

Indeed, if Republicans really wanted to prevent women from having contraceptives, objecting to the President's new directive would not be of any material help whatsoever in accomplishing such a goal.

But there is, in fact, one perspective from which blocking the President's directive would indeed limit women's' access to contraceptives. If one approaches the issue from this perspective – and only if one approaches it from this perspective – then the idea of a War on Women makes logical sense. Furthermore, when we listen to the passionate, heart-felt and indeed almost tearful arguments that are being made by Progressives against the heartless Republicans – vociferously denying that Republicans care anything about religious freedom or constitutional authority, and insisting instead that they only want women to be denied contraceptives – it seems plain that this is, in fact, the perspective which Progressives must necessarily hold.

That perspective is: Anything that constitutes healthcare MUST be provided by government-approved insurance products, since if it is not provided by government-approved insurance products, one cannot legally acquire it.

So, in fact, the controversy over whether religious organizations must provide insurance that covers contraceptives boils down to the notion that people should not have to – and indeed should not be permitted to – purchase healthcare services on their own.

The President's directive on contraceptives, therefore, seems to have been issued in order to establish, once and for all, the essential set of foundational principles for Obamacare, to wit:

1) The government will determine what constitutes healthcare and what does not.

2) If the government says it's healthcare, every insurance product must cover it.

3) If it's not covered by insurance, thou shalt not have access to it.

Women must be provided contraceptives without paying for them NOT because access to contraceptives is so inadequate today that many women going without them. Rather, women must be provided these services without paying for them because we cannot allow women (or any patient) to pay for these services (or any service the Central Authority classifies as "healthcare") out of their own pockets.

All healthcare services must be covered by all insurance products – regardless of which institutions provide those insurance products – precisely because nobody can be permitted to pay for healthcare outside the sanctioned insurance product.

This is the principle which is being established by the President's new directive. This principle, so critical to Obamacare and to the Progressive agenda, is a principle worth fighting for. None of the other explanations offered by proponents or opponents of the President's action make any sense.

SUMMARY

My main point, once again, is that the Central Authority has a deep and abiding need to limit our individual prerogatives when it comes to our healthcare, and has been acting on that need for a long time. The basis for these limitations on our individual liberties – the principle of social justice – has already been established, and has survived court challenges.

Extending these limitations on personal liberties to Obamacare, and broadening their usage, will not require any major changes in direction, or principles, or policy, but will merely require an expansion of already existent – and even "venerable" – rules, rules which have been an established part of Medicare for many years.

Such restrictions by our government on such fundamental individual liberties are a very big deal indeed, and, in fact, signal an end to the Great American Experiment.

When I have expressed this conclusion in the past, many critics have admonished me that I make far too much of it, and that our government, in its benign wisdom, is just doing what's best for us. I beg readers to forgive me if I see, in such a reply, even more evidence that the only nation in the history of mankind to be founded on the principles of individual freedom is well on the way to abandoning those exceptional principles, for the sake of the same, soothing-but-empty blandishments that have been offered, throughout human history, by well-meaning people who end up producing – or becoming – tyrants.

CHAPTER 8 - THE REAL INFRASTRUCTURE OF OBAMACARE

"Today, this isolated relationship [between doctor and patient] is no longer tenable or possible. . . . Traditional medical ethics, based on the doctor-patient dyad, must be reformulated to fit the new mold of the delivery of health care. . . . The primary function of regulation in health care. . .is to constrain decentralized individualized decision making."
- From the ominously titled *New Rules*, Donald Berwick, MD and Troyen Brennan, MD

In 2009, while the Obamacare legislation was being debated, opponents put together various, very scary "flow charts," to show how utterly convoluted and inherently dysfunctional our healthcare system would become under this new plan. These charts incorporated the scores of new federal agencies, panels, commissions and bureaus that were to be created by Obamacare, and attempted to demonstrate their complex interlinkages with meandering flow lines, making evident, for instance, numerous opportunities for procedural endless loops. And on these charts, invariably doctors would be positioned on one distant corner, and patients far away on some other distant corner, and the astounding bureaucratic morass in the middle made it plain that they might as well be on separate planets.

In other words, the main point of these flow charts was to show how getting medical services under Obamacare would become an ungodly mess.

This remains an important thing to understand about Obamacare. Still, if you are an American who has attempted to get healthcare services out of the pre-Obama healthcare system, it would not be surprising if your reaction to such news is, "So what else is new?"

In fact, it seems likely that many Americans regard the prospect of Obamacare thusly: "Yes, Obamacare will almost certainly become a bureaucratic nightmare. Those charts do look a little scary. But really, all that means is that we'll be trading one bureaucratic nightmare for another. And if Obamacare gets a lot more people health insurance, and offers coverage for pre-existing conditions, and stops the evil insurance companies from killing people, it still might be a good trade."

Such flow charts, as nicely as they may illustrate the bureaucratic complexity of Obamacare, nonetheless fail to tell the real story. They fail to show that Obamacare is, in fact, fundamentally different from anything that has come before. That fundamental difference is in the complete, top-down, centralized, command-and-control organization it will bring to American healthcare. This top-down structure will systematically destroy the role of individual physicians in making medical decisions, and as a result their patients will be reduced to faceless members of a herd.

THE REAL STRUCTURE OF OBAMACARE

As we have seen several times, in order to control American healthcare it is absolutely imperative to control the behavior of American physicians. And fundamentally, the infrastructure of Obamacare is set up to do just that.

The scores of new federal agencies that show up on those flow charts, of course, will hamstring doctors in various useful ways. Each agency will have its own regulatory structure, and each will establish hundreds of new rules, regulations, and guidelines, and therefore, will produce hundreds of novel opportunities for doctors (and anyone else working in the healthcare system) to commit healthcare fraud. This will help to achieve the useful goal of placing doctors into a risk-avoidance frame of mind, rather than a patient-care frame of mind. But still, the large majority of these new agencies can be considered as nothing more than mere annoyances – sort of a swarm of flies buzzing around doctors' heads as they plod along, trying to perform the main task.

It's that main task – the real structure of Obamacare – that's important.

Obamacare is set up primarily to eliminate the opportunity for doctors to make individual decisions. Important medical decisions will be made centrally, and will be transmitted, through the new healthcare structure, to the doctors on the ground.

Over the years, healthcare bureaucrats have come to understand that just telling doctors what they are supposed to do will not be sufficient. Doctors may or may not obey, and policing the millions of individual decisions that are being made by doctors every day will be next to impossible.

So fundamentally, Obamacare is designed to incorporate doctors into new organizations that will be established to deliver efficient, high-quality healthcare, as defined by the Central Authority. And here I use the word "incorporate" in its literal form – to merge bodily into a larger structure, and to become fully a part of that larger structure.

To maintain their viability, these new organizations must require their physician-components (and all their other organic components) to function in what is usually referred to as an "integrated, team-based decisional paradigm," that is, to give up any idea of independent decision making. Rather, for the survival of the whole, each entity within the organization will need to closely follow formally established "best practices."

These new organizations – which at the moment are being called Accountable Care Organizations (ACOs) – will likely consist of hospitals, doctors, and legions of "non-physician providers," such as nurse practitioners, physician assistants, and care coordinators. All medical care will be delivered by "patient care teams," and, spearheaded by these teams, the organizations will go "at risk," accepting pre-determined bundled payments to deliver care to a pre-defined population of patients.

For such organizations to work, doctors will have to cease being independent agents. They will have to follow to the letter the care directives established by the "team." The viability of the entire organization will depend on doctors' full compliance with this collective prime directive. Fortunately, since there is no need (or allowance) for independent thought or action on the part of physicians in such a system, one doctor is pretty much the same as another, so doctors are entirely interchangeable. The non-compliant ones can be culled out and replaced as needed.

These ideas are not really new, of course. HMOs tried similar things in the 1990s. The difference is that now there is nowhere else for doctors to go. Private practice is rapidly becoming unfeasible. Direct-pay practices (for as long as they continue to remain legal) are really only suitable for primary care. Specialists, who require lots of expensive stuff – things like gamma cameras, operating suites, catheterization laboratories, hordes of highly trained medical technicians, etc. – generally find it exceedingly difficult to function as independent operators. It is no longer the 1990s; if doctors want to practice medicine, joining an ACO will soon be their only option.

Once doctors are fully absorbed into these new "team-based" entities, it becomes relatively easy for the Central Authority to control things. The ACOs will only be paid if they follow the directives that are handed down by the various panels, bureaus, etc., created by Obamacare, and the ACOs will only remain viable if the imbedded doctors spend less money than the ACO takes in. Since the decision not to spend all that money will have been disseminated among numerous members of the "team," and since team-based decisions will be mindful of "social justice," doctors will be at least partially absolved of the crime of withholding useful healthcare. And since the Central Authority is merely handing out the money (along with a few helpful "guidelines"), it can plausibly deny that it is telling doctors how to practice medicine.

WE ARE THE BORG

Knowing that many American doctors will find this arrangement odious, Ezekiel Emanuel from the White House's Office of Management and Budget, and Nancy-Ann M. De Parle, Mr. Obama's Czar of Healthcare Reform, co-authored an article in the *Annals of Internal Medicine* in 2010, to help change hearts and minds. It is a message directly from the White House to American doctors, appearing in a prestigious peer-reviewed medical journal no less, explaining why joining up with the new ACOs will be to their great benefit, and indeed, that it is an offer they cannot refuse. After reminding doctors of all the glorious accomplishments of Obamacare, they articulated why there is a duty to comply:

> "*[Obamacare] will unleash forces that favor integration across the continuum of care. Some organizing function will need to be developed to track*

quality measures, account for and manage shared financial incentives, and oversee care coordination. . .As physicians organize themselves into increasing larger groups — patient-centered medical home practices and accountable care organizations — they are, out of necessity, investing in the acquisition or development of management skills that could provide these organizing functions efficiently for physicians groups. . .For physicians, this means a profession that is more rewarding, more productive, and better able to realize its moral ideal."

For readers who become somewhat mind-numbed by this kind of policy-wonk jargon, here is the correct translation:

"Physicians! You have been neglecting your moral obligation to the collective, in favor of your archaic devotion to the individual patient. Under Obamacare you will need to join organizations which are devoted to the proper collective goals, and which therefore will guarantee the proper moral ideals. You must function not as individual decision-makers, but as integrated cogs in a vast healthcare continuum, which will stretch from the centralized bastion of gleaming moral authority (from which we pen this message) all the way down to the humble tip of your stethoscope. You will be rewarded for your cooperation, or suffer for your resistance (resistance, of course, being futile). So rejoice for the health of the collective, and for your own well-being, and prepare to be assimilated!"

Doctors, and all other healthcare workers, are to be integrated into localized, healthcare delivery collectives, which will dance to the ever-changing tunes set by the Central Authority. Everything in these ACOs will be shared collectively, including the financial risk, the medical decisions, and even the ethics of those medical decisions. The notion of doctors working as independent professionals, answerable only to their professional standards and to their patients, is to be abolished once and for all. In an Accountable Care Organization doctors do not owe the featured accountability to their patients, but rather, to the ACO itself, and to the Central Authority that regulates it.

This, then, is the fundamental structure of Obamacare. It finally puts doctors into their proper place. They become interchangeable cogs in an integrated healthcare machine, a machine which is tied irrevocably, flesh to flesh, to the Central Authority.

Under this structure patients will lose their personal advocates once and for all. They will finally be reduced to the position that Progressive healthcare requires of them. They will no longer be individuals whose doctors owe them a duty. They will be members of a herd which an ACO is charged with husbanding at the lowest cost possible. And so, assimilating doctors into the Borg is the final step. It removes the last remaining obstruction to the widespread implementation of herd medicine.

Everything else about Obamacare – all those new agencies and all that new bureaucratic complexity – is just details.

How This Structure Facilitates Cost Control

As we saw earlier (Chapter 1), in any system in which healthcare costs are shared collectively, truly controlling the cost of healthcare will require withholding useful medical services from many patients who would benefit from them. But so far, despite all the coercion that has been applied to the medical profession, and despite the troubling extent to which doctors have caved in to that coercion, not enough healthcare is being withheld, and costs continue to accelerate. Physicians still have not been sufficiently controlled.

Reducing physicians to members of an integrated "healthcare team" which makes decisions collectively is a brilliant move. Any vestiges of professional responsibility that may remain to some of the newly-integrated physicians will be washed out by the other members of the team, who will outnumber the doctors and who never have had such a professional imperative. For these others, a moral responsibility to the needs of the collective, i.e., to social justice, will likely be the obvious overriding imperative. And furthermore, it will be an imperative that is strongly reinforced at every turn by the agencies of the Central Authority which will decide how much money the team is going to receive for its efforts. So the integrated teams will be exquisitely sensitive (and even sympathetic) to the needs of the Central Authority.

Obamacare provides countless ways for the Central Authority to influence the integrated healthcare teams to withhold medical services, from imposing outright rules, to influencing treatment philosophies, to threatening (overtly or subtly) prosecution. For the most part, however, these can be reduced to two main efforts: the imposition of expert-generated guidelines, and the imposition of payment caps.

Guidelines - A Tyranny of Experts

A major thrust of Obamacare will be to create numerous panels of experts, appointed by the Central Authority, which will – in an entirely disinterested and objective manner, of course – publish clinical "guidelines" which will suggest to physicians what medical services they ought to offer patients with specific medical conditions. In concept, clinical guidelines are a perfectly fine idea, and indeed are often helpful to practicing physicians. This is why professional organizations have published and updated numerous sets of clinical guidelines for decades.

But the guidelines published by the GOD panelists (Government Operatives Deliberating) will be something new. These guidelines will be treated as sacrosanct rules, which must not be broken, the violation of which might lead to criminal prosecution. We already have examples of criminal investigations based on alleged guideline violations.

I will be devoting much of the remainder of Part II of this book to the tyranny of experts which is about to be unleashed upon American doctors and patients, through the medium of "guidelines," so I will say no more about it here. I will simply note that the structure of Obamacare, wherein it is an integrated team (instead of individual doctors) deciding whether to follow "suggested" sets of guidelines, will render this tool immensely more powerful than it has ever been before.

THE INDEPENDENT PAYMENT ADVISORY BOARD

Perhaps nothing in the Obamacare legislation embodies the top-down, command-and-control nature of Progressive healthcare more than the Independent Payment Advisory Board (IPAB), a 15-member panel of "experts" to be appointed by the President. There are three particular features of the IPAB that illustrate this fact: The IPAB will control all healthcare spending, public and private. The IPAB has been awarded near-dictatorial power. And the IPAB is designed to be a nearly immutable entity.

THE IPAB WILL CONTROL EVERYTHING

While the IPAB has several duties, the chief among these is to impose a final, insuperable cap on healthcare spending.

Obamacare hands the IPAB the authority to cap not only public healthcare spending, but also private healthcare spending (thus demonstrating, once again, that Progressives do indeed mean to restrict private healthcare spending). This particular feature of the IPAB is one of the more difficult-to-tease-out aspects of the Obamacare legislation, so it is fitting that the IPAB acquired this sweeping authority in a suitably convoluted and sneaky way.

Anyone who paid attention to the remarkable process that brought us our new and transformational healthcare system might recall that Obamacare was not passed in the usual manner. It began typically enough; there were separate House and Senate bills, each of which passed in their respective chambers (though without any Republican votes). Normally, the next step would be to send those two bills to a Joint Conference to hash out the differences, and then off to a final vote. This did not happen with Obamacare.

The main hang up occurred in the Senate. There, the President needed 60 votes to assure final passage of his bill. And in the way of negotiating for those necessary 60 votes, five or six Democrat Senators went behind closed doors to cobble together a list of amendments to the original Senate Bill – the so-called Managers' Amendments. It is in the Managers' Amendments that one can find such famous niceties as the bribes paid to Nebraska and Louisiana in order to entice their respective Senators to support the bill. Some of the deals made behind closed doors were so outlandish that even the Managers themselves (according to many reports at the time) did not expect them to survive the Joint Conference that everyone assumed would take place.

The original Senate bill, before the Managers' Amendments were added, never created anything called an Independent Payment Advisory Board. Rather, in Section 3403 it created the Independent Medicare Advisory

Board, whose powers (appropriately) were limited only to federally funded healthcare programs, such as Medicare. It was the Managers' Amendments which re-empowered the IMAB, and re-christened it as the IPAB.

Specifically, Section 10320 (in the Managers' Amendments portion of the legislation) grants the IPAB, beginning in 2015, the authority to limit all healthcare expenditures, that is, all healthcare expenditures, and not just expenditures by Medicare or government-run programs.

To emphasize this expanded authority, Section 10320 changes the name of the "Independent Medicare Advisory Board" to the "Independent Payment Advisory Board." It directs the IPAB, at least every two years, to "submit to Congress and the President recommendations to slow the growth in national health expenditures" for private healthcare programs. Furthermore, it designates that these "recommendations" may be implemented by the Secretary of HHS or other Federal agencies "administratively" (that is, without any action by Congress).

The justification for this mind-boggling expansion of the IPAB's authority, to the extent that any justification was offered, appeared to be that controlling private healthcare expenditures will directly impact Medicare, since the "target" Medicare growth rate (which the IMAB was originally charged with achieving) will be determined by overall healthcare expenditures. Therefore, it is necessary to control all healthcare expenditures, public and private. (More practically, if Medicare patients are subjected to arbitrary cost-cutting measures that do not affect younger Americans, we Old Farts are likely to become inconveniently rowdy.)

Once the Managers had devised sufficient paybacks in the Managers' Amendments to get the needed 60 votes, and the Senate bill finally passed, President Obama and his Congressional allies, Mr. Reid and Ms. Pelosi, determined that allowing the new law to go to Joint Conference would be counterproductive. Support among Democrats in the Senate was so tenuous that party leaders realized the bill would never survive another Senate vote after a Joint Conference. It would be easier, they calculated, to ram the Senate bill, fully intact including the Managers' Amendments, through the House of Representatives, employing the always-useful reasoning that passing the law right then was a manifest emergency. So that is what they did. And while the vote was also a much closer call than Democrat leaders would have liked, the Senate bill finally passed in the House. And in this way, to the astonishment of many, the Senate bill, Managers' Amendments and all, became law.

However convoluted the process may have been, the fact is that Obamacare grants the IPAB, a non-elected entity within the federal government, the authority to limit all healthcare spending, including private spending.

THE IPAB'S AUTHORITY IS NEARLY DICTATORIAL

A quick reading of Section 3403 might leave one with the impression that the IPAB is a sort of Mr. Rogers of healthcare – a mild-mannered, friendly, always-helpful, but ultimately undemanding agent for good. This is the impression imparted by the first few paragraphs of the Section, which paint the new entity as an "advisory" board, whose main task is to develop "proposals" and "advisory reports," which "proposals" and "advisory reports" would solely consist of various "recommendations," that ought to be "considered" for the purpose of cost reduction.

Nothing could be further from the truth. This language is simply another example of supplying a new law, which is far more radical than the authors would like people to know, with a soothingly misleading introductory paragraph. The IPAB is actually designed to be as all-powerful as it's possible to be.

Each year, once the Medicare's Chief Actuary determines that the projected per capita growth rate for Medicare exceeds the designated target growth rate (which is an inevitability), the IPAB is required to submit a plan which will cut healthcare costs sufficiently to bring the growth rate back in line; which is to say, the IPAB will determine what will be paid for and what will not. Then, the Secretary of HHS is required to implement the IPAB's plan in its entirety, without exception – unless Congress acts to block implementation. However, the ability of Congress to do so is severely limited. The representatives of the people are forbidden from taking any action "that would repeal or otherwise change the recommendations of the Board," unless it: a) votes to halt the IPAB mandates with a supermajority of the Senate; and b) devises its own specific cost cutting scheme that will achieve equivalent results. If Congress had the will to do such a thing, however, we never would have needed Obamacare in the first place.

So, in practice, the cost-cutting "recommendations" which the IPAB will "propose" for "consideration" by the Secretary and by the Congress will be implemented in their entirety, automatically, without revision, and will be backed by the full authority of the Federal government.

For all practical purposes, the IPAB will become a new agency of the executive branch with near-dictatorial authority to cut healthcare spending, public and private, where and when and for whom it sees fit.

THE IPAB IS DESIGNED TO BE IMMUTABLE

Section 3403 also contains some remarkable language that likely has never been seen before in American legislative history. To wit:

> "It shall not be in order in the Senate or the House of Representatives to consider any bill, resolution, amendment, or conference report that would repeal or otherwise change this subsection."

So the designers of Obamacare, recognizing that the arbitrary cost cutting that the IPAB will impose on all those ACOs and other integrated healthcare teams (as they happily toil away in the new healthcare worker's paradise) is sure to create significant political blowback, has sought to immunize the IPAB from any revisionary lawmaking that might result.

And as astounding as it may sound, the IPAB and all its designated dictatorial functions are designed by law to be in force for perpetuity. Our Congress has passed legislation that purports to bind all future Congresses from altering it in any way.

We have heard from the President and others that the IPAB is a very important feature of our new healthcare system. This "immutability clause" ought to convince us just how important they believe it to be. This clause necessarily implies that the IPAB is not only the most important innovation in Obamacare, but indeed, it apparently is most important legislative provision ever written. We know this because no other provision has ever received such extraordinary protections from any future alterations whatsoever.

One can only bask in the utter audacity of our Progressive leaders, who are so sure they know what's best for us that they were willing to engage in all manner of legislative legerdemain to pass Obamacare, not only against the apparent expressed will of the people, but also (as it turns out) against the objections of any future American Congress that is sent to Washington by those people.

Not even our Constitution itself – a document that attempted to establish a government for all time – was as audacious as this. For the Constitution, at least, provided a mechanism for its own alteration.

One wracks one's brain to think of the last time a law was promulgated with such audacity – not with the audacity of hope, but the audacity of perpetuity. Even monarchs who purported to reign under Divine Right understood that future monarchs, who would also rule under the same God-given right, might thus alter any laws they made.

I believe we need to go all the way back to Moses, coming down from Mt. Sinai and holding aloft his awesome Tablets filled with divine writ, to find a law or set of laws that, from the moment they were written, were decreed to remain in force for ever and ever.

Only God has ever tried this before.

THE STRUCTURE OF OBAMACARE IN A NUTSHELL

So now we can see clearly the entire skeletal infrastructure of Obamacare. Actual medical care will be parsed out by integrated healthcare "teams." There will no longer be any "doctor-patient relationships," dedicated to the welfare of the individual patient. Instead there will be "team-patient relationships" dedicated to the ethic of social justice. These teams will receive from the Central Authority, via expert panels whose work product is "guidelines," the clinical rules under which they are to determine who gets what healthcare, when, and how. And they will receive from the greatest GOD panel of all – the IPAB – the budgets which will determine how much of that allowable healthcare they can actually deliver.

Individual patients who are cut out and who want to use their own resources to guard their personal welfare will be guilty of the crime of encouraging an unfair, two-tiered healthcare system.

So go ahead, if you must, and amuse yourself with those organizational charts about Obamacare published by Republicans and other troublemakers. They are indeed disturbing.

But if all you get out of those charts is that Obamacare will become a bureaucratic nightmare – sort of a DMV on steroids – you are missing the greater point. Obamacare does far worse than merely add a few more layers of ossified bureaucracy onto an already difficult-to-navigate healthcare system.

It fundamentally changes the structure of American healthcare, centralizing control, eliminating the doctor-patient relationship once and for all, and subjecting individual patients to the decisions of "integrated teams" that will be overtly dedicated to collectivist goals.

This structure will finally systematize the practice of herd medicine in America.

CHAPTER 9 - AN INTRODUCTION TO HERD MEDICINE

Farmer Jones has 10,000 head of cattle in his beef herd. He prides himself in staying up to date on all the latest methods, so he knows that adding a certain antibiotic to his cattles' feed will reduce the incidence of intestinal infections, and will increase his annual overall yield, measured in pounds of beef, by 7%. He also knows that, unfortunately, roughly one in 200 of his cattle will experience a likely fatal allergic reaction to the antibiotic. It is possible to do a blood test to determine which specific members of the herd are allergic, but the test itself is quite expensive, and the logistics of separating the allergic cattle at feeding time and providing them with their own antibiotic-free feed would be so costly it would entirely negate his potential savings. What should Farmer Jones do?

———

Obviously, the cost-effective solution is for Farmer Jones to give antibiotic-treated feed to all his cattle, accepting the loss of a few head as the necessary price for an impressive overall gain in productivity. He would be an ineffective and incompetent rancher indeed if he were to pass up this golden opportunity to achieve cost-effectiveness.

THE HAZARDS OF HERD MEDICINE

If you are a patient or a potential patient (and who is not!), you ought to be especially concerned about two particular hazards that are intrinsic to herd medicine. First, as demonstrated by Farmer Jones, medical decisions that are made on a collective basis rather than on an individual basis may succeed in improving the overall outcome for the herd, but often only at the cost of doing predictable – and avoidable – damage to certain individuals within that herd.

Second, since it is the overall health of the herd which is important, there will always be individuals within the herd whose very existence is seen by Farmer Jones as counterproductive. Individual cattle that are too scrawny, too old, or are otherwise unlikely to prove profitable, are still consuming valuable resources and taking up valuable space. So under any system of herd medicine there will always be a natural temptation to cull instead of cure certain inconvenient individuals.

It is extraordinarily politically incorrect to mention this second point, and so I must apologize right away for having done so. Sorry.

In fact, Obamacare, so far, seems to have taken no overt steps in the direction of actively "culling the herd." But the history of Progressivism, sadly, is not reassuring in this regard. Early Fathers (and Mothers) of Progressivism enthusiastically embraced eugenics as an attractive, science-based method for reducing the sort of undesirable citizens who so obviously hinder the achievement of a perfect society. Certain Progressive societies – led by doctors – have conducted the "humane termination" of people with various disabilities. And collectivist governments (admittedly usually out of frustration at the recalcitrance of human nature than out of any scientific zeal) have been responsible for the deaths of millions of people over the last century. So, if only to keep on the safe side, we members of the Obamacare herd ought to remain alert to any tendency toward culling behaviors. If our Progressive friends are as filled with the milk of human kindness as they insist, our vigilance in this matter may waste some of our time, but otherwise should do no harm. And accordingly, to help focus our vigilance (in order to render it more cost-effective), in later chapters I will point out certain aspects of American healthcare that seem particularly likely venues for culling activities.

In this chapter, however, I will concentrate on the less sinister but more universal hazard inherent to herd medicine – causing predictable and avoidable harm to individuals by insisting on making medical decisions collectively.

A Herd Medicine Hypothetical

Let us imagine that a large clinical trial has shown that a new cancer drug increases the mean survival in women with metastatic breast cancer by three months. Unfortunately, the drug also causes some very nasty side effects, including some that can be fatal. And again unfortunately, this is one of those fancy designer drugs that cost over a billion dollars to develop, and is very costly to manufacture – so it is quite expensive.

A panel of experts, after carefully studying all the evidence, concludes that, given the relatively short improvement in mean survival, neither the risk/benefit ratio nor the cost/benefit ratio justifies approving the drug. The news media, while expressing sadness and compassion for breast cancer patients, solemnly concurs that the experts, of course, are right – that, while the drug has shown promise, it's just not effective enough to justify the risk of side effects, or the cost of the drug. So better luck next time, with the next drug.

I think we must agree that it cannot be society's duty to buy this new drug for all women with breast cancer. Under any publicly funded healthcare system that is run in a fiscally sound manner (at least sound enough to avoid causing a catastrophic financial collapse), some line will need to be drawn, somewhere, regarding what expenses public funds can bear. And very possibly, a cancer drug that only extends the mean survival by three months may not make the cut.

In Chapter 4 we discussed the four possible methods for running a fiscally sound healthcare system. If we were under a Method Three healthcare system, where public spending is strictly limited but where individuals have the option of supplementing the public system with their own private insurance products, or even paying for desired healthcare services themselves, then many individuals would still have access to treatments like this new cancer drug, if they wanted to try it.

But under a Progressive, Method Two healthcare system, public funding is all there is. In this case one centralized coverage decision must fit all, and the result is herd medicine. Under herd medicine the new cancer drug cannot be approved, for anyone, once a panel of experts determines that its herd effect is insufficient to justify approval.

But determining the herd effect of a therapy (i.e., the average response to that therapy across a herd of patients), does not really tell the whole story.

Going back to our hypothetical, if you look at what actually happened in the clinical trial with our imaginary cancer drug, it turns out that very few of the women with breast cancer actually experienced three additional months of survival. Instead, some had a truly remarkable response to the drug, and are still alive a year or more after their predicted demise. In fact, it appears that a few might even have been completely cured. Some women, on the other hand, had very bad experiences with the drug, and side effects hastened their deaths. When you average all of these responses together, you get a mean benefit of three months.

But "three months additional survival" is not actually what we would expect to happen with most individual women who take this drug, and in fact this happened with relatively few of them.

In general, the reason people with cancer subject themselves to the ravages of chemotherapy is not to gain a few more weeks of life. The chemo itself often produces several weeks where life is barely worth living, so that would be a bad trade. Rather, they subject themselves to chemo on the hope – often a slim hope – that by doing so they are gaining some realistic chance at surviving for a long, long time.

If you were to give women with metastatic breast cancer – an incurable disease that invariably causes death – the option of taking our hypothetical new cancer drug, some would opt for it and others would not. But in making their decisions, most of these women would not be thinking about the average of three additional months. Rather, most would be considering the fact that this new drug offers them some chance to beat back their cancer for substantially longer than that. They would be hoping to beat the average. They would be making the same calculus that cancer patients always make.

This new cancer drug represents a new chance at long-term survival, and faced with a fatal disease that is difficult to treat, taking that chance would have been a reasonable choice for many women – even though the drug produces only a tepid herd effect.

Herd medicine removes this option. When our hypothetical panel of experts decides not to approve this new drug – for anybody – what they have concluded is that, because the drug does not produce a sufficiently favorable effect across the herd, individual women should not have the option of using it. This is the only thing expert panels under a herd medicine paradigm can do.

They cannot deal in nuances. They must determine whether a new therapy merits application to the entire herd, or to nobody.

Furthermore, if the answer is "nobody," then the message the experts must convey – the only acceptable message they can convey – is that the new therapy simply doesn't work. Either they will say it is ineffective, or that its modest average effect is completely negated by the risk of side effects. They cannot let on that the actual data suggests that some individuals will have a truly remarkable benefit from the drug, and that on an individual basis, deciding to take the drug despite the risks would not be unreasonable.

It is worth noting that as a general rule, progress in cancer treatment has been a slow, painful and incremental process. Very few therapies have been devised that have single-handedly led to major gains in survival. Rather, progress has come from a long series of small steps – improving the average survival by three months with this drug regimen, then adding another six months with another drug regimen, and so on. Once expert panels begin deciding that adding another three (or six, or nine) month increment to the average survival of the herd does not meet the threshold for approval – that is, once it becomes evident that only "home run drugs" are sure to be approved – then drug companies will become quite reluctant to invest in the development of new cancer drugs. And medical progress will slow drastically.

Herd medicine will remove individual choice, will take away hope, and will stifle the slow, steady progress we have made in treating some of the most deadly diseases we face.

PATIENTS, WIDGETS AND THE AXIOM OF INDUSTRY

The hallmark of herd medicine is that it systematically and officially devalues the worth of the individual, essentially declaring that patients can be treated all alike, as if they are interchangeable members of a homogenous group. This devaluation of the individual, however, was not produced out of whole cloth by the Obamacare legislation. Rather, it is something that has been in the works for several decades, the natural, evolutionary result of a philosophy of healthcare that was all the rage until just a few years ago, but which – mysteriously – we seem to hear very little about these days. I refer, of course, to managed care.

Like many of the travesties that have taken place within our healthcare system, managed care began with a pretty reasonable idea; namely, to apply certain management principles to the healthcare system that have been used successfully in other industries, thereby injecting logic, organization, and accountability to what had been a bastion of disorganization and inefficiency.

The unifying idea behind managed care boils down to one word: standardization. Standardization is virtually a synonym for industry. In industry, standardization is the primary means of optimizing the two essential factors in any industrial process: quality and cost.

This proposition can be stated formally as the Axiom of Industry:

The standardization of any industrial process will improve the outcome and reduce the cost of that process.

If you had a widget-making factory, you would break your manufacturing process down into discrete, reproducible, repeatable steps and then optimize the procedures and processes necessary to accomplish each step. To further improve the quality of your finished product (or to reduce the cost of producing it), you would reexamine the steps, one by one, seeking opportunities for improvement. You would need to understand the process thoroughly, and you would need to collect data about how well the process works. But with the right information, you could almost certainly identify a few minor changes to improve the manufacturing process. The beauty in such a system is that you have only to make one change — to the process itself — and every widget that comes off the line after you make that change will be improved.

So standardization is good. It leads to higher quality and lower cost. Conversely, variation is bad. It reduces quality and raises cost.

Proponents of managed care argued that standardization should be just as useful in healthcare as it is in other industries. As medical care has traditionally been individualized, highly variable, and without any semblance of standardization, there must be a huge opportunity to improve the processes of care and to make them both cheaper and more effective. There is obvious merit in such an idea.

Perhaps the most direct, and the most successful, application of managed care practices to modern medicine was the adoption of "critical pathways" in the 1990s.

Critical pathways are blueprints for delivering standardized care to patients with specific medical problems. Consider a critical pathway for hip replacement surgery. The critical pathway is a specific schedule laying out which services are to be provided for the patient and when, from the date of hospital admission until the date of discharge (which is, of course, predetermined). Checklists are created itemizing which laboratory tests to order and when, which medications to administer at which times, and which specific complications to check for. Everyone involved in the patient's care has their own relevant checklist. From the moment of the patient's hospital admission, the critical pathway predetermines when to take vital signs, when to get the patient out of bed, when to begin physical therapy, and when to provide standardized instructions to the patient before discharge. Every vital medical service is included, and all extraneous medical services are omitted.

A "case manager" monitors the care each patient receives under the critical pathway. Every deviation from the prescribed procedure is tabulated as a "variance." Variances are tracked not to decide who to punish, but to identify areas of the process that need improvement. If too many instances of a particular variance are seen in a critical pathway, then either medical personnel need to be retrained on following the pathway appropriately, or the pathway itself should be changed to reflect more realistic expectations.

Critical pathways, in fact, proved to be extremely helpful in managing many medical conditions. But of course there were some drawbacks and limitations.

First, critical pathways are only useful for delivering medical services, like elective surgery, in which the process of care can be broken down into a predictable series of discrete, reproducible tasks that generate reproducible results. In other words, industrial management tools only work when the process of care is similar to the process of making widgets.

Critical pathways are almost worthless when you are dealing with medical illnesses in which neither the diagnostic procedures nor the treatments that may be employed can be predicted or, therefore, standardized. For instance, it has proven impossible to develop workable critical pathways to manage patients with congestive heart failure (CHF). Knowing only that a patient has been admitted to the hospital with CHF tells you nothing about whether that patient will require cardiac catheterization, a stent, bypass surgery, valve replacement, a pacemaker, an implantable defibrillator, a mechanical ventilator, a prolonged and complicated stay in the intensive care unit, or just a couple of diuretic tablets and overnight observation. No two patients with CHF are exactly alike; and there is no such thing as a standard patient. Unfortunately, most non-surgical medical services fall into this category.

Second, it turns out that when you are taking care of patients, the Axiom of Industry simply does not hold true. Standardization does not always improve outcomes and reduce cost. The reason for this is: Patients are not widgets. And while in theory everyone seems to agree that patients are not widgets, the implications of this fact appear to escape many of our public health experts.

If you're a widget maker, deciding between two manufacturing processes is a matter of simple economics. Nobody expects you to consider the widget itself. The outcome by which you are judged has nothing to do with how many individual widgets get discarded during the manufacturing process or even the quality of the widgets that pass final inspection. Instead, it's the bottom line: how much profit you make in relation to whatever level of quality you put into the widget. So the quality of the widget is not necessarily maximized, instead it's optimized, tuned to the optimal quality/cost ratio as determined by the market forces of the day. This is why, for a widget maker, the axiom holds: standardization, by rooting out variability, reduces the cost of making the widget (at whatever quality level you choose). This automatically improves the outcome, because the outcome the manufacturer cares about is overall profit.

If instead of running a widget company you're practicing medicine, the calculus is supposed to be different. You're supposed to be more interested in how things turn out for individual patients than you are in the bottom line.

So an expensive process that yields a better clinical outcome is one most people (patients, at least) would expect you to use, even though it only gets you a healthier patient and doesn't help your bottom line. A process that increases patients' mortality rate by five percent is one you should disregard, even if it is substantially cheaper than the alternative. The clinical outcomes experienced by patients — the measure of success you're supposed to be concerned about — may move in the same direction as costs, or in the opposite direction. But because you're dealing with patients instead of widgets, the Axiom of Industry doesn't hold – and outcomes and costs do not always move in the same direction.

So the push to strictly apply managed care techniques to healthcare created a dilemma for doctors. Doctors – the widget-makers in this scheme – tried diligently to apply standardized procedures such as critical pathways to the care of their patients. But the more un-widget-like the medical services they were providing, the more often they were compelled to make variances to the prescribed standardized process, in order to best serve their individual patients.

Such variances are a legitimate and valued aspect of any industrial process. In the widget-making world, variances reveal that the process needs to be tweaked to make it more usable. Variances lead to further iterations and refinements of the process, and a steadily improving result. Exceptions are what allow these industrial processes to become self-correcting.

But in the messy world of patient care, the variances revealed instead that industry-like standardization only works for a minority of medical services. No amount of tweaking can standardize the management of complex patients with complex combinations of illnesses.

It did not take long for doctors to simply stop attempting to use critical pathways for un-widget-like medical services. They did this because they actually cared about what happened to the individual widgets in their charge.

Similarly, it did not take long for our public health experts to recognize the same problem. From their standpoint, however, the problem was not that patients are not widgets. The problem was that the doctors on the scene cared about the widgets. Further analysis revealed that the root of the problem was that classic managed care techniques like critical pathways were administered locally, and therefore the misguided loyalties of the doctors on the scene were allowed to hold sway.

The reason we don't hear about managed care anymore is that such terminology refers back to those locally-administered, iterative, self-correcting, continuously improving industrial processes. And our public health experts have now realized that this model does not work, and must no longer be encouraged.

The solution to the widget-makers dilemma is to remove the dilemma. Since a dilemma requires one to choose between two options, any dilemma can be resolved by simply removing the choice. And this is what has now been accomplished.

There is no dilemma for physicians any more. Clinical decisions are now to be made centrally, by expert panels appointed by the government, through the mechanism of what is euphemistically called "guidelines." Guidelines are sacrosanct rules that will determine precisely who is to get what, when and how. Doctors are now enjoined, both by law and by their new medical ethics, to follow those "guidelines" to the letter, without exception.

So instead of the locally-controlled, iterative, self-correcting quality improvement processes like critical pathways – the same kind of processes that have so significantly improved American automobiles over the past three decades – under Obamacare we are reverting to a central-directive-style of management, far more reminiscent of the old Soviet collective farms.

WHY THE EXPERTS INSIST THEY'RE RIGHT THIS TIME

Complex systems controlled by expert-generated centralized directives have never worked and never will. The fact that experts always seem to espouse such systems – apparently under the theory that they are so much more clever, or have better information, or better systems, than those other experts who tried before and failed – is just one of the reasons we should always be afraid of experts.

And sure enough, the experts who are going to determine which medical care we in the herd will receive (and not receive) do indeed have a new and infallible system – a magic bullet – upon which to base those decisions. They call it "evidence-based medicine," which certainly sounds like a useful thing. And further, the "evidence" featured in this new formulation, virtually by definition, must come from a specific kind of rigorous study called the randomized clinical trial, or RCT.

Bias in clinical trials has long been recognized as a problem. All clinical trials are inherently biased. A research study is biased from the moment it is conceived. And those who conceive of, plan, conduct, and analyze the clinical study have every advantage. (This, indeed, is the very reason why everyone is so indignant about the studies conducted by medical industry and their minions in the medical academy.) That advantage of bias is now, under law, defaulting to the government's expert panels.

The formulation which our leaders would have us believe is that first, such government panels will be completely objective and unbiased, and second, even if they were biased, the fact that they are basing all their decisions on RCTs will eliminate any possibility of acting on that bias.

The idea that government-controlled expert panels will be unbiased, of course, is absurd. The reason these panels exist in the first place is to control healthcare costs. Since the main mechanism by which these experts will drive a reduction in spending on medical services is through the application of clinical trials – whose results the experts themselves will officially interpret –

panelists obviously will be strongly biased toward interpreting those results in a way that will justify withholding expensive medical services.

And while they are busily spinning the results of RCTs, the same experts will be assuring us that RCTs provide a guarantee against bias. For, according to the Gospel of the RCT, the chief advantage of this sort of clinical trial is that it eliminates bias altogether, and produces a completely objective result. So, in order to do the right thing, one merely needs to follow the results of RCTs.

This gospel is incorrect. An RCT, like any clinical trial, is inherently biased from the very beginning.

Many clinical researchers believe in their hearts and souls that bias can be eliminated through the use of RCTs. In such trials, "like" groups of research subjects are divided randomly into two or more groups, and each group receives (for instance) a different therapy, whereupon differences in outcomes among the groups are attributed to the different therapies to which they were randomized. Indeed, the widespread belief that RCTs are the necessary and sufficient means to achieve "clinical truth" has become so deeply ingrained within the medical establishment that when anyone (such as your humble author) suggests otherwise, he immediately reveals himself to be a scientific Neanderthal.

The widespread belief in RCTs has become nearly a Cult in the medical establishment, whose creed can be reduced to three main tenets:

1) Data derived from randomized clinical trials represents Truth.

2) Data derived from non-randomized trials represents Falsity.

3) If you don't believe this, you are a heathen.

Objective observers should find it at least a little ironic that an attempt to claim the scientific high ground has so obviously resulted in a new religion, replete with its own dogma.

The sad truth is that the results of RCTs are invariably dependent on the bias built into their design, and even if internally they are statistically legitimate, their interpretation can usually be twisted to suit one's preconceived notions – and for these reasons RCTs, like any clinical trial, can often send us down the wrong path.

Those who design RCTs (the smart ones, at least) know this. Like smart trial attorneys, they know the answer before they ever dare to ask the question. So they tailor their "question" in such a way as to yield the answer they want to get. Indeed, if a lawyer should end up asking a question in court that produces an unexpected answer, he or she is completely incompetent and ought to be sued for legal malpractice. In more cases than one might think, the same is true for those who design RCTs.

For instance, if you are an insurance company and want to limit the use of an expensive therapy, you design your RCT so that patients likely to respond favorably to the therapy are diluted within a broad population of enrolled patients, many of whom are less likely to respond favorably. This tactic will tend to make the average response of the whole population quite unimpressive. (In many instances the clinical characteristics of the likely responders and the likely non-responders will be reasonably apparent to the study designers.)

On the other hand, if you are a drug company that wants to encourage the use of your expensive new product, you design an RCT that preferentially enrolls the relatively small subset of patients who are most likely to respond favorably. Once your product has gained approval through the results of your RCT, you can then trust the marketplace (with a tweak from your direct-to-consumer advertisements) to "extrapolate" the results to broader categories of individuals.

So it is immediately obvious that RCTs do not eliminate statistical bias, as the dogma suggests. Rather, they simply offer an opportunity to control the statistical bias in your favor.

Sadly, it is often child's play for interested parties (both government and private) to twist and spin RCTs to create the desired impression. The conceit of Obamacare – that industry-sponsored research is invariably biased, while government-sponsored (or government-interpreted) research is entirely objective, and therefore, that the only thing we need to assure accurate clinical research is to have it all controlled by the government – is dangerously wrong.

Since all clinical research entails bias, the appropriate way to approach any clinical problem would be to acknowledge that neither RCTs nor any other kind of clinical trial will reliably distinguish between Truth and Falsity, and that no (inevitably conflicted) group of experts should be given the exclusive authority to interpret clinical results. Then, given the possibly competing results from various studies – which often will not yield a firm "answer" – the individual doctor and individual patient can weigh the evidence and review list of risks and benefits most pertinent to that patient, and determine the optimal course of action given that patient's particular circumstances and proclivities. Driving such a process, in fact, is what doctors are supposed to do.

But herd medicine does not allow for such individualized decisions, nor does it allow that there may be grey areas in clinical medicine, or that what's right for one patient may not be right for another. Instead, it insists that RCTs must yield the Truth, that panels of very smart experts can discern that Truth, and that these panels can determine the one Right Answer that is applicable to the entire herd.

In the next few chapters I will demonstrate more specifically how expert-driven herd medicine can cause extreme harm to individuals, and to our society. I will finish this chapter by showing a recent example of how an RCT, even a straightforward one, can be twisted quite easily into a pretzel by biased interpreters.

Spinning an RCT In Order To Shed Inconvenient Results

In 2010, the *Archives of Internal Medicine* published four (four!) articles assaulting the legitimacy and the importance of the JUPITER trial, a landmark clinical study published in 2008, which showed that certain apparently healthy people with normal cholesterol levels had markedly improved cardiovascular outcomes when taking a statin drug.

Superficially, at least, the JUPITER study appears to have been pretty straightforward. Nearly 18,000 men and women from 26 countries who had "normal" cholesterol levels but elevated C-reactive protein (CRP) levels were randomized to receive either the statin drug Crestor, or a placebo. CRP is a non-specific marker of inflammation, and an increased CRP blood level is thought to represent inflammation within the blood vessels, and is a known risk factor for heart attack and stroke. The study was stopped after a mean follow-up of little less than two years, when the study's independent Data Safety Monitoring Board (DSMB) determined that it would be unethical to continue. For, at that point, individuals taking the statin had a 20% reduction in overall mortality, a dramatic reduction in heart attacks, a 50% reduction in stroke, and a 40% reduction in venous thrombosis and pulmonary embolism. All these findings were highly statistically significant.

This study is noteworthy because it was the first large randomized trial to show that taking a statin can markedly reduce the incidence of some very harmful cardiovascular outcomes in people who are considered to have "normal" cholesterol levels.*

_____

* Notably, typical LDL cholesterol levels among primitive hunting/gathering cultures is around 50 mg/dL, instead of the 100 – 120 mg/dL we consider to be normal. These primitive folks have an extremely low incidence of cardiovascular disease, so maybe humans' optimal cholesterol level is much lower than we now think. On the other hand, the low risk of cardiovascular disease among hunters/gatherers may instead be related to the fact that many more of them than of us are consumed by various species of carnivores before they're 30.

_____

To be sure, the JUPITER trial was far from perfect. Because of its design, it could not (and did not) tell us whether the beneficial outcome is specific to Crestor, or is a class effect of all statins (which seems very likely). It did not tell us whether reducing CRP levels is itself beneficial, or even whether using CRP as a screening tool is actually helpful. (The people enrolled in this trial tended to have several other risk factors, such as being overweight, having metabolic syndrome, and smoking, and it is not clear how much additional risk elevated CRP levels really added in this population.) And this trial did not tell us the risks of lifelong, or even very long-term, Crestor therapy.

But JUPITER did tell us something that is very useful to know, and with a very high degree of statistical surety: Giving Crestor to patients similar to the ones enrolled in this study can be expected to result in significantly and substantially improved cardiovascular outcomes, and in a relatively short period of time.

If medicine were practiced the way it ought to be – where the doctor takes the available evidence, as imperfect as it always is, and applies it to each of her individual patients – then the incompleteness of answers from the JUPITER trial would present no special problems. After all, doctors never have all the answers when they help patients make decisions. So, in this case the doctor would discuss the pros and cons of statin therapy – the risks, the potential benefits, and all the quite important unknowns – and place the decision in the perspective of what might be gained if the patient instead took pains to control their weight, exercise, diet, smoking, etc. At the end of the day, some patients would insist on avoiding drug therapy at all costs; others would insist on Crestor and nothing else; yet others would choose to try a much cheaper generic statin; and some would even opt (believe it or not) for a trial of lifestyle changes before deciding on statin therapy. In other words, there is an entire range of reasonable options given the limitations of our knowledge, as there often is in clinical medicine. As time goes by, more scientific evidence is often brought to bear and clinical decisions can become more informed. But whatever the state of the evidence, doctors and patients can generally get by without violating too severely any ethical or medical precepts that would cause objective and neutral observers to complain very much.

But this kind of individualized give-and-take between doctor and patient, in which the pros and cons are discussed in light of the patient's own leanings, is no longer how doctors will practice medicine. Instead, they will practice herd medicine. Expert panels will decide whether people ought to take Crestor, or some other statin, or nothing – and that decision must apply to everybody.

And this makes the stakes very high when it comes to a clinical trial like JUPITER. For herd medicine does not permit a range of actions tailored to fit individual patients (consistent with the uncertainties inherent in the results of any clinical trial). Instead, under herd medicine the results of clinical trials generally cannot be permitted to remain imperfect or nuanced or subject to individual application, but must be resolved by a central panel of government-issue experts into a binary system – yes (do it) or no (don't do it). In the case of JUPITER, the guidelines which some expert panel is going to have to produce will have to say whether or not to recommend Crestor to patients like the ones enrolled in the study, at a potential cost of several billion dollars a year.

It should be obvious that the answer which would be more pleasant to the ends of the Central Authority, and by a large margin, would be: No, don't adopt the JUPITER results into clinical practice.

However, the expert panels which are called for by Obamacare had not been formulated when JUPITER was published. So, still subject to all the duress which is created by unfortunately-resolved clinical trials like this one, the FDA, somewhat reluctantly, approved the use of Crestor for JUPITER-like patients in late 2009. That approval, of course, is subject to review by the new expert panels, once they are actually in operation.

This, I submit for your consideration, is likely what instigated the almost violently anti-JUPITER issue of the *Archives*. It might even be suggested that the production of this extraordinary issue indicates that we may be dealing here with a bunch of wannabe federally-sanctioned experts, auditioning for positions on the expert panels. What better way to get the Central Authority's attention than to let them know that you are of the appropriate frame of mind to assiduously seek out scientific-sounding arguments to discount the straightforward and compelling, but fiscally unfortunate, results of a well-known clinical trial?

Of the four papers appearing in the *Archives*, three are more-or-less legitimate academic articles that make reasonable points, but do no harm to the main result of JUPITER. The fourth is a straightforward polemic, which has no place in a peer-reviewed medical journal, and whose very presence, I believe, strongly suggests that the editors of the *Archives* themselves may be auditioning for spots on an expert panel.

We can make short work of the three reasonably legitimate articles. One pointed out that JUPITER did not tease out the real importance of CRP levels, or whether lowering those levels is useful. This is true, but that fact does not touch the main conclusion of JUPITER. The second article was a meta-analysis which incorporated several other primary prevention trials using statins, and concluded that there is no overall benefit to statins in primary prevention patients. Aside from the usual problems inherent in meta-analyses, a) the JUPITER study looked at a specific sub-population of primary prevention patients unlike those addressed by these other studies, so whether these studies can be legitimately pooled is an open question, and b) since JUPITER is the first study to show a benefit in using statins for primary prevention, it is a foregone conclusion that if you assemble enough of the previous, negative studies and lump them together with JUPITER in a meta-analysis, you will be able to dilute the results of JUPITER sufficiently to achieve an overall negative result. Actually doing such a meta-analysis, then, is merely an exercise in math, not in revelation.

The third article criticized the JUPITER DSMB for stopping the trial earlier than originally planned. The DSMB, however, had no real choice in the matter – ethically or legally – given the striking statistical significance of the benefit seen with Crestor. When a patient signs an informed consent agreement to participate in a clinical trial, part of that "contract," a part required by law, is a statement to the effect that if information comes to light during the course of the study that might impact a patient's willingness to continue participating, that information must be made available. The fact that the Crestor branch of the study was found to have markedly and significantly improved survival, fewer strokes and heart attacks, etc., than the placebo branch, clearly constitutes such information. Indeed, it is the job of the DSMB to monitor the study for this kind of information, and to stop the study whenever it becomes certain that continuing it would expose study participants to unreasonable risks. This is why independent DSMBs exist in the first place – to protect the rights and welfare of the research subjects under the fiduciary agreement that comprises informed consent. Stopping the study when they did was not "premature;" continuing the study would have been illegitimate, unethical and illegal.

This same argument – that RCTs should never be stopped prior to the original stopping point – has been raised in the intervening years by several other experts. It is a viewpoint one perhaps ought to expect from purveyors of herd medicine. The DSMB, after all, is an artifact from a time when the patients agreeing to be enrolled in an RCT were considered to be individuals, who of their own free will volunteered to participate in a clinical trial where some aspect of their therapy would be determined by chance, and whose interests, accordingly, ought to be protected. The notion that a trial ought to be driven to its pre-set conclusion, even after it is shown that doing so will cause predictable and measurable harm to individuals in one arm or another of the trial, derives naturally from a herd medicine paradigm. Such a notion ought to give anyone pause before agreeing to participate in an RCT today.

The fourth article is more striking (and more fun) than the other three. Interestingly, it was categorized by the *Archives* as an "Original Investigation," despite the fact that it describes no investigation of any kind whatsoever – original or derivative. It merely revisits the data from JUPITER (in a spectacularly biased manner), and offers a spate of ad hominem attacks, alleging bias to the point of corruption, without any supporting evidence, against JUPITER's sponsor, its investigators, and most astoundingly, the chair of the DSMB (who is a well-known and highly respected figure, especially known and revered for his complete objectivity and lack of bias). If such an article has any place at all in a peer-reviewed medical journal – which I doubt – it ought to be clearly labeled as an opinion piece, and not as a piece of original research. Whatever it may be, it's not that.

But the most delicious aspect of this fourth article is that two of its authors, including its lead author, are members of a fringe medical group known as The International Network of Cholesterol Skeptics (THINCS), whose stated mission is to "oppose" the notion that high cholesterol and animal fat play a role in cardiovascular disease. Members of THINCS also take an extraordinarily strong position opposing statins for any clinical use whatsoever. (One might actually assume that, since JUPITER shows that cardiovascular outcomes can be improved by statins in people with normal cholesterol levels, the THINCS would embrace the study as evidence that perhaps cholesterol is not as important as it's cracked up to be. But apparently, this argument is completely negated by the fact that statins were the vehicle for making it. Many in the anti-statin crowd would object to statins even if they were proven to cure heart disease, cancer, baldness, and obesity AND produced fine and durable erections upon demand.)

The best part of all this is that the astounding anti-cholesterol, anti-statin bias of the authors was not disclosed in their article – whose main thrust, again, was to criticize the disclosed biases of the JUPITER investigators.

The venerable Pharmalot blog noted this irony, and contacted Dr. Rita Redberg (editor of the *Archives*) and Michel de Lorgeril (THINCS-master and prime author of the fourth article) to ask them why the association with THINCS was not disclosed.

Redberg: "I'm not clear this is an undisclosed conflict. The policy mentions a personal relationship that could influence one's work. I think that could be a big stretch. My initial impression is the group has an intellectual message, but doesn't fit as a personal relationship that could effect the authors' work."

de Lorgeril: "[While it is] very important to disclose financial conflicts of interest that can influence our way of working and thinking about cholesterol and statins, there is so far no obligation to provide a CV each time we publish anything...May I underline the fact that being a member of THINCS – not a group of terrorists, mainly a club of very kind retired scientists with whom I have interesting and open discussion – is not a conflict of interest?"

I may be old fashioned, but I think that being a member of an "out there" group like THINCS, which appears to advance selected and distorted data on its own website aimed at furthering its stated mission of "opposing" (not investigating or questioning) the cholesterol hypothesis and the use of statins, might make one prone to a bit of bias when writing a broadside critiquing a study like JUPITER, and loudly criticizing anyone associated with that study for *their* bias.

The irony here is amazing. The lack of embarrassment is astounding.

This sort of bias (demonstrably rooted in a willingness to select/ignore/distort data in order to make a preconceived point) is likely to be as strong as any that might accompany, for instance, receiving a stipend from a statin company for participating in clinical research. Membership in THINCS may not preclude one from writing such an article, but I think the association at least ought to be disclosed, just as financial relationships must be disclosed.

I have a hard time explaining how this can happen with a prestigious medical journal like the *Archives*. But as Sherlock Holmes says, when you have eliminated the impossible (such as, the idea that this article deserved to be published in its current form), whatever remains, however improbable, must be the truth.

And this is why I am forced to suggest that several of the authors appearing in that issue of the *Archives of Internal Medicine*, along with its editors, may be in the mode of ingratiating themselves to the sundry officials and czars within the government who will be assembling the expert medical panels which will be making the momentous decisions that will determine the flow of hundreds of billions of dollars, and (forgive me) of life and death.

Admittedly the issue of the *Archives* I have been discussing does not accurately reflect the general tenor of criticism the JUPITER trial has engendered in the academic community, which has been far calmer and less polemical. The fact is that the implications of this trial, when straightforwardly interpreted, are very disturbing to payers, both private insurers and the government. So in the years since this study was published there has been a general effort to diminish its results, from several fronts, that, taken together, should give future expert panels plenty of legitimate-sounding resources with which to deny its application to the herd.

This larger group of critics of the JUPITER trial all come from the legitimate medical establishment, and are proponents of using RCTs to make medical decisions. They claim to be willing to follow the data from RCTs to wherever they may lead.

For these critics, it seems pretty clear that the chief concern regarding JUPITER is its cost implications. That is, these people feel strongly that it would simply be too expensive to follow the results of the JUPITER trial to their logical conclusion. This, indeed, would be a very reasonable position to take – as long as their argument went something like this: "Yes, the JUPITER trial shows that many lives would be saved if people like those enrolled in the study would take Crestor, but it's just too expensive to buy Crestor for all these people."

But this sounds like rationing, and Americans don't ration. So instead critics, even those pure thinkers in the academy, have tried to attack the results of JUPITER, arguing that the results of the study actually do not support the use of statins in these patients.

Unfortunately, turning aside the results of a statistically definitive RCT can be a challenge. In fact, the need to discount the results of JUPITER leaves critics little choice but to engage in statistical legerdemain. There are several useful techniques they can employ to this end.

Many of the arguments that have been ginned up in this effort have derived not from data published in the JUPITER trial itself, but instead from statements made in an editorial written by Dr. Mark A. Hlatky, and published in the same issue of the *New England Journal of Medicine* in which the JUPITER study itself appeared.

Most of Dr. Hlatky's editorial is measured and reasonable. But along the way – either inadvertently or slyly – he threw in a key summary sentence that has been greedily grasped by those who would discount the JUPITER results, to wit: "The proportion of participants with hard cardiac events in JUPITER was reduced from 1.8% (157 of 8901 subjects) in the placebo group to 0.9% (83 of the 8901 subjects) in the rosuvastatin [Crestor] group; thus, 120 participants were treated for 1.9 years to prevent one event."

This statement, at least taken at its face value as a stand-alone analysis, is statistically naive, and fundamentally wrong.

In a long-term clinical study in which the endpoints are events that can occur at any time (such as heart attack, stroke or death), then the probability that an enrolled patient will reach an endpoint during the trial increases the longer he/she has been enrolled. But in virtually all clinical trials, the length of time different people are enrolled varies greatly. This is because it often takes years to enroll people in clinical trials, so that when the trial ends, some will have been in the trial for many years, others for only a little while. This means that the risk exposure of each research subject is different, and is proportional to the total time they were enrolled. Not uncommonly, the enrollment process is not smooth – there are periods of more rapid enrollment, and periods of slower enrollment – so if all you do is average the enrollment time (as was done by Hlatky – 1.9 years) you are likely to get skewed results. So it is simply not statistically legitimate to do so.

There is a legitimate, well-known and universally accepted method for analyzing these kinds of longitudinal outcome statistics, and it's called the Kaplan-Meier method. And indeed, the authors of the JUPITER trial presented in their paper a complete Kaplan-Meier analysis of their data, and the results look quite a bit different from Hlatky's summary statement. The Kaplan-Meier analysis reveals that the risk of heart attack, stroke, and death all increase steadily through at least four years, so that at four years after enrollment the risk of reaching one of the "cardiovascular event" endpoints was about 8% (not 1.8%). Further, the Kaplan-Meier analysis shows that the protection imparted by Crestor persists through at least four years, and that indeed the magnitude of protection (i.e., the difference in outcomes between the treated group and the placebo group) increases throughout that entire duration. So, four years after enrollment in the study, the placebo group had roughly an 8% event rate, compared to roughly a 3% event rate for the Crestor group – an absolute difference of about 5% (not 0.9%). This is a far greater benefit than is suggested by Hlatky's shorthand summary.

Suffice to say, then, that Hlatky's summary statement apparently ignores the appropriately analyzed data which is clearly presented in the JUPITER paper itself, and which documents that the clinical benefit of Crestor was substantially more impressive than his widely-quoted summary statement suggests.

But as misleading as this summary statement may be, let us accept it at face value for a moment just for the sake of discussion, since that's the data the JUPITER critics have chosen to latch on to.

Taking these numbers, the critics make the following argument: While the relative reduction in "hard cardiac events" is 50% (1.8 to 0.9), the absolute reduction is only 0.9%, which, anyone would agree, is a pretty small number. So, they conclude, the real benefit imparted by Crestor is actually quite small.

That's a very interesting argument. Let's look at it in a couple of ways.

So we've got a population of patients whose risk of heart attack, stroke, bypass surgery/stenting, or death is about 2% after about two years, and by giving them a pill we can reduce that risk to about 1%, and we're arguing that the absolute drop of 1% is not very much to crow about. Well, OK. But what if we found a pill that reduced their risk to zero at two years? That is, it completely wiped out the risk of cardiovascular catastrophes altogether. Would that be a good thing? Or would we say, "It's just a 2% drop, really not much greater than the 1% drop we had with Crestor, so it's no big deal?" I think not. I suppose we would think that totally eliminating all cardiovascular risk would be a very big deal indeed.

When you're starting at a 2% risk, then any drop in risk is going to be an "absolutely" small number. And if we're not going to pursue improvements in outcome of such a small magnitude, then why the heck are we worrying about preventative medicine in the first place? Once you get past the big things (drain the swamps, don't drink the water downhill from the outhouse, etc.) then all preventative medicine tends to consist of small, incremental improvements in outcome. Popular pronouncements to the contrary notwithstanding, preventative medicine is largely the art of spending a lot of money for this magnitude of incremental improvement. If we Americans decide we shouldn't do this anymore, then I would find it unfortunate but understandable. But it hardly seems reasonable to arbitrarily focus on this one, particular improvement in preventative cardiology, and (within a healthcare system that insists it is not rationing care) pronounce that this is the one we're not paying for.

Another way of looking at this "the benefit is too small" argument is by considering that 7.4 million Americans fit the entrance criteria for JUPITER. By giving all these people a statin, we would be preventing about 66,600 major cardiovascular events over a two year period. If you're going to say that 1% is a small number, I will counter by arguing that 66,600 is a big number. So do statins offer a substantial benefit or not? It depends on whether you choose to focus arbitrarily on the 1% or the 66,600.

(I understand that you may not be focusing at this moment on the 66,600 cardiovascular catastrophes that could be prevented, but on the 7.4 million people who will be taking a drug that costs $120 per month. But we're not talking about cost yet, we're only talking about whether the drug does some good. If we decide it does, then we'll need to link that "good" to a procedure that measures whether the "good" is worth the money we would need to spend to achieve it. The critics of JUPITER try to avoid talking about cost – since that would admit they're rationing – by insisting that there's just not enough "good" to bother with. I am simply pointing out that such an argument – that preventing 66,600 very bad outcomes is not enough to bother with – is on its face absurd.)

Another argument invoked by critics is based on the "number needed to treat" (NNT) analysis. Again they rely on Hlatky's unfortunate summary of the data: "120 participants were treated for 1.9 years to prevent one event." This number – which the critics insist is just too high – is misleading for the reasons already discussed. The real NNT, based on more legitimate statistical analysis, is plainly laid out in the JUPITER paper itself. It turns out that the longer patients in this trial were treated with Crestor, the lower the NNT became. So: At two years, the NNT was 95; at four years, it was 31; and at five years, it was projected to be only 25. Whether you think it is reasonable to treat 25 people with a pill for five years to prevent one of them from having a heart attack, stroke, or death is, I suppose, a matter of opinion. But based on NNT analyses for many widely-accepted therapies in medicine today, it looks pretty good.

All these arguments, of course, are merely distractions. The fact is that JUPITER showed a pretty striking reduction in some very nasty cardiovascular events over a pretty brief period of time, and the only real reason there's any controversy at all is because of the cost of Crestor.

That cost is what makes us want to withhold Crestor, even though it is imparting at least some (and, I am arguing, quite a bit of) clinical benefit. In other words, the high cost makes us want to ration Crestor. The fact that we can only ration covertly, instead of openly, is what makes us want to bastardize the science and do a Kabuki dance with the statistics.

If we worked under a Method Three healthcare system, where the strict limits on public spending were determined openly, then we could do an objective, full-bore cost-benefit analysis on the use of Crestor in JUPITER-like patients, using legitimate and not ginned-up statistical analysis, and taking into account not only the cost of the drug, but also the cost that would be incurred by failing to stop preventable heart attacks, strokes, etc., and then determining where the overall cost-benefit result fell within our coverage criteria. If it met the criteria we would cover it, if not, not. This decision would not be arbitrary. It would be a fully transparent process, so that if the sponsor did not like the results, they would try diligently to find a way to reduce the cost of Crestor (I think they would succeed) to a value that would be compatible with their staying in business. (And for the first time, the price of medical products would be determined by a Laffer-like curve, where a price that was too high – like taxes that are too high – would reduce revenue, instead of increase revenue. Companies, being fairly rational, would ratchet their prices down to the optimal price point.)

But since we insist on doing our rationing covertly, I am sorry to say that we're destined to keep making spurious arguments, and using dumbed-down statistical analysis to back them up. The JUPITER trial, while it is imperfect and while it does not answer every question, really is pretty straightforward. That we get so wrapped around the axle trying to fold such clinical trials into our covert rationing paradigm is simply another demonstration of the fact that covert rationing corrupts everything it touches.

The fact that so many respected academics are making such spurious statistical arguments is disconcerting and discouraging. Among other things, it means that the Central Authority will have many, many fully-domesticated experts to choose from when they assemble their all-powerful expert panels.

Summary

Herd medicine will follow naturally from any centrally-controlled Progressive healthcare system. Unless you are lucky enough to be included in the expert class, or are a part of the government leadership that controls the expert class, this is not a good thing.

Medical services that give substantial benefit to a minority of people will not be offered to any people, since the "herd effect" will likely be below an arbitrary cut-off value. Medical services that do make the cut will be prescribed for everybody, even though (since herd medicine is tuned to the average response across the population), something like half the population will respond less favorably than average. Herd medicine will stifle medical progress. And herd medicine will entice medical experts, who need to curry the favor of Progressive leaders in order to be recognized as legitimate experts, to abuse the science and the statistics of clinical trials.

It is important to note that while those of us who reside within the herd will find these features of herd medicine problematic, for our Progressive leaders herd medicine – which offers the centralized control they find absolutely necessary – is an unalloyed boon.

CHAPTER 10 - A TYRANNY OF EXPERTS

...as the complexities of the new systems increased, with their rewards of abstract power for those who succeeded, the new elites began to develop a contempt for the citizen. The citizen became someone to whom the elite referred as if to a separate species. "He wouldn't understand this." She needn't know about that." ... "She panics easily, so unpleasant news should be held back." The inability of governments to discuss in a coherent manner the political and economic difficulties in which we are mired today is a prime example of their contempt.

- John Ralston Saul, *Voltaire's Bastards*

Experts are critically important in modern society. Over the past 500 years, human knowledge has expanded well beyond the point where any one individual can understand all of it. So Western civilization requires experts – people who have a deep understanding of some circumscribed area of knowledge – simply in order to function.

But experts are humans, and they turn out to be subject to all the foibles of human nature. For instance, their thinking tends to be insular and parochial (since their expertise is, by definition, confined to a small area of knowledge); they tend to be secretive and jealous (since their special knowledge is what distinguishes them from lesser individuals); and they tend to stifle ideas that are new and different (since new ideas often threaten their positions of expertise).

So, the benefits provided by experts come with a fair load of baggage. But considering everything, most of us would say that the cost-benefit calculation of living in a modern society, and therefore being dependent upon experts, in general has been positive.

Still, during the past half millennium of our "enlightenment," there have been discrete times and places where our reliance on experts has been a net negative. These intervals, almost always, have occurred at times when selected experts are backed by the full force and might of some sovereign authority, such that the experts' word becomes law.

The herd medicine we will see under Obamacare promises to be such a time.

HOW SCIENCE PROGRESSES

Scientific progress works like this: A new theory is advanced to explain some phenomenon, usually thought up by a whippersnapper of one variety or another. The entrenched experts, whose career, reputation, social status, income, and sexual fulfillment are based on the old theory, find the new theory to be absurdly wrong (or in some cases heretical), and probably dangerous. Since preserving the "truth" is the highest calling of all, the established experts engage in every device they can muster (from "controlling" the peer-review process to burning heretics at the stake) to see that the truth (as they define it) prevails, and that the young upstarts are put down.

To the uninitiated – and certainly to the upstart whippersnappers – this process seems most primitive and unkind. But actually it is quite useful and practical, and in the long term is very beneficial to mankind. It is a process that allows us to enjoy the benefits of relying on experts, while also allowing for human knowledge to progress beyond the "comfort zone" of those experts, albeit at a purposefully slow and stately pace.

To understand the genius of such a system, we first need to understand that most of the new theories thought up by whippersnappers are, in fact, garbage. In order to break through the imposing barriers of bias constructed by the entrenched experts, the novices have to believe deeply in what they are espousing, and their new theory, ultimately, has to actually offer some substantial improvement over the currently accepted one. The whippersnapper, if very lucky, finally prevails, thus becoming the foundation of a new generation of experts – and the process begins all over again. Hence, science progresses. This process is geared toward the gradual discovery of truth, and not toward the nurturing and vindication of whippersnappers. And eventually, truth always does prevail – and often it does so within just a few generations.

In the short term, of course, this process can look very messy and unfair. It is certainly subject to great bias. In fact, we take pains to set up the accepted experts with lots of grant money, prestige, titles, etc., precisely to make sure they'll develop bias and exercise it, and do everything they can to preserve the status quo. We do this because when the paradigm actually shifts, we want it to shift because the merits of the new paradigm are sufficient to overcome all that useful bias and institutional inertia – and not because of a whim. This process keeps science – and society – on an even keel, and keeps it from being whipsawed this way and that.

And so, while the upstarts will always disagree, it is overall a system that is quite sound.

EXPERTS IN POWER

This time-tested process breaks down when a powerful outside influence – say, a religion or a government – firmly takes a side in the scientific debate, and uses its inherent authority – that is, the authority to administer excommunication, inquisition, incarceration or execution – to sanction the actions of one particular set of experts.

When a group of experts is entrenched within the power structure of a Central Authority, the process of advancing human knowledge becomes corrupted. The opinions (that is, the bias) of the selected experts invariably becomes more than just deeply entrenched – it becomes "settled science," with the weight of the Central Authority fully applied to the settling. No further evidence to the contrary is admissible – no matter how dedicated the dissenters, or how sound their arguments might be. And the upstarts are not suppressed any longer by mere peer pressure and propriety, but rather, by whatever threats of legal violence the Central Authority decides to bring to bear.

Furthermore, acting upon those settled expert opinions now becomes a matter of immediate importance for the Central Authority; time is always of the essence, and any obstructions to those necessary actions must be cleared away by whatever means are necessary.

Galileo famously ran into the problem of settled science, as espoused by experts favored by the chief Authority of the day. The experts sanctioned by the Church did not rely on mathematics, but upon Scripture. And Pope Urban VII (who, prior to his investiture had been a friend to Galileo, and had encouraged his scientific efforts), simply could not afford to let Galileo get away with espousing a system that would call Scripture into question. So, even though the Pope apparently understood that Galileo was right, Galileo had to suffer.

The global warming experts provide another example. It seems apparent that most of the world's governments, including ours, find that the bias of the global warming experts very nicely aligns with the historical bias of governments, which is to say, accruing ever more power over the endeavors of the people. These experts insist that global warming is real; that it is man-made; that it requires immediate action; and that controlling it fully justifies whatever means are necessary. And so governments have thrown in – body and soul – with this side of the debate, to the extent that "global warming" has now become largely sacrosanct. Man-made global warming is officially deemed to be "settled science," and is beyond reasonable question. No new scientific evidence to the contrary is admissible. Competing viewpoints are, in fact, heretical.

The methods utilized by experts in power are not mysterious or new. They were first laid out by Machiavelli 500 years ago, at the very beginning of the Age of Reason, in *The Prince*. Experts in power (to Machiavelli, "enlightened leaders") do not seek answers; they know the answers. They know because they are the experts. If they were to be seen seeking answers, they would not be considered experts any longer, and their power would slip away. Experts in power should operate under a cloak of secrecy, because transparency threatens them in several ways. Too much openness invites non-experts to believe they can make their own decisions; it makes the pronouncements of the experts seem less oracular; it invites second-guessing; it undermines their authority. Experts must control the language; they are the experts, so they get to say what things mean. They must define terminology that is sometimes charged, sometimes soothing, sometimes complex, but that always discourages what the masses would call common sense, and that allows the experts to make their arguments in terms that are too bland or too meaningless to dispute.

The true work product of experts in power is process. They must create complex systems and tangled infrastructures whose purpose and organization only the experts themselves can pretend to understand. Any outsiders who happen to breach their walls will thus find themselves unmanned within a structure that is incomprehensible, and whose denizens speak some alien tongue.

If secrecy, language control and complex processes are insufficient to protect their power, experts will resort to whatever means prove necessary to maintain their status as experts. This prerogative, of course, is the main advantage of having power in the first place.

The methods of expertise laid out by Machiavelli were noted even his day for their utter independence on underlying ideology. They were applicable to any enlightened leadership, whatever the content of their enlightenment. These methods have been employed profitably by authoritarians of every variety for half a millennium - by monarchs, dictators, priests and mullahs. Notably, Progressivism - an ideology that simply aims to develop a perfect society - is so devoid of actual content (i.e., of a fixed ethical underpinning) that it has become a virtual ideology of expertise itself.

And anyone who has studied Obamacare will recognize all the hallmarks of a classic expert-controlled system.

As we enter into a new era of healthcare, where medical decisions will be taken out of the hands of imperfect physicians and entrusted to panels of federally-sanctioned (and thus pretty much infallible) experts, we ought to keep in mind the problems we might create by removing selected experts from the (admittedly imperfect) give and take of scientific discourse and setting them up as experts in power, with the full backing of the Central Authority.

In the next few chapters we will have a look at some of the damage that is likely to occur under the new expert panels that are being established under Obamacare. But the tyranny that occurs when selected medical experts are backed by the Central Authority is a problem that has existed for decades, well before anyone ever heard of Obamacare. Obamacare merely institutionalizes, systematizes, and streamlines the process.

To get a flavor of what's likely in store for us, let's have a brief look at three examples of the travesties that have been perpetrated upon the public by government-sanctioned healthcare experts, even before Obamacare.

MEDICAL EXPERTS AND DIETARY FAT

The Central Authority is quite exercised at the moment over the obesity crisis they perceive – a crisis which we in the herd have brought upon ourselves through our sloth and gluttony, to the great inconvenience of our enlightened leadership. What the Central Authority fails to note (publicly at least) is their own central role in creating the obesity problem. They did it with their war on dietary fat.

An association between dietary fats and coronary artery disease was first noted in the 1950s. In 1957, the American Heart Association (AHA) published its first, tentative recommendations for limiting the consumption of saturated fat. The recommendations were pointedly aimed only at people who had a strong genetic predisposition to heart attacks or strokes, or who already had heart disease. An accompanying editorial by Herbert Pollack, in the August, 1957 issue of *Circulation*, specifically warned against the widespread application of any policy restricting saturated fat:

> *"Altering the dietary habits of a large population group is fraught with a great many dangers. Our knowledge of nutrition is not sufficient at this time to anticipate what ultimate results would happen if the public were encouraged to alter radically their basic dietary patterns."*

The AHA's recommendations regarding saturated fats received sparse attention for nearly 20 years. Then in 1977 our government, having won the war against hunger, turned its attention to the opposite problem (where it remains to this day). At that time, during another notably Progressive administration, the Senate's Select Committee on Nutrition and Human Needs, chaired by George McGovern, nationalized the question of avoiding dietary fat. After holding a series of hearings on the relationship between fat consumption to heart disease, the Committee published the first "Dietary Goals in the United States," advising all Americans to cut back on all fat consumption. With this report, the US government for the first time officially endorsed a particular type of diet – a low-fat diet – for everyone.

The Committee took this stance (on behalf of the Central Authority) despite warnings that were raised at the time by several nutritional scientists, who pointed out that the data establishing a causative role of animal fats in coronary artery disease was circumstantial at best, and further, noted that even if saturated fats turned out to be "bad," there were plenty of other fats that were healthy, and which Americans should take pains to consume. But the official experts who were advising the Committee strongly objected to any such warnings, and insisted that the science on the matter was sufficiently settled to justify universal dietary guidelines for the whole population. Furthermore, they said, trying to educate the bovine masses on the differences between good fats and bad fats (assuming there was such a thing as good fats) would obviously be impossible. The public was too dim for such subtleties. The Senate Committee followed their experts, because experts know the answer. Accordingly, the Committee opted for the far-simpler "fat is bad" message that you can sell even to gun-toting Bible-thumpers.

The anti-fat movement got its next big push in 1983, when the Framingham study published a landmark paper tagging obesity as an important risk factor for cardiac disease. This new evidence allowed the experts to reason thusly: If the people are getting fat, it must be because they are eating too much fat. It is therefore plain that that low-fat diets will prevent heart disease both directly (as they had already decreed in 1977), and now, indirectly (by preventing obesity).

Accordingly, in 1984 the NIH assembled a group of scientists and experts which subsequently issued a Consensus Statement entitled "Lowering Blood Cholesterol to Prevent Heart Disease." This document was an all-out, government-sanctioned, expert-led attack on dietary fat. Again, several of the scientists the NIH had invited to the conference argued that there was a lack of convincing evidence demonstrating that low-fat diets would be healthful. But the true experts, seeing an epidemic of heart disease which must surely be due to fatty diets, carried the day, and the Consensus Statement was voted into publication.

Shortly thereafter the AHA also endorsed this Consensus Statement. Finally, everything was in place for a major campaign across the land for low-fat diets for everyone.

The great low-fat diet era was ignited. Prestigious medical organizations spurred a campaign of public service announcements and media blitzes promoting the need to avoid fats in the diet. Influential magazines (that is, magazines read by women) began a prolonged onslaught of low-fat diet tips, articles, and human interest stories emphasizing the deadly nature of dietary fat. The food industry, which was at first very skeptical (just like the banks were when subprime mortgages were initially foisted upon them by government policy), finally jumped in with both feet (again, like the banks). A massive new product line of low-fat and no-fat snack foods was invented. These, of course, were just packed with carbohydrates, and also with the supposedly "healthy," man-made trans fats (more on this in a moment). This tsunami of change in America's processed foods has been referred to as the "Snackwell phenomenon." And, as if to put an exclamation point on the utter goodness of it all, the AHA, tapping into a lucrative new revenue source, began officially certifying these low-fat, high-carb products (including items such as Frosted Flakes and Pop-Tarts) as being "Heart Healthy."

Americans, however, are filled with the milk of human nature. So they largely ignored the ubiquitous pleas to abandon their burgers, pizza and tacos in favor of broiled, skinless, sauceless, saltless chicken breasts and broccoli. But they did begin scarfing up all those the new-age low-fat snack foods in massive quantities, having been assured that, as long as the snacks contained no fat, they could eat as much as they wanted.

There are a few physiological facts about dietary carbohydrates that the experts chose to largely ignore during the low-fat era. First, the body greedily converts dietary carbohydrates into massive stores of adipose tissue, so indeed you can readily become fat by eating carbs. Second, gorging on the refined carbohydrates found in these new "healthy snacks" causes big spikes in insulin levels (insulin being a key factor in converting excess carbohydrates to fat). When the insulin levels suddenly drop a couple of hours later, that drop produces insatiable hunger. So, two or three hours after enjoying a fat-free Pop-Tart or a Snackwell cupcake, one finds oneself desperately ripping through the cupboards to find another carbohydrate fix. By thus inducing a continuous-snacking mode, the new high-carb snack foods increased the overall caloric intake of many of the people who began eating this stuff, far beyond the additional calories listed on their labels. Third, diets high in refined carbohydrates increase triglyceride levels, reduce HDL cholesterol ("good" cholesterol) levels, and in general create lipid profiles that are likely quite damaging to the arteries.

So, while few people actually stuck to a strict low-fat, controlled-calorie diet (and to this day we still don't know whether doing so is actually a particularly good idea), many more people became addicted to the AHA-endorsed refined carbohydrates that were officially associated with low-fat diets, and as a result, they became obese.

It has only been in the past ten years or so that the low-fat dogma has begun to moderate, largely thanks to the (now mercifully faded) low-carb craze that struck at that time. We now hear somewhat more reasonable advice about good fats and bad fats, and good carbs and bad carbs. But much of the damage has been done. The damage occurred because public health experts made a conscious decision to change Americans' dietary habits, despite clear warnings that the evidence for doing so was shaky at best. At least partly because of the major push for low-fat diets, we Americans are fatter and less healthy today than we used to be.

The Central Authority's low-fat diet policy amounted to a massive public health experiment, with the research subjects being us. Our government and our expert-led medical organizations have yet to apologize for subjecting all of us to this travesty.

THE TRANS FATS TWO-STEP

In the 1980s, coincident and associated with the adoption of the low-fat diet policy, experts also saw to it that the "deadly" saturated fats in processed foods were replaced with the completely benign, inert, man-made variety of fats known as trans fats.

Almost all the trans fats we find in our in food is man-made. Trans fats come from an industrial process that partially hydrogenates unsaturated vegetable oils. The process of partial hydrogenation solidifies liquid vegetable oils, and makes them stable for long periods of time. (Liquid vegetable oils go rancid relatively quickly, and are not suitable for processed foods with a long shelf life.)

For many decades trans fats in American diets were largely limited to the use of Crisco, a shortening used for baking. Trans fats did not replace saturated fats in processed foods, for the most part, until the 1980s. It happened in the 1980s, of course, because of experts.

When the Central Authority declared its holy war on fats in 1984, an organization of food experts and food activists dedicated to stamping out saturated fats – the Center for Science in the Public Interest (CSPI) – took that as a signal to launch a major (and apparently well-funded) campaign to coerce the food industry to abandon saturated fats in all processed foods, in favor of trans fats. Trans fats, the CSPI experts declared, were entirely harmless, and by insisting on using deadly saturated fats instead of trans fats, the food industry was killing us all. The food industry largely capitulated to the CSPI's campaign in 1987, and rapidly moved almost entirely to using trans fats.

The actual safety of trans fats in humans, however, was questionable even then. Indeed, because certain scientists were attempting to call experts' attention to data suggesting that trans fats are actually quite harmful to vascular health, in 1988 experts at the CSPI felt compelled to write a major defense of trans fats in an article called "The Truth About Trans." This article strongly defended trans fats as being completely safe for humans, despite growing warnings to the contrary. The CSPI widely distributed this article to experts and decision makers (such as legislators), and for a year or two the organization seemed very satisfied with itself.

Unfortunately clinical data continued to accumulate showing that trans fats, far from being benign, likely caused more vascular damage than saturated fats. By 1993 the CSPI could no longer ignore this mounting evidence, and did a complete about-face. It launched an indignant campaign demanding that the food industry remove these deadly trans fats from all food products. Their turnaround was artful. It was accompanied by a whitewash of the CSPI's very recent history relative to trans fats (i.e., that they were largely responsible for the widespread use of trans fats in the first place). A sympathetic press (sympathetic because the CSPI was, as always, attacking evil corporations for killing Americans in the name of profit) let them get away with their revisionism.

We can give the CSPI experts credit for being willing to shift course so soon after their seminal victory. But we should also note that they displayed stereotypical expert behavior during this episode. In 1987 they insisted they had the right answer, despite warnings from scientists who had credible evidence that their "answer" was wrong. And, once the experts at the CSPI reversed course in 1993, they never again acknowledged their pivotal role in having trans fats placed in our food supply, nor did they express any remorse for it. Likely, they never felt any remorse. Rather, they almost certainly believed they were successful both times – when they wanted trans fats placed into the food supply, and again when they wanted them removed. For experts, process (and not content) is the important thing. And the process worked well on both ends of the trans fats episode.

This orientation toward process is very convenient for experts. When the content of their endeavors turns out to be a horrible mistake, they simply re-orient their processes and move on as if the mistake had never happened.

To outsiders it appears that when you are an expert, history always began 10 minutes ago. But to the experts, their history is simply a parade of one success followed by another.

SALT WARS

The misbegotten experiments that health experts foisted upon all of us by pushing low-fat diets on us, and by demanding that trans fats be used in processed foods, cost billions of dollars, needlessly transformed large swatches of American industry, and likely produced significant harm to the citizenry. Far from being chastened, however, the experts are determined to continue inflicting us with their expertise, to the great benefit of us all.

Accordingly, without missing a beat, these same experts have now launched yet another experiment that recruits each of us within the herd as unwitting research subjects. And once again, it is an experiment that has a realistic chance of producing serious harm (despite the experts' assurances that the science is settled and that only good can come of it). I speak, of course, of the new dietary guidelines regarding sodium.

Those new guidelines have been promulgated on the basis of these established "facts:" Sodium is bad. We all get too much of it. And if we restricted our salt intake to a much lower amount than we are likely getting today, we will all become healthier and live longer. Relying on this received wisdom, the new guidelines call for us to cut back to 2300 mg of sodium per day – unless we are 51 or older, or African-American, or hypertensive (and the majority of Americans fall into one of these three categories), in which case we are to restrict our sodium to 1500 mg per day.

For anyone who strays from eating only fresh fruits and vegetables, this kind of restriction is likely to prove a challenge. A nice bowl of dry cereal, for instance, even before you add milk, may give you up to 1000 mg of sodium.

Some Americans might consider such severe restrictions to be merely a statement of an ideal, as if the Central Authority were saying, "It sure would be nice if you could keep your sodium intake down to these levels. It might do you some good. So please do the best you can." But this is not at all how the Central Authority is viewing the matter.

The experts over at the Institute of Medicine, for instance, recently published (in conjunction with the new Guidelines) its "Strategies To Reduce Sodium Intake In the US." Noting that public health experts have tried in vain for decades to get Americans to cut back on salt, the IOM says the time for persuasion and education has passed. The great unwashed are proved to be recalcitrant, yet again, to reason and science. It's time to take the gloves off. So the IOM calls for the US government (specifically, the FDA) to use its regulatory firepower to enforce – once and for all – the kind of sodium restriction that the public welfare demands.

Specifically, the IOM calls for the FDA to reclassify "salt" from a food ingredient categorized as GRAS ("generally regarded as safe," i.e., items which have been used for millennia in food preparation without regulatory oversight, such as pepper, parsley, or vinegar, and which are accepted as being harmless), to a "food additive" (i.e., a substance which is certifiably harmful, and for which strict, enforceable rules must be promulgated regarding its use). Re-classifying salt as a food additive will give the FDA the authority it needs to enforce its usage (as with any other regulated substance) in the food processing industry, in restaurants, and even, one must assume, in the home. With this new designation, the FDA (and other government agencies) will be able to deploy whatever regulatory and enforcement muscle they must, in order to assure that the Guidelines for sodium are at last realized.

This is serious stuff. The Central Authority seems dedicated, as never before, to actually implementing a significant sodium restriction for all of us within the teeming masses. All, of course, for our own good.

You might think, if you have not been paying attention, that in order for experts to insist on such a severe across-the-board sodium restriction, the scientific data to support this action must be pretty airtight. But if you have been paying attention, you will not be surprised to hear that the actual advisability of restricting dietary sodium across the entire population is anything but settled. In fact, it remains very controversial among scientists.

There are at least three outstanding questions regarding the advisability of a universal salt restriction. Until these questions are addressed, the implementation of a generalized and severe sodium restriction across the population would seem, to any objective observer, to be quite ill-advised (and, of course, incredibly arrogant).

1) Does Sodium Restriction Really Do Any Good?

Books have been written addressing just this one question. Here I will simply summarize the problem.

The question hinges on the relationship of salt intake to blood pressure – that is, does higher salt intake cause the blood pressure to increase? This turns out to be a difficult question to answer with any scientific precision. The studies are difficult to conduct, and difficult to interpret. Accurately measuring sodium intake in any sizable population of patients is nearly impossible; and even measuring blood pressure (which varies tremendously from minute to minute, depending on activity, stress, and many other factors) in a reproducible way within a population of patients is extremely difficult.

Scores of studies have been conducted to try to address this question. And one can assemble from these a large group of studies which will show that salt intake correlates nicely with blood pressure. On the other hand, one can also assemble from these a large group of studies that shows it does not. And for decades, the salt vs. blood pressure question has been divided into two camps, each of which have major conflicts of interest*, and each of which invariably point to only those studies that tend to support their point of view.

———

148

* In one camp are the National Heart, Lung, and Blood Institute, the National High Blood Pressure Education Program, the Institute of Medicine, and academic experts on hypertension whose careers have been based on funding from these organizations, and whose reputations and academic standing rely on sodium intake being a major determinant of blood pressure and health. In the other camp are the Salt Institute, the big manufacturers of processed foods, and sundry academic experts on hypertension whose careers have enjoyed funding from these sources. Take your pick.

―――――

My own reading of the medical literature suggests that the population itself is divided into (at least) two types of people with regard to sodium and blood pressure: "salt sensitive" people, in whom sodium intake significantly influences blood pressure; and "salt insensitive" people, in whom it does not. Most folks appear to fall into the latter category. So, if we really wanted to use salt intake as a tool for controlling the populations' blood pressure, it might be a good idea to recommend salt restrictions for "salt sensitive" individuals, but not for the majority. But it is inconvenient and impractical to determine people's salt sensitivity, and besides, doing so would go against the principles of herd medicine. So the experts, in their wisdom, appear to have determined that the best way to restrict sodium in the people who are salt sensitive is to restrict it in everybody.

To see just how deeply politics is involved in the salt controversy, I highly recommend an article called "The (Political) Science of Salt," by Gary Taubes, which appeared in 1998 in *Science*, and which outlines the incredible machinations that have been employed by the various interested parties in interpreting some of the complex studies that have attempted to correlate salt intake with blood pressure.

Our imaginary objective observer can only conclude that, at the very least, this is not a settled question.

But even if it were a settled question, and sodium intake did indeed correlate nicely with blood pressure across the whole population (and even legitimate herd medicine would require this minimum criterion before enforcing a universal sodium restriction), the degree of blood pressure reduction predicted by even the most vociferous sodium-restriction-enthusiasts, even employing drastic sodium restrictions, seems trivial. Most experts predict an average reduction in blood pressure of only 1-2 mmHg. The experts defend their universal salt restriction by arguing that this tiny reduction in blood pressure, on a worldwide basis, would save over 100,000 lives per year. But this argument is (scientifically speaking) hogwash. Such estimates are merely calculations made from strings of assumptions piled upon assumptions, and have little or no bearing on reality.

The fact is that we just don't know what effect it would have on the population's health to significantly restrict salt intake in everybody. We don't know the magnitude of blood pressure reduction it would achieve, or the improvement in clinical outcomes that would follow such blood pressure reduction.

We could find out if we really wanted to – by doing a large, randomized clinical trial to test the hypothesis. But the experts have determined that such a randomized trial is not necessary because the science is settled, and besides, time is of the essence. (Astute readers will have noticed that when you are an expert, the science is always settled, and time is always of the essence.)

Our health experts would rather conduct a non-randomized experiment that enrolls every living American as an unwitting research subject. Then, in a couple of decades (reminiscent of the low-fat diet "experiment"), maybe we could figure out how it all worked out.

2) Does Sodium Restriction Cause Harm?

Here is a question that the health experts, who have revealed to us that salt restriction is an unalloyed good, really object to. For it questions their infallible pronouncements. It is, indeed, criticism. So they tend to get downright nasty when anyone brings it up.

But, as it happens, it is a legitimate question.

Sodium is extremely critical for any living creature. For any living cell to function normally, it must exist in an environment that contains, within a narrow range, just the right concentration of sodium. Consequently, living beings have evolved a complex series of mechanisms to assure an adequate sodium concentration under any and all circumstances. So, if animals are made to survive on a severely sodium-restricted diet, these homeostatic mechanisms are called into play to restrict the loss of sodium from the body. The stimulation of these sodium-retaining mechanisms can have many secondary effects.

In states of sodium depletion, tissues are more susceptible to injury from ischemia (lack of oxygen), a condition seen in heart attacks and strokes. Kidney damage caused by many types of medication will occur much more readily in states of sodium depletion. The way the kidneys handle various drugs is also altered when sodium intake is reduced, leading to potentially harmful changes in the blood concentrations of certain medications. The renin-aldosterone system is activated under salt restriction, which can have several adverse effects. (In fact, a major therapy for several medical conditions, such as heart failure and – ironically – hypertension, centers around suppressing the renin-aldosterone system.) Adrenaline levels and LDL cholesterol are increased when sodium is restricted. And at least one study, disturbingly, has correlated sodium restriction with an increase in cardiovascular mortality.

Calling attention to these kinds of findings just makes the sodium-restriction experts angry, and they usually respond by pointing out that so-and-so got a grant from the Salt Institute. (As noted, there are conflicts of interest on both sides of this fight.)

In 2011 alone, five new studies were published which question the safety of salt restriction for the whole population. One in particular, published in December 2011 in the *Journal of the American Medical Association*, suggests that when you compare cardiovascular events (such as heart attack and stroke) to sodium intake, the incidence of those events follows a "J" curve. That is, cardiovascular events are lowest at an "optimal" level of sodium intake. But if sodium intake goes above that optimal level – or if it goes below it – the incidence of cardiovascular events increases.

According to this study, the "optimal" level of daily sodium intake is 4000 – 5999 mg of sodium per day. Cardiac outcomes worsen for those with sodium intakes above or below those values.

As we have already noted, health experts are insisting on sodium intakes far below the 4000 mg threshold. Their recommendations would place everyone on an unenviable portion of the J curve, and (if this new study has any merit) would risk exposing all of us to an excess of cardiovascular disease.

Whenever a study appears that calls into question the advisability of a universal sodium restriction, the experts are quick to respond. In response to the "J curve" study, Heartwire (an online news source for cardiologists) elicited the following response from Dr Graham MacGregor of London's Wolfson Institute of Preventive Medicine (and a major sodium restriction guru): "[These new studies] are a minor irritation that causes us a bit of aggravation, and we have to talk to journalists about it, because they are not interested in news saying salt is dangerous." MacGregor went on to insist that the need for a global sodium restriction remains a settled issue: "What [these irritating investigators] fail to understand is that the FDA is not asking for evidence about why salt should be reduced, they are asking how it should be reduced." So new data is not needed, nor will it be heeded. It is all a settled matter.

At the end of the day, we have conflicting sets of observational data that can be interpreted to say different things. It may be true that a severe population-wide salt restriction would be a huge boon to mankind. But it may also be true that it would harm more people than it would help – or that it would harm and help about the same number, so the overall results would be the same.

The fact is, we just don't know.

3) Is It Even Possible To Change Sodium Intake By Public Policy?

As we have noted, maintaining the proper sodium concentration in tissues is critical to life, so living creatures have evolved a complexity of mechanisms to assure that the concentration of sodium in the body remains within the proper range.

Among these mechanisms, it now appears, is an inherent "sodium appetite" enjoyed by all humans and all animals, an in-born mechanism that determines how much sodium an individual will ingest each day to help keep just the right sodium "set-point." This sodium set-point is maintained by a complex neural network that is still being sorted out, involving several regions within the central nervous system, as well as inputs from the peripheral tissues. The bottom line is that one's own physiology naturally regulates one's sodium intake to satisfy the body's needs.

Furthermore, studies of sodium intake across a wide array of human populations, living under a wide variety of conditions and dietary constraints, also show that the range of salt consumption humans take in to achieve their set-point is remarkably universal, and is maintained within a fairly narrow range. That is, not only do humans consume the proper amount of sodium as determined by the body's needs, but across the diversity of humanity that "automatic" sodium intake is maintained within a remarkably fixed range. (Sodium intake moves within that range to maintain the body's proper sodium set-point.)

As it happens, the lower limit of that universal, naturally occurring, "optimal" range of sodium intake is roughly 2300 mg/day.

By pure coincidence, this natural lower limit, determined by our physiology, is the same as the the upper limit our Central Authority would have many Americans consume. (The rest of the Americans will be consuming only up to 1500 mg/day, which is far below the natural lower limit.)

In other words, by decree, our government would have every American consume an amount of sodium that is below the apparent optimal range (or at best, barely touching the optimal range), as determined by actual human physiology. Almost by definition, anyone living under the recommended guidelines would likely be unable to maintain proper sodium concentrations through sodium intake alone, and would need to recruit the secondary, sodium-retaining, potentially-harmful physiological mechanisms (such as the renin-aldosterone system) to keep sodium concentrations at an adequate level.

Furthermore, it seems to me that if we have a deep physiological need to satisfy our "sodium appetite," and if the only food we can get will be (by the Central Authority's decree) low-salt, then the only way we can satisfy our sodium appetite will be by eating more of it. In other words, an enforced policy of sodium restriction seems likely to worsen our obesity epidemic.

It is apparent that even if a universally-applied policy of significant sodium restriction was proved to be safe and effective, it may not be possible to make people comply with such a restriction. This kind of restriction will be fighting our inherent "sodium appetite" that has been forged through millions of years of evolution. This kind of restriction would appear to fly in the face of our human physiology.

We need salt, dear readers, we truly do. The only reason the Founders did not include an additional paragraph in the Second Amendment (to the effect that, "A palatable diet being necessary to the health and well-being of a free People, the right of the People to bear salt shall not be infringed,") is that it never occurred to them that any government, anywhere, would ever attempt to restrict such an inherent physiological necessity.

Of course, anyone who has observed the Central Authority at work – as it attempts to implement policies that require fundamental changes in human nature, or that require the repeal of the basic laws of economics – should not be surprised at the notion that our Progressive leaders would also try to repeal human physiology.

We have already seen the harm that can be done when we allow public health experts to launch major, population-wide dietary changes, before adequately studying what their effects will be. Especially given the increasing evidence of the harms that might be done by it, we are nuts if we allow the arrogant expert class to enforce a salt restriction program on all of us, before we have completely studied its likely results.

A Tyranny of Experts

A major thrust of our new healthcare system is to implement herd medicine. Fundamentally this means empowering the experts to practice medicine, from a distance, upon the whole population. Urging caution or even a certain amount of circumspection on this newly-empowered expert class, as it begins exercising its much-sought and hard-won right to dictate American healthcare on a collective basis, is destined to be a futile exercise.

The health experts hold the high ground. For they are experts in a system that, if it worships anything, worships experts. They are the ones with the answers. Woe unto anyone who would stand in their way!

They are the ones who will give directives to doctors on the front line, and direction to the sundry health-related agencies of enforcement wielded by the Central Authority. Once they have formed an expert opinion the issue is settled, and it immediately becomes time – backed by the power of the Central Authority – to sweep aside any opposition, and implement the process.

As long as the process itself is successful, actual results visited upon members of the herd are not that important. Therefore, as far as the experts are concerned, their implementation of low fat diets was successful. Their incorporation of trans fats into our food supply was successful. With these fresh triumphs under their belt the experts have been validated, and they move confidently ahead to implement their new sodium restriction policy.

Armed with their infallible answers, they know only one word (a word we have heard before, and one that is being adopted again as a call to arms): "Forward!" If the herd suffers because of it, the experts will pretend not to notice.

For the herd will always be there, and the experts can always try again.

CHAPTER 11 – PREVENTING PREVENTIVE MEDICINE

"Prevention, prevention, prevention—it's about diet, not diabetes. It's going to be very, very exciting."
- Nancy Pelosi

"Although different types of preventive care have different effects on spending, the evidence suggests that for most preventive services, expanded utilization leads to higher, not lower, medical spending overall."
- Douglas W. Elmendorf, Director of the Congressional Budget Office

Back in 2009, when the Obamacare legislation was being debated, we in the herd were given frequent assurances by our Progressive leaders that turned out to be misleading. We were told that we could keep our own health insurance if we liked it. We were told that Obamacare would reduce costs and increase the quality of our healthcare. We were told that anyone who opposed Obamacare most certainly wished to see the cemeteries filled with the sad remains of uninsured children and neglected old people.

But when we were told that Obamacare was all about prevention, that was probably the biggest whopper of all.

Speaker Pelosi, in particular, liked to remind us that if Obamacare signified anything, it signified "prevention, prevention, and prevention." Indeed, it was by providing the funds and the systems for disease prevention that Obamacare would achieve the twin goals of creating a healthier citizenry, and creating the cost reductions necessary to rescue us from the healthcare system's fiscal black hole.

And when spokespersons for the Progressive leadership, such as Citizen Pelosi, were marched out before the microphones to say so, they implied they were talking about providing services such as mammograms and other screening tests that would detect serious illnesses at a time when they were still treatable, and providing medications that would reduce our risk of developing this disease or that. In other words, we were led to believe they were talking about preventive medical services. Indeed, it seems likely that these high profile spokespersons were actually talking about this very thing.

If so, then even the spokespersons were kept innocent of the truth. For the unnamed framers of Obamacare understood "preventive medicine" in a very different way, and they designed the new law to advance their own, very circumscribed, concept of preventive medicine – and to stifle what the rest of us would consider preventive medical services.

The authors of Obamacare actually never intended to increase spending on the kind of preventive medical services everyone thought they were talking about. Rather, they intended to reduce spending on such preventive medical services as much as possible, and wrote into the legislation the mechanism for doing so.

They did this because they fully understood a fundamental truth about preventive medical services, a truth that they were obligated to act upon, but which they could not speak out loud. Namely, that preventive medical services – virtually every preventive medical service you can name – invariably will cost the healthcare system far more money than they can ever save.

This being the case, then under any publicly-funded healthcare system that is serious about keeping costs down, preventive medical services will have to be, well, de-emphasized.

I must hasten to add that there are, of course, preventive measures that turn out to be cost-effective. And to demonstrate that this is the case, and as a public service, I will now conduct these preventive measures, in their entirety: Don't smoke. Eat a sensible diet. Keep your weight down. Get plenty of exercise.

There you are. And the only reason these measures are cost-effective is that it costs the system very little to utter them.

And to the extent that Obamacare will be serious about disease prevention, finding ways to entice, cajole, embarrass, or force American citizens into what our leaders consider to be healthier lifestyle choices will constitute the bulk of it. This is why we are seeing a great acceleration in the efforts by the Central Authority to regulate what we eat, and why obese Americans have joined the short list of identifiable groups (along with conservative blacks and conservative women) whom it is entirely acceptable, and even laudable, to demonize publicly. This is what our Progressive leaders really (and secretly) mean by "prevention." We will be addressing this variety of preventive medicine in a later chapter.

Here, my intent is to demonstrate how our new healthcare system has established the mechanisms for preventing the very kinds of preventive medical services most of us thought Ms. Pelosi was talking about a few years ago.

WHY PREVENTIVE MEDICAL SERVICES ARE TOO EXPENSIVE

While it may initially seem counter-intuitive to think that preventive medical services will invariably cost the healthcare system far more money than they can ever save, a few moments of thought will demonstrate the truth of it:

a) The preventive measure itself costs money.
b) The preventive measure may not be very effective.
c) Many "preventive healthcare services" consist of some kind of screening test for "early detection," and these screening tests almost always produce more false positive results than true positive results – leading to the need for more definitive, more expensive, and often invasive confirmatory tests.

d) "Early detection" of any medical condition often detects "occult" disease, that may or may not have become manifest if it had remained undetected.

e) Treating the diagnosed – and often occult – medical condition is often very expensive, produces expensive complications, and/or is ineffective.

f) Early treatment of many medical conditions will not lead to a cure, but rather, may convert what would likely have been a relatively short and fatal disease to a much more chronic, much more expensive disease.

g) Spending money to successfully prevent a particular medical condition simply gives the beneficiary the time to develop some other medical condition – possibly a much more expensive one – in the future.

h) If the patient whose life is saved by the screening test and subsequent therapy is an Old Fart (like your author), that patient will persist, for several more years, to soak younger, worthier Americans for Social Security and Medicare payments.

Q.E.D. The healthcare system will spend far more money by offering these preventive services than if it did not offer them.

This result should not be very surprising. It is the natural result any time healthcare services are to be paid for with pooled funds. Consider what would happen if smoke detectors were regarded as a preventive medical service. Smoke detectors clearly save lives here and there – we have all heard anecdotes about a family being aroused to safety by a smoke detector. But we cannot show any real data proving that the overall survival of people who have smoke detectors is significantly higher than of people who don't. So if it were society's job to buy smoke detectors for every individual, then society would – rightly – determine that the cost is not worth the insubstantial benefit.

The only reason most people have smoke detectors is that it is NOT society's job to pay for them. The individual does. And the individual does not care that smoke detectors cost $1.2 million per life saved. They only care that the life saved, potentially, is theirs, and that owning the smoke detector that might just save their life does not cost them $1.2 million, it only costs them $19.99.

Therefore, I am not arguing here that preventive services are useless or undesirable. Often they are quite useful and very desirable. Rather, I am simply pointing out that, even when a preventive medical service works exactly as designed, all you get is a healthier patient; in the long run, at least, you have not actually saved any money. In fact, if you must provide that preventive service to everyone, you will necessarily lose money. The people who will be running Obamacare understand this, and further, understand they will have to find a graceful way to stifle preventive medical services.

This fact ought to prove embarrassing to our leaders, who have spent the last few years assuring us otherwise. Indeed, we cannot overemphasize the extent to which they have doggedly insisted that not only are preventive healthcare services cost-effective, but also it is precisely because of such preventive services (delivered in the remarkably efficient manner which will be achieved by our new healthcare system) that we will enjoy tremendous cost savings over the next decades.

However, the fact that preventive services are simply too expensive to provide is not news to our leaders. They understood it all along. And accordingly, in the Obamacare legislation they took pains to provide themselves with the tools they will need to accomplish this feat. Their chief tool will be the United States Preventive Services Task Force.

THE NEW ROLE OF THE USPSTF

Under Obamacare, the job of determining which preventive services are to be available to Americans and which are not has been assigned to the United States Preventive Services Task Force (USPSTF), a panel of experts appointed by the administration.

The USPSTF has been around for a very long time, and traditionally its job has been to periodically review available data pertaining to various preventive medical services, and to issue recommendations regarding those services – who ought to receive them and when. Its recommendations have been generally respected by American physicians, but were never intended to be binding, and have never been treated as if they were. In fact, most medical specialists in America have been more likely to pay attention to recommendations on preventive services issued by their own professional organizations (such as the American College of Cardiology).

This all changes under Obamacare. The USPSTF is to become the one and only arbiter of preventive medical services. The new law gives the USPSTF final say in which preventive services are to be covered by private insurers (Section 2713), by Medicare (Section 4105), and by Medicaid (Section 4106). If the USPSTF awards a preventive service a grade of A or B, it must be covered. If it awards a preventive service any other grade, it cannot be covered. The recommendations of the USPSTF (including the ones they have issued in the past, prior to Obamacare), are now to be binding – for everyone.

And as we have seen (Chapter 7), if a service is deemed by this expert panel not to be a covered service, it very likely will not be available at all, even if you are willing to pay for it yourself.*

---

*While Chapter 7 makes the case that Progressive healthcare systems will always tend to restrict individual prerogatives, this is especially true with preventive medical services like screening tests. For, if a self-paid screening test turns out to be positive and a new diagnosis is made, it will lead to expensive confirmatory tests and/or treatments that the healthcare system itself will have to pay for.

THE USPSTF AND MAMMOGRAPHY

It is likely that the first time most Americans will recall ever hearing about the USPSTF was when this panel, in the fall of 2009 as the fight over Obamacare was reaching a crescendo, chose that moment to release its controversial new "recommendations" on breast cancer screening.

Many American women were stunned at these new recommendations, most particularly because the USPSTF determined that most women under 50 no longer need screening mammograms. Women were shocked because they had been urged for over a decade by various cancer societies, by the government, and by their doctors to get regular mammograms beginning at age 40. They had been told this screening was important because the early detection of breast cancer was the best way not to die from breast cancer.

The outcry by women was so great that, apparently, our Progressive leaders feared the controversy would cause people to actually begin reading the proposed Obamacare legislation. If people had done so, they would quickly learn that Obamacare was converting the heretofore mild-mannered and unobtrusive USPSTF into an all-powerful final arbiter of which preventive services would be available to Americans and which would not. Furthermore, they would learn that all of the prior recommendations ever made by the USPSTF would become retroactively binding once the new law took effect.

Damage control was required. Accordingly, Secretary Sebelius quickly issued a statement telling Americans that the mammography recommendations of the USPSTF were merely that – non-binding recommendations – and that women should continue getting their screening mammograms as they and their doctors thought best. Then, in order to remove her hasty statement from the category of "lie," the Secretary quickly caused specific language to be inserted into the pending Obamacare legislation exempting the new mammography recommendations from the law, thus making that one set of USPSTF recommendations - and only that one set - non-binding.

That special new language can be found in Section 2713, which addresses private health plans. Similar language, however, does not appear in the Medicare or Medicaid sections (4105 and 4106), so it appears that patients covered by these two programs will indeed be subject to the USPSTF ruling on mammography.

The mammogram controversy stirred up by the USPSTF subsequently died down, and apparently without anyone noticing that, new mammography recommendations aside, for the rest of the preventive healthcare services that exist in the universe, only those that have achieved a grade of A or B by the USPSTF will henceforth be covered, or even available.

When we look a little deeper, we find that the USPSTF's new recommendations on breast cancer screening reveals to us something else that is quite important. It reveals the surprising extent to which the experts in the government's medical panels are willing to engage in scientific legerdemain, in order to settle upon the answers that are most soothing to the Central Authority. This revelation stems from the fact that the methodologies used by the USPSTF in making its new recommendations on mammography were fundamentally unsound. This is a disturbing observation, since it sets a precedent for future decisions which this and other expert panels will be making for all of us in the herd.

In rendering its decision on breast cancer screening, the USPSTF helpfully published a document laying out in detail the specific clinical studies it relied upon, and the rationale it used, to synthesize concrete recommendations. And by analyzing the USPSTF's own written justifications, it is possible to derive at least four new "rules" – new precedents – upon which this and similar panels of experts can rely in the future.

1) The USPSTF now recommends that breast cancer screening should no longer be done for most women under the age of 50. But by the panel's own words, screening mammography in women in the 40 – 49 age group appears to be just as effective at reducing mortality as it is in women 50 and older, and the panel indicates this fact several times within its own document. And as nearly as I can tell, the panel's only concrete rationale for dropping mammography for women under 50 is that it has found "a new systematic review, which incorporates a new randomized, controlled trial that estimates the 'number needed to invite for screening to extend one woman's life' as 1904 for women aged 40 to 49 years and 1339 for women aged 50 to 59 years."

This rationale implies the following rule, Rule 1: If you have a preventive measure which is equally effective across a large population of patients, you can withhold that preventive measure from any arbitrary subgroup within that large population, when performing the effective measure in that arbitrary subgroup is more costly than it is for some other arbitrary subgroup.

2) In its public justification for withholding mammogram screening for women aged 40 – 49, the USPSTF did not emphasize cost savings, but rather, emphasized the fact that screening in this age group results in more false positive tests than for older age groups, and thus in more unnecessary biopsies, along with the potential for more unnecessary emotional trauma. While this is certainly true, the traditional response to such a circumstance would be for doctors to carefully review the pros and cons of screening with each woman, so as to allow the individual to decide whether the possibility of needing an unnecessary biopsy outweighs the possibility of diagnosing breast cancer while it is still curable.

But instead, the panel established Rule 2, the herd medicine rule: Rather than allowing individuals to apply their own values when weighing healthcare decisions which reasonable people could decide either way, it is legitimate for expert panels to make those decisions from on high for all patients; and furthermore, it is legitimate for the panel to make different decisions for different and arbitrary subgroups of patients (e.g., one decision for women 40 – 49 years of age, another decision for women 50 or older).

3) The USPSTF now recommends that women not be taught breast self-examination. In point of fact, since most doctors stopped teaching self-examination a long time ago, this recommendation will probably have little actual impact. But the panel came to this recommendation based on clinical trials conducted in backward, 3rd world healthcare systems (Russia and China), where the treatment of breast cancer is far less advanced than it is in the U.S., and where clinical outcomes in patients with breast cancer have little to do with outcomes in the U.S.

Perhaps more to the point, a similar tactic was used in deciding to withhold mammogram screening for women under 50. That is, the "new randomized controlled trial" the panel invoked to justify this decision was conducted in England, where outcomes for the treatment of breast cancer are substantially – and famously – worse than they are in the U.S.

So Rule 3 is established: It is legitimate to take the results of clinical trials conducted in backward countries with poor healthcare systems, or in less backward countries which nonetheless have demonstrably inferior outcomes, and directly apply those results to coverage decisions affecting American patients who are being treated in the American healthcare system. This is like performing a careful statistical analysis of outcomes from a Pee Wee football league, then telling the New England Patriots to abandon the forward pass, because the percentages just aren't there.

4) The USPSTF now recommends that women 75 and older not get any breast cancer screening at all, despite the fact that (from the panel's own words) breast cancer is the leading cause of death among women in this age group. The panel justifies this recommendation by noting that there are insufficient data from randomized trials in these elderly patients, and further, that "women of this age are at much greater risk for dying of other conditions that would not be affected by breast cancer screening."

It is, perhaps, convenient that very few randomized clinical trials assessing preventive measures have ever been conducted in elderly populations, and further, that if such trials were conducted, any actual benefit that might accrue to the subset of relatively healthy older people who might benefit from preventive medicine would be diluted by the inclusion of large numbers of less healthy elderly patients. And, while doctors usually have little problem identifying those healthy 75-year-olds who are likely to survive another 10 – 15 years, and in whom detecting early breast cancer would likely be beneficial, the large, long-term, randomized clinical trials "proving" to the satisfaction of the USPSTF that these women deserve screening will, for all practical purposes, never be done.

So, Rule 4: Preventive measures should not be offered to old people, because they're probably going to die pretty soon anyway.

160

Whether or not you agree with the substance of the USPSTF's actual recommendations on breast cancer screening, it should be pretty obvious that the methodologies the panel used to reach those recommendations, and the four new rules those methodologies have established, are dangerous for all of us. Perhaps worse, the methods used by the USPSTF reflect an unfortunate mindset that seems apparent among members of this expert panel, in particular, regarding to what extent such panels may be willing to employ (for want of a better term) creative analytics, in order to produce recommendations likely to be pleasing to the Central Authority.

THE USPSTF AND PROSTATE CANCER SCREENING

More recently, the USPSTF created another hub-bub when they released their latest, updated recommendations on whether men should routinely have PSA testing for the early detection of prostate cancer. The USPSTF's recommendation was simple and straightforward: No.

Proponents of PSA testing immediately complained because prostate cancer kills many men, and its early detection makes it easier to treat. Without PSA testing, the early detection of prostate cancer is difficult and often impossible. But those siding with the USPSTF point to randomized clinical trials showing no significant reduction in mortality in populations of men who have had PSA screening, and further, that men who have PSA screening end up having a lot of very unpleasant and expensive medical procedures which can leave them with life-altering side effects.

The document published by the USPSTF in justifying its PSA recommendation points out two major findings which it has gleaned from the extensive medical literature on PSA screening. First, when PSA screening is applied to large populations of men, it is difficult to demonstrate a reduction in overall mortality. Of two large clinical trials comparing men randomized to PSA screening to those randomized to "standard care," one found that PSA screening yields a relatively small but statistically significant reduction in cancer-related deaths, but the other showed no mortality benefit. So, given a large population of men eligible for screening, doing PSA testing appears to yield a benefit that is either small or non-existent. And as a result, from a public health standpoint a recommendation to do widespread PSA screening is simply not justifiable based on current evidence.

This finding fully accounts for the USPSTF's new recommendation to withhold PSA screening.

But the second major finding revealed by the medical literature (which the scientists on the USPSTF faithfully report, but then apparently discount) is that, for men in whom screening has actually detected early prostate cancer, subsequent treatment indeed significantly reduces mortality. This second finding addresses one of the big questions that has often been raised about early detection of prostate cancer, namely, whether the cancers detected by PSA screening actually require treatment. Many of these early cancers apparently never cause death, so many have speculated that "watchful waiting" might be a reasonable course of action rather than aggressive prostate treatment. But the USPSTF's review of the relevant studies shows that when early-stage prostate cancer is identified, the best clinical trials available show a significant reduction in cancer-related death and all-cause mortality with treatment.

As the backdrop for its negative conclusion on PSA screening, the USPSTF's document strongly emphasizes the drawbacks of screening. PSA screening often leads men to experience some very bad outcomes from prostate biopsies, or from therapy for prostate cancer. The very nasty complications resulting from these procedures are all too frequent, and are very difficult to even think about let alone experience. Furthermore, pursuing all those positive PSA tests with biopsies is extraordinarily expensive for the healthcare system. The reasoning offered by the USPSTF in making their new recommendation to withhold PSA screening relies heavily on the price which men must pay, in terms of complications, if they have to pursue the results of a positive PSA test – and on the financial cost to the healthcare system of doing so.

I have long been disturbed by the state of the art of both prostate cancer screening and prostate cancer treatment, by the lack of obvious progress in improving these things, and by the seeming complaisance with which many urologists seem to accept the status quo. PSA screening appears far too sensitive (too many false positives, leading to too many biopsies). Prostate biopsies often yield both false positive results (detecting cancers that are probably clinically meaningless) and false negative results (missing cancers that are clinically important). And the numerous treatments available for treating prostate cancer (all of which tend to be very unpleasant) have not been rigorously compared, leaving the various "camps" of urologists to argue that their pet treatment is the best one, and all those other urologists have their heads up their nether regions.

All this confusion and uncertainty places the individual faced with the prospect of whether to have a PSA test, or worse, with newly-diagnosed prostate cancer, in a complete quandary, and apparently with no objective means to resolve what he ought to do next. But despite all these shortcomings, the urology community has aggressively turned PSA screening and the cascade of uncertainties (and resultant procedures) that flow from it into a burgeoning industry, to the extent that one must wonder how badly these specialists really want to clarify the current muddle. And for this reason, it is difficult to take the loud objections being made by the American Urological Association against the USPSTF's new recommendations very seriously.

So from a herd standpoint, the USPSTF recommendations on PSA screening may seem quite reasonable.

Still, one must consider carefully the second major finding from the USPSTF's own analysis of the medical literature on prostate cancer screening:

Even with all the drawbacks associated with PSA screening, and even with all the conjectures about whether these early prostate cancers really need to be treated after all, it turns out that if prostate cancer is detected by some screening technique, then treating that cancer saves lives. And we must further note that while the USPSTF dutifully describes this result in the body of their report, they do not mention it in the Abstract of their report, and they do not seem to have given it much weight, if any, in their final recommendations.

But clearly this is an important result, and ought to be taken into account. It should not be simply brushed off as irrelevant, or unworthy of notice. It begs to be explained.

How can it be that, on one hand, offering PSA screening to a large population of men does not seem to result in much overall mortality benefit, whereas on the other hand, if you do find prostate cancer when you screen for it, then treating that cancer significantly reduces mortality?

Most likely the explanation lies in the dilution effect. The moderate (but statistically significant) benefit of treating early prostate cancer is washed out when those patients are diluted within a much larger population of men who are eligible for screening, and who may or may not have prostate cancer, which may or may not be detected adequately by current screening techniques, and if it is detected patients may or may not opt for treatment.

To see how such a dilution effect might operate, let's consider seat belts. Everyone knows that seat belts save lives. So how could we devise a study to prove it? One way would be to compare the mortality rates of people who are in automobile accidents, according to whether they were or were not wearing seat belts. Odds are it would be fairly easy in such a study to show a mortality benefit with seat belts. But now instead let's imagine a study comparing the mortality rate of all drivers, over, say, a 5-year period, according to whether they routinely wear seat belts, regardless of whether or not they are in an automobile accident. I do not think you would be able to demonstrate an overall mortality benefit with seat belts in this second study.

The PSA screening studies that the USPSTF relied on to make their PSA recommendations are analogous to this second seat belt study. The prostate cancer treatment studies that did show a mortality benefit are analogous to the first seat belt study.

Please note that I am not directly comparing PSA screening to wearing seat belts. Wearing seat belts does not lead to a lot of unnecessary expense, nor does it create life-altering side effects. PSA screening, given the state of the art, is neither inexpensive nor benign.

But despite its major drawbacks, PSA screening does detect early prostate cancer. And if you measure outcomes from the point where the prostate cancer is actually diagnosed (instead of from the point where you decide to do PSA testing), survival is measurably increased by its early detection and treatment.

So the dichotomy is explained. From a herd standpoint, where you have to decide what the result will be on a large population of individuals if some screening test is implemented, it does not make sense to do PSA screening. But if you are an individual who might have prostate cancer, in whom the early detection of that cancer might save your life, then it might make sense to do the PSA screening. (Whether it does make sense or not depends on how you, the individual, assign relative weights to the notion of dying from prostate cancer vs. the inconvenience, expense, pain, and possibly horrible side effects from PSA testing and the procedures it might lead to.)

So while from a herd standpoint it would be a mistake to recommend widespread PSA screening, from an individual standpoint either decision – to have or to forgo PSA screening, depending on how you yourself weigh the tradeoffs – would be entirely reasonable.

But under our new healthcare system, individuals are not allowed to decide this for themselves. The USPSTF will make one decision for everybody. And while in the particular case of PSA testing, many of us may not be particularly sorry to see the new USPSTF recommendation, I submit that given the general nature of medical screening tests, it is child's play to set up a clinical trial that would "prove" (given the expense of the test, the false positives, the false negatives, the side effects of the test itself, the side effects and expense of the follow-up tests needed to see whether a positive screening test is truly positive, the expense and side effects of the treatment that will be used if the diagnosis is actually confirmed, the relative efficacy and inefficacy of that treatment, not to mention the dilution effects of having to screen a large number of individuals to find the relatively few who actually have the condition of concern and will benefit from its treatment) that just about any preventive screening test will fail to produce an overall benefit to the population.

The whole process makes me wonder why we can't just stop pretending that Obamacare is all about prevention, disband the USPSTF altogether, stop funding any screening tests whatsoever and any research to develop new ones, and call it a day? That would be much more transparent, not to mention cheaper, than stifling preventive medicine in the painfully slow and deceptive way we are doing it today.

THE MEDIA JUMPS ON BOARD

I am fairly cynical about the mainstream media, particularly when it comes to reporting on medical matters. So I have fully expected the brilliant people in the media to continue to be extremely surprised and disturbed each time some heretofore sacred preventive medical service is suddenly discovered by the all-powerful USPSTF to be, after all, useless.

So imagine my surprise when recently (October 29, 2011) the *New York Times* published a "news analysis" which begins to aggressively sell the public on the notion that medical screening tests are, in general, a bad thing to do.

Even I thought the Progressives would be somewhat circumspect about breaking such remarkable and counter-intuitive news to those of us in the herd – especially considering that they have just spent the last three decades teaching us just the opposite. But perhaps it should not be so surprising when you consider the Progressives' smooth, unapologetic and entirely unremarked transition, around twenty years ago, from sounding the alarm about global cooling to caterwauling about global warming, or moving overnight from demanding that trans fats be placed into our food supply to demanding that they be removed. Even I must often remind myself that when you are a Progressive, history always began 10 minutes ago.

And this turns out to be a great convenience.

The *Times* article emphasizes that while medical screening tests do save lives, those lives are saved at great cost. There is the dollar cost, of course, but the main concern is the cost to individuals resulting from false positive screening tests, which often lead to expensive, sometimes dangerous, and often psychologically difficult follow-up testing. Our thinking has to change, the *Times* says, and the paper backs up this new discovery with quotes from sundry healthcare experts who have also seen the light. It turns out that there is a major downside to preventive medical services, a downside which doctors have rarely talked about in their unreasonable zeal to prevent disease, but which, thanks to enlightened thinkers whose voices are at last being heard, are now becoming very important. "[D]octors and patients are stuck in a sort of cancer time warp," the *Times* alleges, and they need to get with the modern way of thinking.

There is, of course, nothing wrong with pointing out the hazards and disadvantages of preventive medical services. They are real, and they do substantial harm to many people.

But I must emphasize, once again, that this whole issue becomes a special problem only when we are forced into a paradigm in which preventive services either must be given to everybody, or must be withheld from everybody. It is usually not very difficult for an individual woman to decide whether the potential benefit of finding breast cancer while it is still treatable is worth the risk of possibly needing what might turn out to be an unnecessary and psychologically difficult biopsy. Individual patients may very reasonably decide either way.

But the "debate" which the *New York Times* suggests is taking place is not whether individuals should or should not opt for certain preventive medical services. That question, implicitly at least, has already been answered, and is not worth even mentioning. Individuals should not be making these decisions at all, but should instead just do what the experts say.

So, the *Times* indicates, the only real question that remains is whether the experts who will be making a universal decision for the herd should relent to the outdated and unreasonable pressures coming from doctors and patients stuck in a time warp, or rather, follow the dictates of good science, and cut back on those preventive services for everyone. The correct answer, the *Times* suggests, is obvious.

When we can only make medical decisions collectively, individual Americans will be systematically and predictably harmed. And that includes, according to the USPSTF's own documentation, several thousand women and men each year whose early, currently treatable, but ultimately lethal breast and prostate cancers will no longer be detected early enough to do any good. This is a necessary result of herd medicine.

But most striking, to me at least, is that the *New York Times* has already "progressed" to a position where it is simply and naturally right that healthcare decisions should be made collectively – even decisions involving preventive medical services. Indeed, the issue is not even worth mentioning in a high-profile article about preventive medicine. I would have thought that the major media, having spent decades loudly selling all of us on the utter importance of preventive medicine, out of simple self-respect might have hung in there a little longer, at least on this particular aspect of Obamacare.

Silly me.

Chapter 12 - Your Duty to Maintain Wellness – or – The Importance of Demonizing the Obese

"A majority of doctors support measures to deny treatment to smokers and the obese, according to a survey that has sparked a row over the NHS's growing use of "lifestyle rationing". Some 54% of doctors who took part said the NHS should have the right to withhold non-emergency treatment from patients who do not lose weight or stop smoking."
- *The Guardian* (UK), April 28, 2012

In the previous chapter we considered the role that preventive medical services will play under Obamacare, which is to say, as little a role as possible. Indeed, preventive medical services, since they will always cost the system far more money than they can ever save, will be de-emphasized at every opportunity, and outlawed when necessary.

So when our leaders promised that Obamacare would be all about "prevention, prevention, and prevention," were they simply lying to us? No. In fact, it appears, they remain very serious about preventing illness. It's just that when they say the word "prevention," they're not talking about preventive medical services like screening tests or prophylactic medications. Instead, they're talking about inducing all of us within the herd to adopt healthy lifestyle choices, such as eating wisely, maintaining a healthy weight, and getting plenty of exercise.

These lifestyle choices would of course undoubtedly be good for us (assuming we could agree on what we mean by eating "wisely," or what a "healthy" weight is, or how much exercise is "plenty"). But I don't think very many Americans realize yet just how serious our Progressive leaders are about correcting our suboptimal living habits and putting us on the right path to good health, or to what lengths they would be willing to go in order to get us there. This is in fact a very serious matter to them, because the way we each live our lives goes to the very core of the Progressive program.

On the broad scale, it is not possible to develop a perfect society if the citizens who live within that society follow their own personal whims, and engage in self-indulgence, overeating, sedentary living, or any of the other myriad of behaviors by which we reveal ourselves not to be working relentlessly for the benefit of the whole.

Focusing more narrowly, a Progressive healthcare system simply cannot function efficiently if the citizens whom it serves do not take every precaution to maintain their own good health. Those who, through their own lack of self-discipline, allow themselves to develop an avoidable illness are affecting more than just themselves. They are robbing their fellow citizens of resources that might otherwise have been theirs, and possibly more importantly, their infirmities will detract materially from the aura, projected by any ideal society, of a happy, healthy, robust citizenry, all working harmoniously for the greater good.

Therefore, under any system like Obamacare, where providing healthcare to everyone is a collective responsibility, maintaining your own wellness is not merely something you ought to do for your own good. It is your sacred duty to the collective.

And if your chosen actions (or inactions) cause you to become unwell, and if your unwellness causes you to consume healthcare resources which otherwise might have been available to more deserving individuals who (unlike yourself) became ill through no fault of their own, and if such faultless individuals subsequently suffered or died as a consequence of your failure to honor your duty to remain healthy, well then, your failure to perform your duty would make you no different from any other common criminal whose selfish actions produce harm to their innocent victims. Maintaining your wellness is not a nice-to-have; it is your non-negotiable obligation.

And the Central Authority, consequently, has an equally sacred obligation to hold you to your duty.

You have been told, by the caring people who will be running our new healthcare system, that your wellness is very important to them. And so it is. This is why you will, by law, be "entitled" to annual, detailed "wellness checks," provided by the dedicated team of healthcare workers which will be assigned to your care, and which will assess (and record) your efforts to maintain your own wellness, and then will give you all the instruction you could possibly need to alter whatever suboptimal behaviors you may be currently displaying. The results of these annual wellness checks will be entered into a federally-approved universal electronic medical record, so that any healthcare provider, anywhere, at any time (or any agent of the Central Authority who finds access to your records convenient to his or her own special purposes) will have a complete record of the trajectory of your state of health over the years – and of the degree of your compliance with the instructions you have received for maintaining your wellness.

Of course, if you elect to forgo the annual wellness checks to which you are entitled, that information (i.e. that you cared so little for your wellness that you couldn't be bothered to do anything about it) will also be maintained in the universal electronic records.

Then, when you become ill 10 or 20 years from now, your health records (along with other pertinent electronic records of your past behaviors, such as your annual purchases of ice cream and salt, the volume of sedentary entertainments you download from Netflix or the App Store, and your relative propensities for purchasing running shoes vs. Barcaloungers) can be consulted to decide to what extent your illness can be considered self-induced. For, when resources are scarce, the only moral thing to do is to distribute them according to who is the most deserving.

I understand this may sound just a bit paranoid. So let us reflect for a while on a particular pattern of behavior already being displayed by our Progressive leaders, regarding a supposedly self-induced medical condition.

THE DEMONIZATION OF OBESITY

In his book *The Amateur: Barack Obama in the White House*, Ed Klein relates Michelle Obama's reaction when Oprah Winfrey asked the First Lady to appear on her TV show to discuss the problem of childhood obesity. According to Klein, Ms. Obama flatly refused the offer, allegedly saying, "Oprah, with her yo-yo dieting and huge girth is a terrible role model. Kids will look at Oprah, who's rich and famous and huge, and figure it's OK to be fat." Ms. Winfrey herself was said to be quite disturbed by this rejection, allegedly complaining, "Michelle hates fat people and doesn't want me waddling around the White House."

An attitude of disdain (if not outright hatred) has been studiously adopted by many Progressives toward people who are obese. Even Saint Oprah – who is dearly beloved by women and men of all races and ages, whose good works in America and abroad are admired by all, whose early endorsement of Barack Obama was arguably the event that ignited his winning the White House, and what's more, who has often and famously striven to lose weight, her mighty and even heroic struggles to do so embodying the tremendous difficulties faced by people above a certain age who endeavor to get their weight down to publicly acceptable levels – is not to be given a pass. Despite everything she has accomplished, Oprah's weight renders her a negative role model.

This, because being overweight is simply too great a sin to be tolerated.

We are, in fact, witnessing a sustained and concerted campaign to demonize the obese. It is a campaign which is being conducted with a great end in mind.

It is not difficult to demonize the obese. In literature and films the obese have long been portrayed as unreasonably jolly (which itself is a great sin in any serious society), or as slovenly and lazy, or as just plain evil. (Hello, Newman!) Nobody likes to sit next to fat people on airplanes or buses. They block the aisles at the grocery store (their favorite haunts). They reduce miles-per-gallon when they ride in our cars, and if they insist on sitting in the same seat every time, they cause asymmetric tire wear and thereby produce automobile accidents. On humid days, they sweat (and thus stink) more than you and me. And, of course, they are unsightly. So, with rare exceptions nobody complains when the obese are criticized and attacked.

It is remarkable that I can write a paragraph like the one I have just done without any serious qualms or concerns about how most readers might perceive my lack of sensitivity. Unless you, dear reader, are yourself fat, I have no concerns about having offended you, for I have said nothing that is not perfectly acceptable in modern American discourse.

Given the current hypersensitivity we see to anything smacking of criticism of various races, ethnic groups, religions, professions, political movements, sexual orientations, immigration status, victims of certain diseases, and scores of other categories of Americans, the obese present us with a refreshingly safe target upon which to unleash vituperation and innuendos. Insulting obesity is not only acceptable but encouraged. We can say about the obese just about anything we like. It is perfectly fine to insist that it is the obese – those lazy, self-indulgent fat people – who are driving our healthcare spending off a cliff. Prominent and respected figures appear to feel no compunction whatsoever against making the most offensive public statements against the obese, and when they do they generally receive applause rather than condemnation.

Demonizing the obese is now such a prominent theme in American life that it has become difficult to satirize. In 2011, when Governor Christie was still entertaining the possibility of a presidential run, I wrote a blog post urging him not to do so because he is just too damned fat. Fat people, I noted, have characteristics we do not like to see in presidents (sloth, gluttony, lethargy, etc.), and allowing a fatty to aspire to such a high position would create the false impression that obese people are worthy of any consideration whatsoever, and would make people think that the obese ought to have the same individual freedoms as the rest of us. Furthermore, I allowed, a Christie candidacy would amount to a serious setback to the Progressive program (which is to say, controlling individual behaviors for the great benefit of the collective). When I further urged the Governor to stay in New Jersey, except perhaps to occasionally cross the state line just long enough to stock up on Philly cheese-steaks, I believed myself to be engaging in the outlandish extremes customary to a master of irony.

So imagine my surprise when, just after publishing this diatribe, an article by Michael Kinsley appeared on Bloomberg also declaring Christie too fat to be president. The reason? Because "a presidential candidate should be judged on behavior and character, not just on policies." Fat people, Kinsley elaborated, are a "perfect symbol of our country at the moment, with appetites out of control and discipline near zilch." In other words, fat people have shown themselves, by their very obesity, to be entirely unworthy characters, and being unworthy, should not aspire to the presidency, or presumably, to any other position of importance. Eugene Robinson of the *Washington Post* shortly thereafter agreed that Christie's weight should prevent him from running, noting that the "obesity epidemic" is costing the government a lot of money, and implying that people like Governor Christie are responsible for the massive federal deficit. This being the case, his candidacy would be entirely inappropriate. So there you have it. Actual Progressives were making the very same arguments for Christie to stay out of the race that I made in what I had thought to be a brilliantly satirical blog post.

A chief advantage for choosing obesity as a prime target for public castigation is that obesity is a condition which is immediately visible to all – there's no need to sew a Star-of-David-like emblem to fat people's clothing. So unlike, say, closet smokers or pedophiles, it is a simple matter to identify, at a glance and at a distance, those obese individuals whose selfishness and laziness are costing the rest of us our healthcare dollars, and thus, potentially our lives.

Fully government-funded and government-controlled healthcare permits – and even demands – that we declare to the obese that their unsightly physiques are no longer a matter of personal choice, but are now a matter of legitimate public concern. The choices they are making – that is, their gluttony, sloth, etc. – are placing unwanted and unsustainable demands on us purer, svelter, fellow-citizens, not to mention placing us in danger of not receiving the healthcare which we (in contrast) actually deserve. Hating the obese has become nearly a patriotic imperative.

THE HAZARDS OF OBESITY - REAL AND BOGUS

There can be no doubt that obesity is a significant health hazard. When you are grossly obese, virtually every organ system in your body is negatively affected, and your risk of developing diabetes, heart disease, vascular disease, kidney disease, and other expensive illnesses increases markedly. Severe obesity is a severe health hazard.

In our public discourse, however, the hazards of severe obesity are being projected onto people who are merely overweight*. But the hazards of being only modestly overweight are much less clear.

------

* The Centers for Disease Control defines weight categories, according to body mass index (BMI), as follows: BMI scores of 20 to 24.9 are considered normal, scores of 25 to 29.9 are overweight, scores of 30 to 34.9 are obese, and scores above 35 are extremely obese.

For instance, in 2002 a report in the *Journal of the American College of Cardiology* examined almost 10,000 consecutive patients who had angioplasty and/or stenting for coronary artery disease, and found that those who were overweight or obese had fewer complications and a lower one-year mortality than those who were thin or of normal weight. Several more recent studies claim to have shown the same thing.

A 2007 report in the *Journal of the American Medical Association* showed that overweight people who were physically fit had a lower risk of death than normal-weight people who were sedentary. Another 2007 report by the National Bureau of Economic Research noted that while Americans were growing fatter, other changes in health behavior (such as reduced smoking and better management of cholesterol and hypertension) more than offset any increase in health risk posed by the population's increase in obesity.

In 2009, a meta-analysis in the *Journal of the American College of Cardiology* concluded that while obesity itself increases the risk of heart disease, obese people who develop that heart disease have significantly better survival than thin or normal-weight people who develop the same kind of heart disease. Some cardiologists have already termed this growing line of evidence, i.e., the general observation that at least in some situations overweight cardiac patients fare better than thin ones, as "The Obesity Paradox." Such phenomena as an Obesity Paradox, however, are too inconvenient to be brought up in public discussions on the hazards of obesity.

In addition, while there is no question that Americans are becoming fatter, the magnitude of the increase in our obesity over the past two decades has been at least somewhat exaggerated by a change in the definition of obesity. When the CDC changed that definition in 1997, as many as 30 million Americans who went to bed at a normal weight woke up the next morning to find themselves overweight if not obese, and all without gaining a pound.

Also entirely ignored in the public discourse is the accumulating evidence that one's weight-related medical risk (like blood-pressure-related risk, and salt-intake-related risk) appears to be "U" shaped. That is, one's risk goes up when one's weight becomes either too high, or too low. Several epidemiological studies have suggested that, while overall mortality rates indeed begin to climb when the BMI exceeds 25, they also begin to climb as the BMI drops below 22.5. If this is true, then a) the optimal BMI lives in a very narrow range (22.5 to 24.9) where relatively few of us are permitted by nature and our genes to dwell, and b) by rights, we should be castigating the underweight with the same vituperations we are encouraged to heap upon the fat.

Finally, the idea that the obese are using more than their share of healthcare resources may be incorrect. An article published in 2008 in the *Public Library of Science Medicine Journal* compared the lifetime cost of healthcare (beginning at age 20) for obese individuals and for smokers to the lifetime cost for non-smokers who maintained a healthy weight. Naturally, the study concludes that the healthy individuals can expect to live longer than the obese and the smokers (84 years vs. 80 and 77 years, respectively). However, the healthy young people will consume $400,000 in lifetime healthcare costs, vs. only $365,000 for fat people and $321,000 for smokers. The cost savings this study discovers with the obese and the smokers are provided courtesy of their premature deaths. Therefore, normal-weight non-smokers, over their lifetimes, appear to cause a bigger fiscal drain than the obese and the smokers – and eliminating obesity and smoking would create an even bigger strain on our healthcare system.

According to the *Wall Street Journal* (August 23, 2006), the CDC has instructed its researchers not to comment on such contradictory research on obesity, in order to avoid creating "public confusion."

At a time when we are studiously ignoring research which sheds at least some doubt on the significance of being modestly overweight, other "research" on obesity, research which by any objective standards seems staggeringly stupid, is being published with great fanfare. I will give two notable examples to demonstrate the point.

In 2009, Professors Edwards and Roberts penned an article demonstrating that fat people are largely responsible for global warming. Their article was published by the prestigious Oxford Press in the *International Journal of Epidemiology*. This paper, which indicts a whole class of individuals with the supreme crime of global warming – a crime which will prove to be of such stupendous proportions, apparently, that even the atrocities perpetrated by Hitler and Stalin will seem mere trifles in comparison – reaches its conclusions without ever offering even one tiny glimmer of actual data or evidence.

Rather, the authors rely (in the style of their apparent forebears in the tradition of Scholasticism) on the already-approved body of scientific work, choosing from that body an array of assumptions based on bits of sanctified data from physiology here (e.g., Basal Metabolic Rate = 11.5 X body weight in KG + 873kcal), and behavioral science there (e.g., that the average daily activities of humans consists of 7 hours sleeping, 7 hours of office work, 4 hours of light home activities, 4 hours sitting, 1 hour standing, 30 min of driving and 30 min of walking at 5 km/h), then applying these bits to an incredible chain of assumptions and estimations, to demonstrate that fat people (and not coal-fired electric plants or cow farts) are the chief cause of global warming. One of their key assumptions, for instance (made, again, without corroborating data) is that fat people, being lazy, travel in cars far more often than skinny people, and that, because they are fat, they purchase very large cars that guzzle a lot of gasoline. Their startling conclusion is that we have the obese to blame for melting the ice caps, killing the polar bears, flooding the seacoasts, and turning our farmland, forests and fields into hot, dry, desert. From this analysis, anyone with a cheap telescope can only conclude that Martians, when they existed, must have been very, very fat.

An equally astonishing piece of scientific analysis appeared in the *New England Journal of Medicine* in 2007, proving that obesity is contagious. This study actually received a fair amount of media attention when it was published (though we have not heard much about it since, one hopes out of embarrassment).

This work came from the studios of the famous Drs. Christakis and Fowler, who have embraced a software package, comprehensible only to themselves, that churns out complex images of "social networks," from which they can derive all manner of heretofore unimagined associations.

Using data from the venerable Framingham database, these pioneers combed through old records for information about the body weight, relatives, and social contacts of individuals who were enrolled in this famous study. They then used their esoteric computer modeling software to create various "animations" depicting the evolving social relationships of the subjects, and the development of obesity, over time. From their own description of their procedure, they iterated their animations numerous times, adjusting their baseline assumptions each time, until they had produced the results that seemed to make the most sense to them. The Scholastics again would be proud.

To summarize the findings they settled upon: A person is far more likely to become obese if a friend becomes obese, even if that friend lives hundreds of miles away. (This finding is really quite remarkable, considering that the only other natural force that acts on bodies instantaneously and at a distance is gravity. This newly discovered force that produces obesity at a distance – shall we call it obevity? - will have to be incorporated, with great difficulty no doubt, into the Grand Unification Theory now being sought by physicists everywhere.) Remarkably, the same effect was not seen when close neighbors became obese, or even (to such a great extent) when family members became obese. Furthermore, if the friendship is mutual (that is, if the fat person considers you a friend in addition to you considering the fat person a friend), the odds of your becoming obese triples. And worse yet, this study shows that even if you wisely avoid the company of fat people yourself (in an attempt to remain acceptably svelte), fat people who are acquainted with your acquaintances may still have an impact on your BMI. That is, you don't actually have to befriend a fat person to be affected; befriending a skinny person who has a fat friend is enough to make you fat. Obesity, then, is a particularly insidious contagion that propagates itself throughout the social network even without direct contact. The obvious conclusion from all this (though mercifully unspecified by the authors) is that obese people, being such extraordinarily virulent vectors for such a dread condition, ought to be culled out from the herd and, perhaps, concentrated in special camps.

One should not have to read any of the critiques that were subsequently published regarding the methodologies used in this study (including one written by your humble author) to understand that the study and its findings are absurd.

The remarkable thing is not that silly studies like these are being produced – such is always the case – but rather, that the editors of prestigious journals of science and medicine are seeing fit to publish them. This fact alone is sufficient to demonstrate just how deeply imbedded in our polity is the project of demonizing the obese.

Harsh Treatment of Witches Is Justifiable

The very publication of such studies suggests that the obese are rapidly becoming the witches of the 21st century. And when you are faced with witches, you are obligated to do everything in your power to stop them while you can.

It is easy for those of us living hundreds of years after the Salem Witch Trials to condemn (or at least laugh at) the folly of those olden and less sophisticated times. I will simply point out that burning witches is an evil act only if you don't believe that witches are real. If you, supported by all the respected authorities of the day, believe that real witches are present in the community, and that they indeed are capable of producing extreme harm to innocent individuals, surreptitiously and at a great distance – kind of like the obese – or are capable of reducing the entire community to a hot, dry cinder – also like the obese – then roasting them slowly over a pile of green faggots is at least reasonable, if not the only responsible thing to do.

By their own selfish actions, actions which threaten the collective far more than merely themselves, the obese have become fair game for whatever manipulations our government can devise to cause them to either lose weight, or pay for their sins.

And especially now that we have so many programs and policies aimed at preventing obesity – putting apple slices in Happy Meals, publishing calorie counts in restaurants, being lectured at by First Ladies and skinny movie stars, etc. – we can reassure ourselves that anyone who still chooses to remain obese despite all this abundant assistance must be especially contemptible.

Our actions against the obese may begin with simple taxes on the calorie-laden foodstuffs particularly favored by fatties, but the sky's the limit. A special "carbon tax" based on their BMI would be legitimate, for instance, since it will always cost a lot of energy to move a fat person from point A to point B, whatever the mode of transportation. The periodic mandatory public "weigh-ins" such a tax would justify would serve the useful purpose of public humiliation, an important incentive to weight loss. And it goes without saying that it would be fully justifiable to simply withhold certain healthcare services if one is deemed too fat. Under the more enlightened culture of Great Britain, the National Health Service (the model to which Dr. Berwick and other of our current healthcare heroes openly aspire), the obese are now being removed from the waiting lists for medical services.* By virtue of their obesity (and the lack of social responsibility their obesity reveals), fat people have forfeited their equal access to healthcare.

------

*Removing fat people from the NHS waiting lists has at least two beneficial effects. It punishes them, of course, for their selfish refusal to maintain their own wellness. But it also reduces the long waiting lists that exist in Britain for medical services, closer to the target waiting times which the government has been promising its citizens for decades.

Demonizing the obese, of course, is its own reward. But it also provides several critical precedents that will come in very handy sooner or later.

Ignored in the general disgust we profess toward the obese is the fact that, for the large majority of people who are seriously obese, their obesity has a very large component of genetic predisposition. For such individuals maintaining a "normal" body weight is virtually impossible. So when we learn to demonize the obese, we are also learning that wellness is your duty even if your genes (or some other force that is largely beyond your control) mitigates against it. In this way we are setting a very useful precedent that will allow us to discriminate against other groups of people who have genetically-mediated medical conditions.

Those who may wonder why this is a big deal need to go back and study the original Progressives, for whom some form of genetic purification was an indispensable step toward achieving societal perfection. This was true not only for notorious eugenicists such as Woodrow Wilson, H. G. Wells, George Bernard Shaw, and Margaret Sanger, but also for the kinder, gentler Progressives we generally revere even today, such as Theodore Roosevelt, Winston Churchill, and even Mohandas Gandhi. This sort of thinking fell out of vogue, for obvious reasons, after World War II. So it is no longer polite to talk openly about genetic cleansing.

But discriminating against people who have a genetic predisposition to gross obesity (in the name of achieving an optimally efficient healthcare system for the purpose of cost saving) would be a start.

Once the Central Authority sets into motion the laws and regulations needed to control the behavior of fat people (or people who might otherwise become fat), they will have established the mechanisms and techniques (and the justifications) for controlling all of the private behaviors that might be useful to control, for all American citizens.

The obese, therefore, are the perfect prototype. Thanks to them, we are teaching ourselves that it is right and proper to disdain any individual who is leading less than an exemplary life. Many of the people whose lifestyles are suboptimal, unlike the obese, may be relatively difficult to spot. But at the end of the day, they will reveal themselves in the ultimate manner – they eventually will fall sick.

And by their diseases we shall know them.

For the past several years, our infallible healthcare experts have been busy declaring more and more illnesses to be "preventable." And if an illness is preventable, and an individual fails to prevent it – well, what more do you need? That person has obviously failed to perform their sacred duty to society, and has forfeited any claim to the healthcare we more deserving people can expect.

The list of illnesses which are officially preventable now includes coronary artery disease, heart failure, kidney failure, diabetes, stroke and many kinds of cancer. And recently Alzheimer's disease was added to the list.

It is possible that in a decade or so, if you acquire an illness from this growing list of "preventable" medical disorders – especially if your annual wellness checks reveal that you have gained weight since high school, or you habitually fail to exercise at least 90 minutes per day, or that you imbibe less than one or greater than two alcoholic beverages per day, or you commit any one of a hundred other lifestyle sins – you may be triaged to some sort of Tier B healthcare, as in Great Britain. Tier A, of course, will be reserved for people who obviously care more than you do about wellness, and about their duty to society (and also, obviously, to the sundry experts and political leaders who are critical to the success of the collective).

Just as obesity does today, the overall state of your health will demonstrate your true commitment to the perfect society to which we all aspire. For, when it is your duty to maintain wellness, the very fact of your illness reveals a grave dereliction of duty.

CHAPTER 13 - AGE-BASED MEDICINE AND END-OF-LIFE HEALTHCARE

"..[T]erminal patients should be allowed to convert projected expenditures on futile treatments, and other benefits, into death benefits if they choose physician-assisted suicide. If death can be voluntarily chosen, and can confer benefits to the still living, the sense of tragedy from death can be lessened and the bond of intergenerational community is strengthened."

- K.K. Fung, Dying for Money. *American Journal of Economics and Sociology*, 1993.

———

In the last chapter, without calling it out, we introduced a new concept of Progressive healthcare – Group Medicine.

Group medicine is a subcategory of herd medicine. Under group medicine, a group of individuals sharing some common characteristic – such as obesity – is culled out from the greater herd for "special treatment." The people included in that group will still not receive individualized healthcare; they will still be treated under the one-size-fits-all principles of herd medicine. It's just that the rules guiding their medical care will be specific for their group.

In this chapter we will address the biggest group of all – old people – and the special problem the individuals included in this group present to a Progressive healthcare system, namely, what to do about end-of-life-care.

WHY PEOPLE THINK OBAMACARE HAS DEATH PANELS

It is unfortunate that one cannot engage in a dispassionate and objective analysis of the Progressives' ideas on age-based medicine and end-of-life healthcare without being immediately accused of invoking "death panels," and thus of displaying the dearth of sophistication, the lack of understanding, and the primitive logic commonly attributed by Progressives to Sarah Palin.

I must remind my readers that I have yet to use the term "death panel" to refer to any of the multitude of expert commissions created by Obamacare, whose charge will be to dispassionately examine the scientific evidence in order to determine which patients will get what, when and how. These bodies, in fact, will be explicitly aiming to optimize the medical outcomes of the entire population (titrated to the amount of money we're allowed to spend on healthcare), and not actively prescribing death for anyone.

Judging from the histories of governments which have adopted a collectivist philosophy, if death panels should appear on the scene they will not be aimed at determining which patients may live or die. That job, of course, will fall to the doctors at the bedside, who will offer or withhold medical services according to the dictates (i.e., "guidelines") handed down by those sundry expert commissions. Rather, any death panels which might eventually materialize will more likely be aimed at keeping those doctors themselves (and any other functionaries whose job is to do the bidding of the Central Authority) in thrall.

So why has the term "death panel" caught on to such an extent that conservatives so often use it as shorthand to express what they see as the "sense" of Obamacare, and Progressives so often use it to accuse rational and mild-mannered critics of Obamacare (such as your humble author) of belonging to the Neanderthal persuasion?

While most would blame Sarah Palin for coming up with this unhelpful phraseology, it is my view that President Obama himself must carry at least an equal part of the blame. For, if Progressives have not created actual death panels, they at least created the environment in which those words, when Ms. Palin first uttered them, immediately caught fire.

One should recall that when, in late 2009, Ms. Palin used the fateful words, "death panels," the Obamacare legislation was being slowly and painfully shoved through a surprisingly reluctant Democrat Congress. And as a result she caused many of our more complacent legislators to abruptly bestir themselves into a higher state of arousal, if not outright agitation. Palin's accusation caught more than a few of them utterly unawares, and embarrassingly flatfooted.

They felt, no doubt, like they were in that dream where you unaccountably find yourself naked in a crowd. But this time, rather than reaching to hide their sadly exposed nether parts, they reached instead for their pristine copies of the monstrous Obamacare legislation which had been laid before them, and which they famously (and understandably) never read. One could almost pity them, desperately rifling through the 2700 virgin pages, muttering to themselves, "Death panels? This damned thing has death panels?"

But in fact, their initial instincts were correct, at least as regarded the advisability of actually reading the legislation. There was in truth no reason for them to waste their time. I myself have subsequently read large swatches of the thing, and I can assure one and all that it was not designed for reading, comprehensibility, or (for that matter) imparting any actual information of any sort. And besides, Obamacare contained no provisions for creating anything called death panels, so had they read the bill they would not have discovered any.

The very notion of death panels seemed to have many supporters of Obamacare nonplussed. How could someone as inarticulate and obviously illiterate as Sarah Palin get away with accusing our highly-educated healthcare reformers of setting up such a thing as death panels? And even more perplexingly, why did so many Americans believe her – even, apparently, millions of Americans who had been enlightened enough to vote for President Obama less than a year earlier?

I believe it is this: When Sarah Palin said, "death panels," she was dropping one last, tiny crystal into a supersaturated solution. Her words took what had been an amorphous and even chaotic sense of unease about healthcare reform, and immediately crystallized it into an organized latticework of directed rage and fear. So the real question is not how Sarah Palin came to be savvy enough to know just the right words. (Progressives know that even a distinguished panel of monkeys, given enough time and enough typewriters, will eventually produce King Lear.) Rather, the real question is: What put the rabble in such a supersaturated state to begin with? Why did the absurd-on-its-face idea of "death panels" so resonate with them? What made those words galvanize their shapeless disquiet into a solid mass of resistance?

I am very sorry to have to tell my friends of the Progressive persuasion the sad truth. For it was President Obama himself who created this circumstance. Sarah Palin may have first named the death panels, but before she ever thought of the phrase the President had already described them in detail.

During his first year in office, President Obama offered several homilies relating just what a "death panel" would look like. He described their function, how they would operate, and who they would target. Perhaps the most instructive example is the one he gave on ABC television during his June 24, 2009 National Town Hall meeting.

I refer, of course, to the famous question put to him by the granddaughter of a 100-year-old woman who had received a pacemaker. The questioner pointed out that her grandmother had badly needed this pacemaker, but had been turned down by a doctor because of her age. A second doctor, noting the patient's alertness, zest for life, and generally youthful "spirit," went ahead and inserted the pacemaker despite her advanced age. Her symptoms resolved, and Grandma was still doing quite well five years later. The question for the President was: Under Obamacare, will an elderly person's general state of health, and her "spirit," be taken into account when making medical decisions – or will these decisions be made according to age only?

President Obama's answer was clear. It is really not feasible, he indicated, to take "spirit" into account. We are going to make medical decisions based on objective evidence, and not subjective impressions. If the evidence shows that some form of treatment "is not necessarily going to improve care, then at least we can let the doctors know that – you know what? – maybe this isn't going to help; maybe you're better off not having the surgery, but taking the pain pill."

I will give President Obama the benefit of the doubt regarding his suggestion that a 100-year-old woman who needs a pacemaker might be better off with a pain pill. Mr. Obama is not actually a doctor, and cannot be expected to understand that using a "pain pill" to treat an elderly woman who is lightheaded, dizzy, weak and possibly syncopal because of a slow heart rate might justifiably be considered a form of euthanasia rather than comfort care. I do not believe the President was intentionally suggesting the old woman's death should be actively hastened by means of a pain pill. Indeed, given that repeated falls from lightheadedness would likely have led to a hip fracture had the pacemaker been withheld, a pain pill might eventually have been just the thing for granny.

Still, President Obama's clear and unflinching answer in this case told us several important things about Obamacare: 1) Under Obamacare, there would be at least one panel, or commission, or body of some sort, that is going to examine the medical evidence on how effective a certain treatment is likely to be in a certain subset of patients. 2) This, let's call it a "panel," will "let the doctors know" whether that treatment ought to be used in those patients. ("Letting the doctor know" is a euphemism for "guidelines," which itself, as we have seen, is a euphemism for legally-binding and ruthlessly enforced directives.) 3) "Subjective" measures ought not to influence these treatment recommendations. Non-objective parameters – such as the doctor's medical experience, intuition, or personal knowledge of the patient; or the patient's "spirit," or will to live, or likelihood of tolerating and complying with the proposed treatment; or even extenuating circumstances that might increase or decrease the success of the proposed treatment in a particular individual – simply cannot be evaluated or controlled by far-away expert panels, and therefore must necessarily be discounted. 4) But since our government is a compassionate and caring one, and wishes to reduce unnecessary suffering, palliative care will be made available in the form of pain control, even while withholding potentially curative care.

What the American public accurately heard the President say was that we will have an omnipotent "panel," acting at a distance and without any specific knowledge of particular cases, that will tell a doctor whether he/she can offer a particular therapy to a particular patient – or whether, instead, to offer a "pain pill." His description of this process, repeated with variations over the next several months in several venues, obviously made quite an impact on the people. Of course, Mr. Obama is widely known to be a gifted communicator.

In any case, all that remained was for Sarah Palin to give the President's panel a catchy name. And when she did, the American people knew exactly what she was talking about. They knew, because President Obama himself had been spelling it all out for them in plenty of detail for six months.

Indeed, it seems to me that, if not for President Obama's having so carefully laid the groundwork, Palin's accusations of "death panels" would have fallen flat. It would have been regarded by most people as the absurdity that Progressives insist that it is, rather than the epiphany it turned out to be.

Progressives who strenuously object to its usage in reference to the expert commissions created by Obamcare can blame Sarah if they want to – but by all rights they should actually be taking up the matter with their dear leader, who is the chief source of the misapprehension, if misapprehension there be.

Whatever you choose to call these expert panels, however, one thing that was very clearly articulated by President Obama is that the directives that are going to be passed down to physicians by these panels, "letting them know" which services they should offer and which they should withhold from which patients, will take the age of the patient into very strong account.

AGE-BASED MEDICINE

That groups of Americans under Obamacare will be culled out from the herd, to receive medical care according to their age, is all but explicit.

In Chapter 11 we saw a particularly well-known example when we examined the recommendations made by the USPSTF regarding mammogram screening. While the ratio of true-positive versus false-positive mammograms is a continuous variable, which gradually increases with age as you begin testing women as young as in their 20s, and while there apparently is no natural age-related threshold or break point where the test suddenly becomes more (or less) accurate, the USPSTF was pleased to offer an arbitrary age-related cutoff (age 50), above which mammograms are to be offered, and below which they are not.

Whether or not you agree with the new USPSTF guidelines, you must concede the entirely arbitrary nature of the age cutoff. The difference in the risk/benefit ratio of doing mammography in a 49-year-old woman vs. a 50-year-old woman, for instance, is immeasurably small. Yet the cutoff is set – arbitrarily – at 50. This arbitrariness is an essential feature of age-based medicine.

"Well, you've got to set a cutoff somewhere," proponents of Progressive medicine will say. And yes, that is true. And if we were merely talking about general guidelines, and not firm rules which must be obeyed in each case, then the "arbitrariness" of age-based cutoffs would not be a big problem. But if instead you're going to practice herd medicine, where everyone is treated exactly the same regardless of personal preferences, and you're going to systematically ignore or disallow the consideration of circumstances that might affect an individual's response to the proposed medical service, then arbitrary cutoffs are indeed a problem. And from the aspect of the patient (those for whom the health care system, ostensibly, exists in the first place), the arbitrary nature of age-based medicine has a great potential to produce harm.

It is therefore important to note that from the aspect of the Central Authority, age-based medicine is not arbitrary at all. It is entirely objective, and is based on clearly-defined principles.

THE FORMAL RATIONALE FOR AGE-BASED MEDICINE

The Central Authority's rationale for age-based medicine was perhaps best described by Ezekiel Emanuel, MD, President Obama's Special Advisor for Health Policy (and brother of Rahm), in an article appearing in *The Lancet* in January, 2009, entitled, "Principles for allocation of scarce medical interventions." In this article, Emanuel proposes an ethical basis for rationing healthcare resources based upon age. He calls it the "complete lives system."

At first blush, if you look at it in a certain way, the complete lives system seems ethically justifiable. In determining who gets what healthcare services it is OK to discriminate against the elderly, Emanuel holds, but not just because they are old and therefore relatively decrepit. Rather, such discrimination is justifiable because every person, over the course of their complete lives, will experience the entire range of healthcare priorities – the high priority of the young, and then, if they are lucky enough to live a long time, the low priority of the old. Thus, all people are treated exactly the same over the course of their lives.

If Emanuel had stopped there, I for one might have grumbled a bit (being an Old Fart myself and thus already dwelling within the low priority stage of my life), but I would have had to admit that, from a certain aspect, the system seems equitable.

But Emanuel did not stop there. Instead, Emanuel went on to elaborate that under his system, it is also perfectly justifiable to discriminate against the very young. Specifically, he says:

> *"Consideration of the importance of complete lives also supports modifying the youngest-first principle by prioritizing adolescents and young adults over infants. Adolescents have received substantial education and parental care, investments that will be wasted without a complete life. Infants, in contrast, have not yet received these investments."*

So, Emanuel holds that it is OK to discriminate against infants, toddlers and young children on the grounds that society has not "invested" a lot of resources in them yet. That is, their worth to society is not very great, and their loss would not be noticed very much by the collective.

This provision against the very young fatally undermines the notion that all human lives are of equal intrinsic value (which, Emanuel says, is the premise of the complete lives system), in favor of the idea that an individual's real worth ought to be determined by their practical value to the state. And so, the state has the right – and the duty – to determine which lives are valuable enough to save, and which are not.

As if to emphasize the objective and scientific nature of his proposal, Emanuel included in his article a graph depicting one's worth to the state as a function of age. The graph plainly shows that one's value to the Central Authority begins, at birth, at a very low level. It then rapidly increases to a peak at around age 20. From there it drops gradually until about age 50 – where it plummets to much lower levels by age 60. One's intrinsic worth to the collective then continues to drop even lower until, at age 75, it returns to the ultra-low levels not seen since birth. The graph precipitously ends, somewhat disturbingly to an Old Fart such as myself, at age 75. (I will have more to say on the magic age of 75 shortly.)

Emanuel's *Lancet* article may be the most explicit statement yet provided by an official of the Obama administration on the ethical precepts underlying Obamacare. It places the Central Authority in the position of assigning intrinsic values to groups of human lives, based on how useful those lives are to the aims of the collective (or, how much society has "invested" in a certain class of individuals), so that healthcare priorities can be distributed accordingly.

If you are a patient, age-based healthcare rationing seems arbitrary. But from the point of view of Progressives it is not arbitrary at all; rather, is based on an entirely objective measure. Groups of people who are useful to the aims of the collective are to receive a high priority when it comes to healthcare. Groups of people who are deemed to be not so useful will receive a much lower priority.

Obviously, the criteria for producing such groups does not necessarily have to be limited to age. In fact, when the chief concern is to protect the interests of the collective, it would be wrong to limit your considerations in this way. Other obvious criteria that ought to be considered in devising various groups for the purpose of determining healthcare priorities would reasonably include your tax-generating potential, your IQ, your disabilities, your likelihood of supporting a Progressive agenda, your BMI, and your genetic makeup.

Explicit groupings based on these other parameters are merely conjecture at this point. Age-based groupings are not. Not only has a rationale for age-based healthcare been published in the peer-reviewed medical literature, but also, steps are being taken to put it into effect.

Devaluing The Very Young

Under Emanuel's scheme, infants and toddlers have very low value to the collective because very few resources have yet been "invested" in them. For this reason, whether they live or die is of little import to the Central Authority, and so their priority for receiving healthcare services ought to be accordingly low.

So far, thankfully, we see very little evidence in our healthcare system that the very young – once they are born, at least – are being discriminated against. Neonatal intensive care units, for instance, are running full bore, and the people who work in them remain extraordinarily dedicated to doing everything possible to help their tiny charges to survive.

Still, the justification for withholding care from the very young, when the time comes, has been established. And while it is difficult to find evidence of the devaluation of young children within our healthcare system, it is not particularly difficult to find it elsewhere.

184

Perhaps the most striking example was provided by an article* written by two medical ethicists in early 2012 entitled, "After-birth abortion: why should the baby live?" Here is the authors' abstract:

"Abortion is largely accepted even for reasons that do not have anything to do with the fetus' health. By showing that (1) both fetuses and newborns do not have the same moral status as actual persons, (2) the fact that both are potential persons is morally irrelevant and (3) adoption is not always in the best interest of actual people, the authors argue that what we call 'after-birth abortion' (killing a newborn) should be permissible in all the cases where abortion is, including cases where the newborn is not disabled."

---

*Giubilini A, Minerva F. After-birth abortion: Why should the baby live? *Journal of Medical Ethics*. March, 2012.

These medical ethicists, in other words, propose to allow parents to kill their young children for any reason they might have invoked to abort that child prior to birth – that is, for any reason at all. The key point being made by these ethicists is fundamentally the same as the point made by Emanuel's article. When they are very young, people have no intrinsic value that really matters to society (they are merely "potential persons"), so what happens to them is of no particular concern.

Within the tyranny of experts which we are establishing to run our Progressive society, the medical ethicists are probably the most dangerous of all.

From the very beginning, as I have pointed out, devaluing human lives that are inconvenient to the aims of the collective has been an intrinsic characteristic of Progressivism. Indeed, the reason I am against elective abortion has little to do with religion. It is, in fact, the very same reason why hard-nosed Progressives are so passionately in favor of abortion. It is that making abortion legal requires experts to define some point, after the fertilization of the egg, that precisely defines "human life."

Such a definition will necessarily be arbitrary, and being arbitrary, will change over time depending on current exigencies. The definition of "human life" has already devolved, over just a few decades, to permit the late-term abortion of babies capable of surviving out of the womb. And now, respected medical ethicists suggest, "human life" does not even include infants, or perhaps even toddlers. Other potential candidates for exclusion from "human life" abound. And today, facing fiscal disaster, the impetus for excluding even more groups from that definition is plainly growing strong.

Even William Saletin, a vocal pro-choice writer for *Slate*, was troubled by the "after-birth abortion" article. He wrote, "The case for after-birth abortion draws a logical path from common pro-choice assumptions to infanticide. It challenges us, implicitly and explicitly, to explain why, if abortion is permissible, infanticide isn't." His ensuing discussion shows clearly, to his own apparent dismay, that there is, in fact, no logical stopping point once "common pro-choice assumptions" are accepted.

People are not yet killing their inconvenient babies, at least not with the full approbation of the authorities. But the ethical groundwork for allowing such actions has been laid, and we in the herd are being desensitized to the idea.

DEVALUING THE OLD - THE AGE-75-CUTOFF

President Obama, in his June, 2009 National Town Hall Meeting, clearly stated that once a person reaches a certain age, that person should not expect even routine healthcare services, such as a pacemaker. He did not identify the threshold age at which he would favor withholding medical services, but indicated that, in any case, that threshold has certainly been crossed by the time one reaches age 100. He wisely avoided indicating that the actual age threshold is substantially lower than that.

But at the time of his Town Hall Meeting, his Special Advisor for Health Policy had already published his article in *Lancet* detailing the administration's age-related priorities for healthcare services for anyone who cared to look at them. To review: once you survive to age 20 your priority for healthcare services is and remains high until around age 50, at which time it drops rapidly to age 60, then drops more gradually to extremely low levels by age 75. After age 75 you drop off the map altogether.

Aside from this graphic evidence supplied in Emanuel's article, there are other indications which strongly suggest that age 75 is to become the magic threshold, above which we ought to stop expecting at least the more expensive varieties of medical care.

The clearest indications come from our friends on the USPSTF, the panel which under Obamacare has the final authority to determine who will and who will not receive preventive healthcare services.

In Chapter 11, we saw that the USPSTF does not want women over the age of 75 to receive any more screening mammograms – despite the fact that breast cancer is the chief killer of women in this age group. For our present purposes the relevant aspect of this recommendation is not the recommendation itself, but the rationale the USPSTF used to arrive at it. That rationale was: a) there are no well-controlled, randomized clinical trials proving that the overall mortality rate of women over 75 is improved with screening mammograms, and b) if such studies ever were to be done, they would likely show no overall benefit anyway, since people in this age group tend to die pretty soon, of something or other.

This should prove to be a very convenient rationale for the Central Authority, since it can be applied to old people for any medical service one can think of. "We are scientists," the expert panels solemnly pronounce, "and we can go only where the science takes us. Because randomized trials have not been conducted that show a survival benefit with Medical Service X in people over 75, our hands are tied."

No broad-based randomized clinical trial, measuring any medical intervention whatever, would ever be likely to show an overall survival benefit in a broad population of old people – and this explains why such trials are not done. Fundamentally this means that under the expert panel paradigm favored by any Progressive healthcare system, it will always be easy to render it inappropriate (and illegal) to provide those "unproven" services to the elderly.

Placing the cutoff at 75 years of age is entirely arbitrary. It could just as easily have been 70, or 80, or some other value. But this is the age which the Central Authority pretty clearly has identified as the threshold for which "routine" medical interventions ought to be withheld. Not only is it consistent with Emanuel's article, but it is also an age that appears in several recent USPSTF directives. Prior to the USPSTF's recent revision of guidelines for screening for prostate cancer (in which nobody is to have have screening any more), PSA screening was to end at age 75, despite the high incidence of fatal prostate cancer in elderly men. Current recommendations for colonoscopy also stops at age 75, despite the continued risk of colon cancer in the elderly.

From available evidence, therefore, it appears likely that the Central Authority has identified age 75 as the time when people ought to stop expecting routine healthcare services, because, apparently, once you reach age 75 your only remaining duty as a citizen is to die.

In any case, it seems apparent that when you turn 75, the Central Authority assigns you to that group of American citizens (possibly along with infants and toddlers) for which it is inappropriate to spend very much money. If I am correct, then we Old Farts should be alert to the sundry mechanisms which the Central Authority is likely to employ in the attempt to withhold our healthcare.

End-of-Life Healthcare

It is a famous axiom of those who decry the waste that takes place within the healthcare system, and who argue for tighter control over the behaviors of doctors and patients, that 60% (or 70%, or 80%, or some other very high proportion) of all healthcare expenditures are made during the last six months of life. This axiom is usually stated with a high degree of indignation, as if doctors can always tell when some Old Fart is fixing to die, whereupon they say to themselves, "This old guff is not long for this world, so if we're going to make any money off him by doing unnecessary medical procedures, we'd better get a move on."

And while there are undoubtedly unscrupulous doctors who take this attitude, the real reason a lot of money is spent in the last few months of life is: people often are very sick during the weeks and months prior to death. And when people are sick, they and their families expect, and doctors believe their duty is to provide, efforts to make them well.

Quite often, even in old people, these efforts are successful – sick people will recover to some reasonable semblance of well-being. Often enough, even very old people who look very sick will recover with appropriate care. And in fact, unless the patient has some obvious, irreversible terminal illness – such as widely metastatic cancer that has failed to respond to therapy, or end-stage heart failure – doctors usually cannot tell with any real precision when somebody has entered into that famous "last six months of life." The only real way to tell is retrospectively.

But when you are trying to cut healthcare costs, the retrospective method will simply not do. You need to devise a prospective method for not wasting all those "last-six-months" healthcare expenditures.

It is my suspicion that the ultimate method of doing so is going to be the age-75-cutoff-method. That is, once you hit 75, any serious illness you may develop after that will be an indication that your six-month-clock has started, and the efforts of your healthcare professionals will turn away from helping you to recover, and toward helping to usher you into the next life as humanely as possible. (After all, there will be no randomized clinical trials proving that the treatment for your condition in people your age improves the overall survival of the group.) I believe that the evidence provided so far by agents of the Central Authority point pretty clearly in that direction; that is, that end-of-life healthcare will be initiated the moment you need any significant healthcare services after age 75.

The beauty of the age-75-cutoff-method is that it will prove to be a self-fulfilling prophesy. That is, if you withhold medical care for elderly patients who are very sick, there is a very high likelihood that they will indeed die very soon. And by tabulating your statistics, before long you will be able to claim that, as a matter of fact, you can determine when that terminal six-month-clock has begun. The ability to determine this milestone prospectively will open up all sorts of opportunities for cost savings.

Our Progressive leaders are probably quite frustrated that our culture has not yet advanced enough that they can simply impose the age-75-cutoff method overtly, today. But they are not just sitting idly by. They are doing everything they can to encourage us Old Farts to "voluntarily" forgo healthcare services.

ADVANCE DIRECTIVES

On January 1, 2011 (that is, on New Years Day, a holiday which many Americans spend in a condition that – thanks to the revels of the previous night – renders them relatively unlikely to pay attention to press releases), the White House announced a new policy that would have paid doctors for discussing end-of-life planning during their Medicare patients' annual "wellness visit." Under this policy, physicians would be paid to encourage their patients to establish an advance directive, which would guide medical care if the patient became incapacitated from illness, and could no longer make medical decisions for him/herself.

But just a few days later, the new policy was suddenly revoked. It was revoked, officials lamely explained, because it had not been implemented using the approved procedures. But, as anyone would know who watched Congress make Obamacare the law of the land, this could not possibly have been the real reason.

The real reason, of course, was that – even through a New Year's haze – this new policy was shaping up to unleash a firestorm. And a public firestorm threatened to energize the House of Representatives, just as it was about to be taken over by the cretinous opposition party.

As keen observers will recall, the Obamacare bill originally included similar language on advance directives. Physicians were supposed to urge their older patients, repeatedly if necessary, to establish advance directives, and their success in extracting advance directives from Old Farts was to be one of the "performance measures" by which doctors would be judged to be in good or bad standing with the Central Authority.

But then Sarah Palin said "death panels," and a furor ensued. The provision on advance directives was quickly removed from the Obamacare legislation, as if Congress was admitting that Ms. Palin had been correct and they had been caught out. (In truth, even if you buy the notion of "death panels," the provision on advance directives was something else entirely.) So the debacle of New Years Day 2011 was the Central Authority's second failed effort to virtually mandate advance directives.

Obviously, advance directives are very important to our Progressive leaders.

In concept at least, advance directives are a good idea. Advance directives allow patients to establish beforehand, usually by a written document, what kinds of medical treatment they would or would not want should they fall victim to a serious, life-threatening illness that leaves them unable to express their wishes. Advance directives are supposed to work by providing guidance to their physicians, who, in their fiduciary capacity, are charged with acting in the patient's best interest.

A well-constructed advance directive allows patients to choose to spare themselves from demeaning, undignified, painful or otherwise undesirable medical procedures and treatments, should they become incapacitated at a later date. "Well-constructed" implies that the advance directives are clearly and concisely written, that they honor the ethical and legal norms approved by society, and that they provide the physician with clear guidance.

But it is more difficult to write a "well-constructed" advance directive than might at first meet the eye. The major problems are two-fold: Advance directives often express imperfect knowledge, and they are often imperfectly expressed. These limitations mean that in appropriately exercising an advance directive, often the physician cannot follow them to the letter, but must interpret them according to the circumstances at hand.

A healthy and relatively robust individual cannot always know how he or she will feel years into the future, when illness strikes and it is time to exercise an advance directive. Every doctor has seen critically ill patients who, despite having advance directives to the contrary, unhesitatingly choose to be attached to a ventilator when the time comes, for instance, rather than face certain imminent death. So experienced doctors know that advance directives do not always indicate what patients will actually choose to do when the time to make a choice is upon them.

They also know that, while conscious patients have the opportunity to repeal their advance directives, unconscious or incapacitated patients do not.* So, in exercising an advance directive, the conscientious physician interprets that directive in light of many other factors, such as, her personal knowledge of the patient, the opinions of family as to what the patient would want done, and the chances of a long-term recovery if the therapy being considered is used. Then she will negotiate with responsible family members an approach that appears to meet the patient's presumed desires.

_____

*Conscious patients can repeal their advance directives in theory. However, I have personally witnessed actual doctors argue vociferously against using a medical therapy that a sick patient now desperately wants, because years ago the patient signed an advance directive expressing aversion to that therapy.

_____

Therefore the advance directive in many cases is an important part of the decision-making process, but it is not the only part. The appropriate use of an advance directive requires the doctor to behave as a true patient advocate, to selflessly place the desires expressed in the directive in context with everything else that might affect the patient's true and current wishes, and then make a recommendation that, to the best of his or her ability, honors those wishes.

Unfortunately, doctors can no longer act primarily as their individual patient's advocate. Indeed, physicians are officially enjoined (by the New Ethics formally adopted by their own professional organizations) to give the needs of society at least equal consideration. And so, as has demonstrably happened with other "guidelines" in medicine, it is inevitable that advance directives will be reduced to a legal edict, which must be followed to the letter if the physician wishes to remain clear of the Department of Justice.

The likelihood that there will be no room for interpretation means that constructing just the right kind of advance directive for yourself – one that will be precisely suitable to any contingency that may occur – has become extremely difficult. If you get the details just a little bit wrong for the circumstances that actually arise, the price you pay may be very heavy. It would be better to have no advance directive at all than to have one that is misleading or ambiguous. Advance directives must be written with extreme care, and only after long, thoughtful consideration.

That is not how the Central Authority would have it, however. For many years now, the Feds, under the Patient Self-Determination Act, require hospitals to inform patients about advance directives at the time of every hospital admission, and to invite them to sign one. To say this is a less than ideal time to implement an advance directive would be something of an understatement. Asking a patient to sign an advance directive at the time of hospital admission, often by including it in the pile of routine and mind-numbing legalistic documents which patients must sign if they want to receive medical care, and often with no more guidance than that provided by the admissions clerk (who might explain, "This tells the doctors you don't want to be kept alive on a machine like a vegetable,") tells us something about whether the true motive for advance directives is to protect the patient's autonomy — or as an excuse to withhold care.

Having the discussion in a doctor's office these days, sadly, might not be much better. The Central Authority knows that squeezing what really ought to be at least a 30-minute discussion into a 10-15 minute office visit already packed with Pay for Performance requirements (while providing the added threat of punishment if the physician fails to extract an advance directive from the patient), will yield, at best, a signature on a boiler-plate document.

But despite the slap-dash method by which such a document may be implemented, it is a document whose language – when the time comes – will be exercised with all the legalistic exactitude of a contract attorney by any doctor who knows what's good for him.

I think that Americans are right in being suspicious of the big push we are seeing to urge advance directives upon us. Invoking "death panels" in this regard is utterly inappropriate, but the end result will suffice. It is good that we have all been given pause.

Still, the concept of advance directives is a good one, and I believe most Americans might do well to have one. Despite the damage that is being done to them, I think advance directives still can be salvaged. To this end, I hereby suggest several steps we can all take in executing an advance directive that will actually do what we want it to do:

1) Don't be pressured into implementing an advance directive by anybody whose career depends on keeping the Central Authority happy. Unfortunately, this likely includes your doctor if you are not paying your doctor yourself.

2) Don't sign a boiler-plate document. These likely will have been drafted with the interests of the Central Authority in mind, with the help of very smart lawyers, and when these documents are called into use in all probability they will be interpreted for the convenience of the Central Authority.

3) Try to keep your advance directive from showing up in an electronic medical record. Write it yourself, and store it where your loved ones can find it when they need it. Give a copy to your spouse, your children, and perhaps (if you have a direct-pay doctor who works only for you) your physician. This way, since your advance directive will not be immediately available to hospital personnel if you are suddenly incapacitated, no unfortunate and irreversible decisions regarding the aggressiveness of your medical care can be made before your loved ones are notified.

4) Write your advance directive as a general guideline, with as few specifics regarding particular types of medical care as possible. You should assume that any type of treatment you mention in a negative light will be withheld under any and all circumstances, including circumstances you may not be aware of in which you would want that treatment.

5) You are not writing your advance directive for the doctors (it is most tragic that we can no longer trust doctors in this regard!); you are writing it to help your loved ones make the right decisions for you, perhaps despite the doctors. So your goal should be to clarify your general desires for your loved ones. Discuss your advance directive with your loved ones after you have written it, or more ideally, before you have written it. Your written words will remind them of your wishes when the time is right.

I have written an advance directive for myself that attempts to follow these rules. The document is stored at home with my important papers. My wife knows where to find it, and knows my general feelings regarding these matters. With the guidance I have provided, I trust her and my children to make these important decisions for me. For anyone who is interested, my advance directive is reproduced here:

MY ADVANCE DIRECTIVE:

If I am able to communicate my wishes by any means whatsoever, then I wish to make my own decisions regarding my own healthcare. If, despite my ability to communicate, my condition makes it inconvenient to fully inform me of my situation and all my treatment options, then until such time as it becomes sufficiently convenient to do so, I want everything possible to be done to sustain my life and effect a recovery.

In the event of an incapacitating illness in which I cannot communicate, the basic guideline initially should be to do everything possible to sustain my life and effect a recovery.

After a reasonable period of time (in general, I would consider a week to be reasonable) if no progress has been made in the recovery of my mental function, and the likelihood of mental recovery is judged to be small, then withdrawal of life-sustaining care should be strongly considered. To help my wife and/or children with this decision, I would like to have an evaluation by a neurologist to help clarify the prognosis.

If improvement in my mental status has been made, then efforts to sustain my life and affect a recovery should be continued.

If at any point in my care there is a period of at least two weeks in which I am persistently unable to carry out meaningful communications sufficient to make my own wishes known (in the opinion of my family members and the neurologist), and the likelihood of mental recovery is judged to be small, then I would consider the withdrawal of life-sustaining care to be a blessing.

So. Advance directives are a very good idea, but unfortunately, have been identified by the Central Authority as a potentially powerful tool for withholding healthcare services, especially in the elderly. Even before Obamacare, certain insurers were refusing to reimburse hospitals or doctors that provided medical care that seemed to go against specific language contained in an advance directive. That, of course, was child's play. Now that the Central Authority has gotten hold of them, advance directives will likely be treated the same way as other guidelines are now treated in medicine, that is, as edicts, and thus as vehicles for the criminal prosecution of medical personnel who deign to "interpret" them.

This means that if you wish to take advantage of the benefits which advance directives can provide, you will have to proceed very carefully.

PHYSICIAN-ASSISTED SUICIDE

In the summer of 2008, the Oregon Health Plan (the Medicaid plan in that state) injudiciously sent a letter to lung-cancer patient Barbara Wagner denying coverage for the expensive chemotherapy her doctor had recommended, and offering instead to cover palliative care "including doctor-assisted suicide."

Despite the fact that there were plenty of distractions at the time (including a presidential election and the world's economy on the brink of Armageddon), that letter unleashed an impressive public outrage. (If you have forgotten the outrage, simply Google the search terms "Barbara Wagner" and "suicide.") Indeed, the outrage was sufficient to penetrate even the dulled sensibilities of the Oregon Health Plan's executives. One Jim Sellers, a spokesman for the plan, admitted to ABC News that "the letter to Wagner was a public relations blunder and something the state is 'working on.'"

It is clear that the Oregon Health Plan executives were at least a little blindsided by the general reaction to their ham-handed denial letter. Denial letters, after all, are a routine activity for health insurers, and they always list (as an aid to the patient) services which the insurer judges to be reasonable alternatives to the denied care. While in this case the denied service which Ms. Wagner sought offered some reasonable hope for prolonged survival, while the service being held out by the Oregon Health Plan as an alternative (to say the least) did not, that's really not so much different from the content of more "routine" denial letters. The difference is one of degree, and not of substance.

So, Oregon Health Plan executives must surely have wondered, "What's the big deal?"

One must try to be understanding of such insensitivity. It is a fundamental task of health plans – whether run by Medicare, Medicaid, or private insurance companies – to deliver unpleasant news to people whose lives are at stake, and it is normal (even necessary) for those who are charged with this task either to grow thick skin or to develop the traditional indifference of bureaucrats. It is perfectly predictable that such thick skin or indifference might dull one's ability to discern subtle differences in degree among various denials of services, subtle differences that might call for more artful phraseologies than those employed in this instance by the Oregon Health Plan. The failure to recognize the need for a more artful denial letter, Mr. Sellers appeared to indicate, was the only problem in the case of Ms. Wagner. The solution, he therefore suggested, is certainly not a substantive change in any policy, but better public relations.

Those who ran the Oregon Health Plan must have been particularly disheartened when even vocal proponents of physician-assisted suicide took pains to criticize their ill-considered denial letter. To so blatantly juxtapose the reality of healthcare rationing with the "option" of assisted suicide seriously undermines the chief argument advanced publicly by the end-of-life movement, namely, that assisted suicide is merely an individual autonomy play, and is not in any way a cost-saving tool. So even proponents of physician-assisted suicide understand that offering it up as a covered medical service at the same time you are denying potentially life-prolonging therapy is both insensitive and unseemly.

Not to mention counterproductive to their cause.

I am not a proponent of physician-assisted suicide. I have two major reasons for objecting to it. On a purely practical level, embracing and systematizing physician-assisted suicide under any healthcare system that is desperate to reduce spending on medical services will almost surely lead to some terrible abuses of the practice.

My second objection to physician-assisted suicide is based on a consideration of ethics. I will admit to being on somewhat shaky ground here because I am not formally trained in ethics, and it appears for all the world that those who are formally trained in ethics have universally concluded that physician-assisted suicide is perfectly OK in every way.

Debating with modern medical ethicists, at least if you are merely a layperson, is mostly a losing proposition. This is not because ethicists are intellectually (or even ethically) superior to the rest of us, but rather because they are adept in couching their arguments in arcane twists of logic and webs of jargon that make their arguments unintelligible to the uninitiated. This technique, of course, places novices like myself in the position of having little choice but to accept the ethical bottom line without really understanding how the bottom line was reached. It reduces medical ethicists to a priesthood, and medical ethics to received knowledge.

But advancing unintelligible ethical arguments is, well, unethical.

In any case, with these caveats I will now present my understanding of the chain of logic by which modern ethicists justify physician-assisted suicide – and its close cousin, euthanasia. I would be delighted to engage into a discussion with any ethicist who is offended by my attempt to reduce their argument to accessible English. Modern ethicists argue as follows:

Point 1: Our society has already decided that the autonomy of the individual patient is the overriding ethical consideration in making end-of-life decisions. We formalized this determination when we decided that an individual has a right to refuse medical treatment even if that treatment is very likely to save their life. Clearly, this determination means that individual autonomy is the universally agreed-upon controlling ethical precept.

And by adopting this controlling precept, we thereby have also firmly decided that passive euthanasia – allowing nature to take its course by withholding treatment at the request of the patient – is ethical.

Point 2: There is no ethical distinction between passive euthanasia and active euthanasia. That is, whether we let death occur by withholding effective medical care, or by actually doing something to help death along a bit, either way we're taking an action that hastens death. Ethically, both of these actions are equivalent. So, once we decide that individual autonomy is the overriding concern, we must also allow for active euthanasia when a patient wishes it.

Point 3: Once active euthanasia is deemed ethical, there can be no further ethical objection to the lesser act of physician-assisted suicide. If it is ethical for a doctor him/herself to bring on the death of a patient who requests it, there can be no objection to doctors preparing the suicide machine and handing the patient the switch.

The striking thing here (to me, at least) is that in establishing the ethical case for physician-assisted suicide, we necessarily also establish – as a veritable pre-condition – the ethical case for physician-provided euthanasia. Whether the patient says, "Help me to take my own life," or "Take my life for me," modern medical ethics supports the physician who replies, "Roll up your sleeve."

For those who don't see a problem with this, I refer you to the Dutch system, where, in full accordance with modern medical ethics, the rules permit both physician-assisted suicide and active euthanasia for patients who request it. Reports on the results of the Dutch system (reports which both sides have used to bolster their respective opinions on either the glories or the travesties of such a system) do point out one striking finding – hundreds of times each year, acts of involuntary euthanasia are occurring. That is, patients are being killed under the Dutch healthcare system at the hands of their doctors, without their explicit permission or even foreknowledge. All these patients, it is claimed, are being euthanized for entirely humane reasons.

What do our friends the medical ethicists have to say about such involuntary euthanasia? Well, it turns out that it's OK with many if not most of them. Ethicists don't like to tell us that their chain of logic doesn't end with Point 3. Once we make the principle of individual autonomy the overriding consideration in determining end-of-life ethical issues, the same chain of logic takes us directly to Point 4.

Point 4: Since honoring the ethical precept of individual autonomy makes voluntary euthanasia available for patients with intractable suffering, it would be unethical to withhold the same benefit from suffering patients who are too incapacitated to give their permission. Their incapacity should not restrict them from a good that is available to others, for to do so would be discriminatory and inhumane. To cure this problem, the boon of active euthanasia can and must be performed, even without the patient's explicit permission, in incapacitated patients whom "reasonable people" would agree are suffering too much. Therefore, involuntary active euthanasia is also ethical.

This conclusion, of course, leaves us in a place where others (i.e., "reasonable people," like doctors or other agents of the Central Authority) can decide for an individual what constitutes intractable suffering, and further, can decide when such an individual is simply too incompetent to know that euthanasia is the best thing for them.

I maintain that under our system of covert healthcare rationing, where doctors are under extreme pressure to do the bidding of the third party payers (both private insurers and the government) who determine their professional viability, and where the payers are under extreme pressure to reduce costs, and have already displayed in numerous ways their willingness to permit suffering and death among their subscribers in order to do so, then opening the door for physician-assisted suicide (let alone physician-administered euthanasia, whether the patient requests it or not), would inevitably lead to some nasty abuses, and would ultimately serve to undermine our civil society. I am too politically correct to use the "other N-word," but I will take this opportunity to remind you that such a thing has already happened, in a country that boasted the world's most advanced, cultured and educated people, within the memory of millions of living people.

I believe that the principle of individual autonomy is vitally important. Indeed, it is the founding principle of American culture. However, no single ethical principle, no matter how important, can be allowed to overrule all other ethical principles in all other circumstances. By nature ethical precepts are often in conflict with one another, creating what is called an ethical dilemma. And (I humbly submit) it is supposed to be the job of ethicists to help us work through those ethical dilemmas, to find the right balance between competing principles, and not to simply declare that no dilemma actually exists, because Ethical Precept A is the only one we need to pay attention to.

Individual autonomy is critically important to American culture, and the fact that we must fight to preserve individual autonomy in the face of

196

Progressive healthcare is indeed a chief underlying theme of this book. But in no other aspect of our culture do we let it absolutely rule. The autonomy of individuals needs to be checked, and we indeed limit it. This is the fundamental reason that governments are necessary in the first place.

The reason we have laws (supposedly) is to make sure that the behavior of individuals acting in their own interest, especially those who have accrued power (for instance, by accumulating great wealth, by acquiring large weapons, or by becoming heads of state), does not abrogate the natural rights of other individuals. Indeed, most of the political fights we have – between Democrats and Republicans or Progressives and Conservatives – are to determine where to place those limits, on individuals and on the collective, to best encourage a robust society that honors individual autonomy but that also encourages reasonably equal opportunities for individual fulfillment (i.e., "happiness"). The main purpose of our public discourse, then, is to find the right balance between the rights and needs of individuals and the rights and needs of society as a whole.

So for ethicists to say, "Individual autonomy is all there is to it, and we have no choice but to follow that principle to wherever it may lead us," is not only completely irresponsible and dangerous, it also flies in the face of our culture's history and our everyday experience. The cost to society not only should but must be taken into account as we consider institutionalizing physician-assisted suicide (let alone voluntary or involuntary euthanasia). In my opinion, ethicists who argue that we need not consider the cost to society in making end-of-life policy have declared themselves unworthy of the title and they ought to be completely ignored.

The cost to our society of institutionalizing and systematizing physician-assisted suicide, especially while we are still covertly rationing healthcare, would be severe. The cost would be paid in the currency of a further devaluation of human life, and a potentially fatal coarsening of our culture.

So far, those pushing assisted suicide insist that they are doing it to preserve individual autonomy and human dignity. And no doubt, many of these voices are entirely sincere. For the most part our Progressive leaders to this point have been content to sit on the sidelines, and let these sincere end-of-life advocates do their work for them. But every now and then our leaders' enthusiasm for the potential cost savings that might be realized through the widespread adoption of assisted suicide bubbles to the surface.

The letter the Oregon Health Plan sent out to Ms. Wagner is one such example.

Here's another example. Writing in *The American Journal of Economics and Sociology* as long ago as 1993 (the last time Progressive healthcare reform was prominent), Professor K.K. Fung pointed out that the healthcare system could save a lot of money by creating incentives to induce sick patients to commit suicide, with the help of their doctors. He blandly called his plan "physician-assisted suicide with benefit conversion." Under this plan, patients (or rather, their estates) would be paid a nice, tidy sum – calculated as a percentage of the projected cost savings the healthcare system would realize thanks to their self-termination – to opt for a painless and dignified death at the hands of their physician.

Physician-assisted suicide as an occasional and extraordinary solution to a rare, intractable clinical dilemma is one thing; institutionalized and encouraged as a routine healthcare option it is quite another. It is not difficult to imagine the promotion of assisted suicide as an attractive choice that any really sick person ought to consider. TV commercials, pop-up ads, and even pamphlets included in your hospital admission packets will remind you that you always have the option of saving yourself, at a time of your choosing, from the suffering, pain, needles, knives and scans with which the healthcare system likes to torture sick people. You have the means of taking control of your own destiny, asserting your autonomy, and removing yourself to a place where, free from all the pain, and enveloped in peace, you can be gently eased into the next life. You no longer have to worry about being a burden to your family and loved ones (or to the collective). You have it within your power to do one last thing for yourself and for the people who care about you. It's your choice, you are told lovingly – and expectantly.

And even if you choose not to listen to this stuff, your children and your grandchildren will. Whether or not they come right out and say it, you'll know what they're thinking: "Well, it's sort of getting to be about that time, isn't it?" And before you know it, your option for assisted suicide will become your duty for assisted suicide.

Furthermore, you should ask yourself whether the Central Authority can really stay its hand for very long when it is facing fiscal oblivion, and at the same time it has both the ethical cover and the capability to direct its agents at the bedside (i.e., your doctor) to perform euthanasia on unfortunate (and unproductive) citizens such as yourself, who are too "incapacitated," or too damned selfish, to understand it's the only thing to do.

When all is said and done, it is deeply ironic that by steadfastly clinging to the ethical precept of individual autonomy to guide end of life healthcare we will very likely completely devalue the inherent worth of the individual.

This outcome, really, demonstrates that our reliance on individual autonomy is in fact not the pinnacle of ethical thought; rather, it is a palliative, a partial and ultimately inadequate (though necessary) compensation for having to live in an imperfect world. Indeed, the attractiveness of Progressivism – the reason so many well-meaning people gravitate to it – derives fundamentally from its recognition of the inherent limits of individual autonomy as an organizing principle.

Especially as we face our final exit from this imperfect world, the palliative of individual autonomy loses much of its significance. To throw all other considerations to the wind, to make some ideal notion of the dying person's autonomy the overriding concern, ignores reality, ignores the other things the dying person needs more than his autonomy, is harmful to society, and calls into question our real motives. Encouraging a rapid exit is no way to honor a dying person's individual worth. There are far more important things we should be doing for the dying patient. We should offer relief from physical and emotional pain, offer help in resolving remaining issues of family or personal conflict, and offer spiritual support. We should let the dying person know that we will not abandon him, that we are embracing him, and not hastening to move him along to the final exit as quickly as we can. It is by such an affirmation of that person's continuing importance that we really honor his value as an individual.

Finally, I am compelled to point out that modern medical ethicists insist on clinging so tenaciously to the precept of individual autonomy only when it comes to end-of-life healthcare, that is, only when doing so happens to justify inducing the expeditious and efficient deaths of inconvenient Americans. In all other questions regarding medical ethics – for instance, the practice of one-size-fits-all herd medicine; the adoption of New Age Ethics by the medical profession, which commits doctors to act primarily for the collective instead of for the individual patient; and the stifling of the individual's prerogative to defend his own health with his own resources – these ethicists totally abandon individual autonomy in favor of achieving "social justice." They are, in other words, utilitarians, who invoke "individual autonomy" only when it suits their desired end, that end being the devaluation of the individual for the benefit of the collective. Ultimately, the ethicists' devotion to individual autonomy at the end of life is entirely cynical.

At least until we solve the fiscal problems of our healthcare system, we simply should not embrace assisted suicide – no matter what we may think of the ethics of the act itself – and we should fight efforts to make it acceptable. Once it is acceptable, the fiscal pressures will soon systematize it, and render it nearly mandatory. And the real cost to our society would be profound.

If people want to commit suicide and if medical ethicists insist that assisted suicide is OK, then let the ethicists do the assisting. I have relatively little to say against ethicist-assisted suicide. But for the love of God keep the healthcare system – and especially the doctors – out of it.

WHAT THE CENTRAL AUTHORITY HAS PLANNED FOR US OLD FARTS

In the next chapter I am going to talk about conflicts of interest within the healthcare system. This has become a hot topic in recent years. And when this topic comes up, it is always framed as a problem of physicians, and drug companies, and medical device companies, all of which may often stand to gain when some product or procedure is recommended for a patient.

But the biggest conflict of interest of all does not involve doctors or the biomedical industry. It involves the Central Authority.

The Central Authority, under our Progressive healthcare system, is to become the ultimate arbiter of who gets what medical services and when. At the same time the Central Authority is facing an existential fiscal crisis, a crisis primarily caused by healthcare expenditures. Therefore the need to cut costs, and specifically the need to withhold healthcare services whenever it can be gotten away with, will necessarily override all other considerations. This is a conflict of interest.

Given this conflict of interest, what does the Central Authority see when it sees an elderly person?

1) It sees a person whose intrinsic value to the collective is vanishingly small, as documented in Dr. Emanuel's 2009 *Lancet* publication.

2) It sees a person who, by virtue of age, is either consuming a tremendous amount of healthcare resources, or soon will be.

3) It sees a person who, each month, is collecting a Social Security check; that is, who is continuously taking away some of the Central Authority's precious resources, which could otherwise be applied to its critically important work.

4) It sees a person who may very well have accumulated a sizable IRA or 401(k), and who, each month he or she continues living, is frittering more and more of that money away on golf or Jazzercise. Assuming that Progressives succeed in reinstituting a sizable death tax, the elderly person who, by virtue of remaining alive, continues spending down his 401(k) is in essence stealing funds that are earmarked for the Central Authority.

Talk about conflicts. We Old Farts don't stand a chance.

From every indication the Central Authority is giving us, the age-75-cutoff looks real. At the very least, the Central Authority has determined that in this age group cancers should go undetected. It seems at least plausible that steps will be taken, likely tacitly, to institute a "last-six-months clock" for people over 75 who become seriously ill. Once that clock is started, aggressive and potentially curative care will be left aside (along with optimistic talk), in favor of palliative care and crepe-hanging. Advance directives – which will have been wheedled out of most of us by our doctors – will be enthusiastically invoked and followed to the letter with the strictest interpretation possible, and (ultimately) assisted suicide will be broached to us, circumspectly at first, but soon enough (as we begin to understand the futility of our position) with increasing urgency.

Laugh if you will, Whippersnappers. Soon enough, all this will be yours.

CHAPTER 14 - STIFLING MEDICAL PROGRESS

> *"Rapid scientific advance always raises expenditures, even as it lowers prices. Those who think otherwise need only turn their historical eyes to automobiles, airplanes, television, and computers. In each case, massive technological advance drove down the price of services, but total outlays soared."*
>
> - Henry Aaron (the economist one, not the home run one)

In 2011, David Brooks – the Progressive who passes as the house "Conservative" at the *New York Times* – wrote a remarkable piece suggesting that the root problem underlying our unsupportable national debt is, essentially, the unreasonable desire of Americans to be cured of their illnesses. This is indeed an interesting and enlightening formulation.

Since the root problem is the unreasonable attitude Americans have toward disease and death, the only possible solution, Mr. Brooks indicates, is for Americans to drastically change their attitude.

Brooks began his piece with a paean to Dudley Clendinen, a former colleague at the *Times* suffering from ALS (Lou Gehrig's disease), who had recently written about his plan to commit suicide before allowing himself to become completely incapacitated by his illness.

Many of us will understand, respect, and even support Mr. Clendinen's plan to commit suicide under these conditions. However, understanding and respecting his plan is not the same as insisting that everyone in his position should feel obligated to do likewise, or that failing to do likewise makes you unreasonable (or worse). But this is exactly Mr. Brooks' position: "[I]t is hard to see us reducing health care inflation seriously unless people and their families are willing to do what Clendinen is doing – confront death and their obligations to the living." In other words, Clendinen is doing no more than his rightful duty. He does not deserve praise as much as people who choose otherwise deserve criticism.

The problem, Brooks indicates, is our unreasonable desire to be cured of illness, and our failure to just accept our ultimate fate, which is death. Those unreasonable expectations are precisely what is driving up our healthcare costs, and therefore are fundamentally threatening to our society.

The exhortation to suicide was merely Mr. Brooks' opening salvo. (After all, the failure of most of us to commit suicide in a timely fashion can be only a relatively minor cause of our unsustainable healthcare spending.) He quickly moves on to his main point, which is that our unrealistic expectations regarding healthcare cause us to concentrate too heavily on medical research in a never-ending attempt to find new cures and new treatments. It is our insistence on continued medical progress, in the face of inevitable death, that is the real problem.

He insists that our sustained drive for medical progress is wasteful and ineffective. Indeed, he asserts, real medical progress is mostly an illusion. The

War on Cancer was declared over 40 years ago, he points out, and has still not been won. And despite all the research we have done, heart disease is still the number one killer. Indeed, the main thing we have achieved with all our monumental efforts in medical research boils down to "devising ways to marginally extend the lives of the very sick." It is time for us Americans to readjust our expectations regarding illness and death, and accept gracefully that both are inevitable, and then cut back drastically on all those wasteful and ultimately counterproductive attempts to achieve medical progress.

As his authority in drawing such a conclusion, Brooks relies heavily on an earlier article which appeared in *The New Republic*, co-authored by the noted medical ethicist, Daniel Callahan. In that article, Callahan set out in detail the problems caused by that which passes today as medical progress (which Callahan describes largely as an extraordinarily expensive chimera), and outlined an approach to fixing those problems. First, he says, Americans need an attitude adjustment: "[T]he public must be persuaded to lower its expectations. We must have a society-wide dialogue on what a new model of medicine will look like: a model that will be moderate in its research aspirations. . ." And then, having had our expectations appropriately reduced, we all will finally recognize that "[t]he only reliable way of controlling costs has been the method used by most other developed countries: a centrally directed and budgeted system, oversight in the use of new and old technologies, and price controls."

And so, relying on this widely recognized, widely revered authority, Brooks – in America's Newspaper of Record – spells out in clear terms a critical aspect of any Progressive healthcare system, an aspect that Progressives only rarely dare to mention publicly. Namely, in any truly Progressive healthcare system, the Central Authority will have to stifle medical progress.

WHILE THE PROGRESSIVES MAY HAVE A POINT. . .

I must interject right away that I am not attempting to defend the status quo when it comes to the current condition of medical research and development. Much of what passes for research and development in the United States today is indeed fundamentally wasteful, and I am in favor of a drastic change in how we move medical technology forward. So when Progressives such as Brooks criticize the rationale under which we strive to find new ways to prevent, cure or ameliorate disease, and when they criticize the effectiveness of such efforts, they generally make some very telling points.

I for one, however, wish the Progressives had discovered this conveniently nihilistic attitude (i.e., that medical progress is an illusion, and we would do well to just accept the fact that we're all going to get sick and die, and stop expecting modern medicine to do something about it) before they went to all the trouble of taking over our healthcare system. Since healthcare itself is futile, Progressives ought now to realize, then so must be is all the time and effort they are wasting on it.

My objections to the Progressive formulation regarding medical progress is threefold. First, while I will not argue that all of our investment in medical progress has been stunningly successful, I will point out that neither has it all been futile. Hundreds of thousands of cancer survivors are leading happy lives today who would have been dead from their disease in 1970. And while the mortality rate from heart attacks approached 20% in 1970, today (in the U.S at least) it is around 2%. So while we haven't cured all cancer or all heart disease, our efforts have still improved and extended the lives of a lot of people. Second, the solution our Progressive commentators recommend is precisely the wrong one. (More on this shortly.) And finally, the very reason medical progress is so often counterproductive has a lot to do with our increasingly Progressive healthcare system itself.

I can summarize what I mean by this last point with a simple, three-statement progression:

A) Under any Progressive healthcare system, healthcare is a right.

B) Since healthcare is a right – and since rights cannot be rationed – anything that is deemed to be "healthcare" must be provided by society to each individual.

C) Anything that can be proven to prevent, cure, or ameliorate any illness, no matter how marginally, must be deemed to be "healthcare," and thus must be provided to each individual.

Under a Progressive healthcare system, therefore, any company that comes up with any new treatment that can be shown, in a clinical trial, to offer some marginal benefit over the currently available treatment, can (theoretically) rely on the healthcare system "covering" that new treatment. The healthcare system has no choice in this regard. Because healthcare is a right, then if Treatment B is demonstrably better than Treatment A, everyone is absolutely entitled to Treatment B. (Progressives, of course, will actually withhold medical care on a par with the most heartless of insurance companies, but they will do so only in secret, or if they must do it in the open, will carefully explain why the withheld care is doing more harm than good.) In any case, this formulation creates a strong incentive for companies to produce low-risk, high-reward medical products, products that advance healthcare only marginally and break little new ground – a new statin, say, or a slightly more rapidly-acting erection enhancer – but (since they are "better" in some way than current products), will have to be paid for. At the same time this kind of system discourages companies from working on high-risk products that are more likely to represent true medical breakthroughs. A Progressive healthcare system intrinsically distorts the direction of medical progress.

Progressive healthcare systems inevitably produce all sorts of other counterproductive distortions as well. As we have seen in earlier chapters, a Progressive system attempts to prevent individuals from spending their own money on their own healthcare. It treats each individual as interchangeable members of a herd. It undermines preventive medicine, demonizes the obese (for starters – other groups ripe for demonization will not be far behind), and attempts to covertly ration healthcare services according to one's value to the Central Authority (manifested by the attempts of Progressives – as is nicely illustrated in Brooks' article – to expedite the demise of our older citizens).

But, as Brooks and Callahan so passionately argue, a top priority of a Progressive healthcare system will have to be stifling medical progress. Not to reformulate medical progress to make it more efficient and effective, but to stifle it.

THE REAL REASONS PROGRESSIVE MUST STIFLE MEDICAL PROGRESS

Stifling medical progress is a critical need for Progressives. There are at least six reasons this is the case.

1) Brooks and Callahan correctly note that the medical progress we have enjoyed over the past 60 years is the very thing that has so drastically driven up the cost of our healthcare. If doctors were still treating heart attacks with 10 days of bed rest, or depression by telling people to buck up, or cancer with sad looks, we would not have had a fiscal crisis in the first place. The new treatments that medical science develops are virtually always far more expensive than the "treatments" they replace.

2) It is only rarely that medical progress helps the people who are in the Central Authority's "sweet spot," that is, the people between 20 and 50 years of age who (as agents of the Central Authority have written – see Chapter 13), are really worth an investment of healthcare dollars. Rather, most medical progress has been made in fighting the heart disease and cancers that affect the far-less-worthy older population, or in treating certain congenital disorders, genetic defects or infectious diseases that affect very young (and thus also relatively worthless) people.

3) As Brooks and Callahan emphasize, it has been the general nature of medical progress that advances in healthcare have tended not to cure or eliminate diseases, but rather, have tended to convert relatively brief (and thus relatively inexpensive) fatal illnesses to the much more chronic (and therefore much more expensive) medical conditions especially enjoyed by our rapidly burgeoning population of older citizens.

4) A large proportion of medical progress has come under the category of "preventive medical services" – items such as the expensive imaging tests we use to screen for cancer and heart disease, or the use of statin drugs to reduce the risk of heart attack and stroke, or the development of implantable defibrillators to prevent sudden death. We have seen (Chapter 11) how preventive medical services always cost the healthcare system far more money than they can ever save.

5) Medical progress is largely unpredictable, that is, despite the best efforts of medical scientists to pursue progress in an organized and predictable manner, the real medical breakthroughs are all too often fairly serendipitous. They often come out of left field, from where you least expect them.

Because medical progress is largely unpredictable, it is largely uncontrollable – you cannot titrate medical progress, or determine ahead of time either its speed or the direction it will take. And when the operational model of Progressive healthcare utterly depends on centralizing the control of the entire system, then allowing medical progress to simply proceed in its own direction and at its own pace presents a huge threat to the system. Just think of the havoc that would result if, for instance, suddenly and without official permission, some independent group of researchers finally developed a practical, fully implantable artificial heart. The healthcare budget would explode overnight.

6) This is the most important reason. The general direction of medical progress during the past decade has passed a critical inflection point, one that presents an existential threat to the Progressive healthcare model. In a word, fundamental advances in medical research, combined with a convergence of wireless technologies, have turned us down the path toward individualized medicine. New therapies are on the horizon that will be targeted toward individual patients with specific needs, and not toward the entire herd. New diagnostics are now feasible that can be accessed and interpreted by almost anyone, that will tend to "democratize" and decentralize the management of medical conditions. I will have much more to say about individualized medicine in Part 3 of this book, as I believe it may offer us our last, best hope to vanquish the herd medicine model that is so critical to the Progressives. But for our present purposes it is enough to note that if medical progress is left unfettered, it promises to undermine and perhaps even destroy the one-size-fits-all Progressive healthcare system – and ultimately, the entire Progressive Program itself.

Allowing medical progress to continue in the direction it has begun to take in recent years will be suicidal for Progressives. If they are to permit medical progress to continue at all in any meaningful way, they will need to control it utterly. They will have to subject it to the same top-down, expert-directed, command and control structure they mean to apply to the rest of the healthcare system. There can be no free-wheeling or even modestly independent research. Medical research, such as it is, will have to be taken in hand and controlled centrally.

Brooks has made the emotional argument, and Callahan the ethical argument, for our Progressive leaders to do just that. However, Progressives being Progressives, and the ends justifying the means, our leaders haven't been sitting around waiting for the public arguments to be made in order to act.

Indeed, their efforts have already gone a long way toward stifling medical progress.

INSISTING ON RANDOMIZED TRIALS IN ALL CASES

By insisting that all new drugs and medical devices be "proven" in large, randomized clinical trials (RCTs) before they can be approved, the Central Authority has erected a major hurdle for companies that want to introduce new healthcare products. RCTs, to be sure, have added tremendously to our knowledge over the past few decades, and in many cases they are indeed the only useful way to study the effect of a medical intervention. But as we saw in Chapter 9, RCTs in fact do not separate truth from falsity, as many academics and virtually all regulators seem to insist. RCTs do not even accomplish the one thing they are supposed to accomplish, namely, to eliminate bias from medical research. Rather, RCTs give the designers and interpreters of clinical trials the opportunity to control that bias, and turn it in the direction they wish. And the RCTs which are used to determine whether a medical product can be approved for use are usually designed with the participation of the regulators, and the final interpretation of those studies always is performed by the regulators.

RCTs are often extraordinarily difficult and time consuming to administer, and generally are extremely expensive to run. That expense has increased tremendously in recent years, as the regulators have begun insisting upon enrolling many thousands of patients into these studies. Accordingly, the cost of developing new drugs and clearing them through the regulatory hurdles has become astoundingly expensive in recent years. According to Eric Topol in his recent book *The Creative Destruction of Medicine*, the average cost of bringing a new drug to market in the United States increased from $250 million in 1995 to $4 billion in 2010. Even the big drug companies now have to think long and hard about the risks before attempting to bring new products to market, as one or two failures of that magnitude in a short period of time could bring them down. And for small start-up companies, the expense is simply out of the question.

There are several reasons the pipeline for new drugs has shrunken so markedly over the past several years, but the tremendous cost of gaining regulatory approval – a cost which requires companies to place their bets very, very carefully – is clearly a major one.

Aside from the cost they engender, RCTs are sometimes inappropriate and counterproductive. I will give two brief examples.

In the early 1990s, implantable defibrillators had progressed sufficiently to have become widely applicable in people who had a high risk of sudden death from cardiac arrest. Most cardiac arrests are caused by the sudden onset of a lethal heart rhythm disturbance called ventricular fibrillation, or VF. If a person develops sudden VF, unless the arrhythmia is terminated within a few minutes (usually by shocking the patient's chest with a defibrillator), the odds of death are virtually 100%. Accordingly, the mortality rate of out-of-hospital cardiac arrest is exceedingly high. The reason implantable defibrillators are so attractive is that, once implanted, they successfully terminate VF – by automatically delivering a shock directly to the heart – over 95% of the time. And in non-randomized clinical trials, in which defibrillators were implanted in high-risk patients, it was clearly documented that people who had these devices had an excellent chance (in excess of 90%) of surviving subsequent cardiac arrests.

So clearly, implantable defibrillators were effective, and they saved lives.

But before regulators would agree to cover implantable defibrillators in Medicare patients, they insisted that an RCT be performed, in which high-risk patients would be randomized to receive either the implantable defibrillator, or "best medical therapy," with overall mortality as the end-point. The trial was performed, and indeed showed that people who were randomized to the implantable defibrillator lived significantly longer. Medicare subsequently agreed to cover the therapy. But the RCT was very expensive, took several years to complete, greatly stretched the ethics of medical research (since patients who were known – by any minimally objective observer – to need the implantable defibrillator were allowed to be randomized to have it withheld), and sent a major warning shot across the bow of developers of any new medical technology. That message was: No matter how obviously effective your new product may be, and even if it clearly saves lives, you will not be able to sell it before you demonstrate its effectiveness with an expensive RCT.

A more recent example misusing RCTs involves the treatment of malignant melanoma. Malignant melanoma, even with the best available therapy, is extremely lethal, leading to death within a year in the large majority of people who receive this diagnosis. Recently, however, a revolutionary approach to treating malignant melanoma was developed. The biotech company Plexxicon developed a drug (currently known as PLX4032) which is aimed at a gene mutation (the BRAF mutation) that is present in the tumors of about 50% of patients who have malignant melanoma. In patients with the BRAF mutation, an astounding 81% had a profound and rapid shrinkage of their tumor in Phase 1 clinical trials with this new drug. Furthermore, no toxicity was seen. Nothing remotely like this had ever been observed before with malignant melanoma. The "best" drug available, dacarbazine, produces a tepid response in 15% of patients, and causes lots of nasty toxicity.

Given a remarkable response like this, one would think that a creative approach could be devised to confirm the effectiveness and safety of PLX4032 – using as a control, for instance, the universally poor experience seen with all other therapies, an experience that has been very well-documented in the 68,000 people a year who die from this disease – instead of demanding the typical, large RCT in which half the patients are doomed to "standard" ineffective and toxic therapy with dacarbazine.

But our regulators – and the medical academics whose careers rely on a steady stream of RCTs – would not hear of it. The effectiveness of this new drug will not become official until we have an RCT which has generated two different piles of dead bodies, which the regulators can count.

If parachutes were considered a medical device (and why should they not be, since they are meant to prevent injury and death), before the parachute makers could market them within our current healthcare system, they would have to conduct a few randomized trials, in which a couple thousand people are tossed out of helicopters at 10,000 feet, half with and half without the test article. After all, one is almost as likely to survive an unprotected free-fall (by landing on a sloping snow bank, for instance) as an unprotected out-of-hospital cardiac arrest.

While large RCTs are usually a good idea when testing a new medical product, the mindless requirement to apply them in all clinical situations – even in situations where more creative and less onerous approaches would clearly be better – is a bad idea. Especially in the approaching era of individualized medicine (if such an era is really permitted to develop) more and more therapies like PLX4032 for malignant melanoma are anticipated – treatments that will be tailored (usually based on the individual's genome or their tumor's genome) to a very specific subset of patients with a particular disease. In these cases there will be a reasonable likelihood of achieving relatively dramatic effects. Insisting on large RCTs for this kind therapy will often be inappropriate and counterproductive – especially in "parachute-like therapy," where the outcome without the new treatment is well known and very dismal. An absolute requirement for RCTs presents a broad and sometimes unnecessary hurdle to research efforts. It is, however, a useful approach to inhibiting medical progress – and in particular, to inhibiting individualized healthcare.

INSISTING ON USING HERD MEDICINE STATISTICS

It's not just the requirement to conduct RCTs that present a formidable hurdle to medical progress – it's the way the RCTs are analyzed and interpreted. Fundamentally, the expert panels that will use the results of RCTs to determine whether or not a medical service will be available to doctors and patients will rely on population statistics – the overall effect of the new therapy on the entire herd.

We considered some implications of herd medicine statistics in Chapter 9. There, we postulated the existence of a new cancer drug that, in a large RCT, increased the mean survival of women with widespread metastatic breast cancer by three months. We noted that any self-respecting panel of experts, weighing the rather short improvement in survival against the high cost of the drug, would conclude that the drug simply does not work well enough to justify its expense. Then we noted that, while this decision makes sense from the collective's perspective, it does not make as much sense from the viewpoint of the individual woman with breast cancer. That woman is not looking at the population statistic – the mean extension of life by 3 months – but rather, is looking at the chance this new drug offers her for a much more dramatic response (since 10% or so of the women who received the drug were alive and apparently cancer-free a year or two later). Despite the risk of serious toxicity with the drug, it would be entirely reasonable for a woman with breast cancer to wish to give it a try. Using herd medicine statistics robs these individual women of the opportunity to take a chance with such a drug.

Now look at herd medicine statistics from the aspect of the pharmaceutical executive whose company has developed the cancer drug. You just spent $2 billion developing and testing the drug. The results of the clinical trials looked pretty good to you. The mean survival was increased by three months for the whole group, and a substantial minority of women had truly dramatic responses. This is how the treatment of cancer has traditionally progressed – by coming up with successive treatment regimens that advance the mean survival by a few months at a time. You always hope for the home run, of course – a cure, or prolonging life by a year or more – but those are few and far between. In the meantime, developing and selling "leapfrog drugs" like this one – which incrementally improve the treatment of cancer – has, over time, substantially improved the overall survival in patients with many kinds of cancer. And it provides the funds your company needs for continued research and development.

But this new herd medicine paradigm changes everything. If a $2 billion drug that actually works is rejected because it does not improve the mean survival across the whole group to the (unspecified, arbitrary, and changeable) standards of an expert panel, the risk to your company of continuing to work on cancer drugs has just become prohibitive.

In this way, herd medicine will stifle medical progress.

PRICE CONTROLS, REAL OR THREATENED

Recently, emails have come to light showing that in 2009, the pharmaceutical industry was busily negotiating behind the scenes with the Obama administration regarding its support for the pending Obamacare legislation. In exchange for a substantial reduction in the $100 billion in "rebates" which Obamacare initially required from the drug industry, Big Pharma agreed to support the law. They did this by spending $150 million on a pro-Obamacare advertising campaign, and giving another $70 million to two 501(c)(4) front groups. There is some sort of convention, I believe, that makes this something other than extortion when the Central Authority is doing it.

The threat of a $100 billion "rebate" was scary enough for the drug companies. (Apparently, thanks to their deal, this was reduced to "only" $80 billion). But what really frightened them into cooperating, judging from the email exchanges, was the threat of placing price controls, in one form or another, on the drugs they sell.

It is widely known, among non-Progressive economists, that "price controls never work." And this sentiment is universally true, if by "work" you mean that the product whose price you are controlling actually remains available at the controlled price, for a substantial period of time. In this sense, price controls may "work" for a few days or a few weeks (depending on the product being controlled). But after some relatively short period of time, the people who produce this product are no longer able to produce it, because the price they are permitted to charge for it no longer covers the cost of production. And so two things inevitably result. First, shortages of the product develop. And second, black markets develop. So you can still acquire the product on the black market if you really need it, but the price will be very high – in fact, it will inevitably be much higher than the original price that induced the price controls in the first place. (When you buy a product on the black market, you are paying not only the cost of the product according to a now-very-unfavorable supply/demand ratio, but also you are covering the cost of doing business for the black marketeer – things like "acquiring" the product illegally, paying off sundry officials, and purchasing the various layers of offensive and defensive weaponry that the black market industry traditionally requires.)

This is what always happens with price controls. It happens even within the healthcare system, and even with drugs. We are seeing this right now.

Since 2005, in the United States we have experienced severe shortages of numerous critical drugs. Generally speaking the drug shortages have involved sterile, injectable generic drugs. Sterile injectables are relatively expensive to make, and because the requirement for sterility dictates they must have a finite (and relatively short) shelf life, they are relatively expensive to manage logistically after they are made. We are seeing shortages in some of the more important and critical drugs used in medicine, including "crash cart" cardiovascular drugs, antibiotics, and important chemotherapy agents used for cancer. In recent years increasing numbers of patients with life-threatening illnesses have not been able to receive the drugs they need to optimize their odds of survival, and they have had to receive some substitute therapy, that is, instead of getting the drug they ought to have, they get a drug that is available. When your life is in the balance this is not a pleasant thing.

Hospitals have had to resort to semi-legal "grey markets" to get even a minimal supply of these drugs.

We have all heard the arguments over what is causing these critical shortages. Our friends the experts have studied the problem, and have concluded that the cause is "multifactorial," and includes things like insufficient production space, disruptions in the supply of raw materials, several drug makers opting out of the generic drug business, and a spate of manufacturing quality issues that have resulted in prolonged production interruptions. In other words, we are asked to believe that a series of disparate, unfortunate events suddenly began happening to the drug industry in 2005 (since prior to that there was no particular problem with these drugs), with no underlying explanation, and that all these unwanted happenstances, quite miraculously, mainly affected only one kind of product – sterile, injectable generic medications.

The problem has all the earmarks of having resulted from price controls. But none of the experts who are studying the shortages have mentioned an attempt to control the price of these drugs. So what gives?

What gives is a little-noticed provision – Section 303(c) – of the Medicare Modernization Act of 2003, which strictly limits the price Medicare will pay for "injectable" generic drugs. Prices for these drugs can still rise, but only by 6% or less, and only once every six months. Congress (in its great wisdom and expertise in matters economic) made the judgment that this kind of price rise would be sufficient to balance market forces. But Congress was wrong. This law took effect January 1, 2005, and soon thereafter we began to see shortages of those products whose prices were being controlled.

Progressives often talk about placing price controls on the newer, non-generic drugs that are so often very expensive. (It was largely to stifle such talk, I believe, that induced Big Pharma to support Obamacare back in 2009.) One might think that Progressives simply and stubbornly fail to understand that price controls never "work," and that they inevitably lead to shortages and black markets.

It seems likely to me, however, that at least some Progressives understand perfectly well the mechanics of price controls, and are threatening to institute them on new (on-patent) drugs with a perfect understanding of what the results will be.

For these Progressives, medical progress is the problem. And new drugs – drugs that are not only expensive themselves but that often increase the survival (to at least some degree) of people with expensive diseases – are an important component of medical progress. Enlightened Progressives understand that placing price controls on "new drugs" will lead to a shortage of "new drugs" – that is, it will discourage drug companies from making the incredibly expensive investments necessary to develop new products.

Better yet, since the lead time on new drugs is measured in years, you don't actually have to institute these price controls. You just have to seriously threaten to institute price controls, and the uncertainty you will create (as to whether it will be possible for the companies to recoup their investments in future years) will slow research and development immediately.

Price controls on drugs have been in the air for more than a decade. As we have seen, price controls were actually instituted, on a portion of the drug industry, in 2005. And threats of severe price controls on new drugs have been clearly articulated to the drug industry during the Obama administration, and (judging from the recently released emails) have been heard by the industry, loud and clear.

It may not be a coincidence that the number of approvals of new drugs has fallen substantially in recent years, or that the pipeline for new drugs has largely dried up, or that resources that drug companies might formerly have spent in research and development have apparently been diverted to mergers and consolidation within the industry.

Indeed, it may be that price controls, or the mere threat of price controls, have "worked" exactly as designed.

OUTLAWING DOCTOR-INDUSTRY RELATIONSHIPS

A worldwide controversy is now roiling over the appropriate relationship between physicians and industry. Superficially at least, this controversy has to do with the undisputed fact that a physician's relationship with industry can unduly influence his or her behavior. That is, this controversy is said to be related to the conflicts of interest that are always inherent, to some degree, in such relationships.

I believe there is a deeper, and far more disturbing, reason behind this controversy. I believe that, at some level, it is an effort to stifle medical progress.

Before defending this outlandish claim, we should first talk about conflicts of interest, because it is ostensibly the chief concern that is being expressed regarding physician-industry relationships, and it is in fact a very important issue.

A "conflict of interest" is present when an individual has a primary, fiduciary duty (i.e., a duty of trust) to Entity A, but then develops a secondary relationship with Entity B, which (by creating self-interest, competing loyalties, or even just an inability to be objective), threatens to interfere with the primary duty to Entity A.

Physicians may have (at various times) at least three primary fiduciary duties that must take priority. These are: a duty to patients when practicing medicine; a duty to students (i.e., actual students, colleagues, or the public) when teaching; and a duty to society (and truth itself) when conducting medical research. It is clear that ties with specific companies and their products can easily create important conflicts of interest that may interfere with each of these primary fiduciary duties, and it is equally clear that physicians have commonly allowed this interference to happen.

Far more often than we like to imagine, doctors have allowed bias to creep in when recommending a course of action for their patients, in imparting knowledge to trainees, colleagues or the public, or when designing, analyzing or reporting results of clinical trials. And typically, most doctors who exercise inappropriate bias have convinced themselves that they are really acting in the best interests of their patients, students or society at large. For it is quite difficult to be objective about one's own conflicts of interest.

And there is no question that industry has become adept at the gentle art of creating conflicts among physicians (subliminally whenever possible), and have carefully incorporated the creation of such conflicts into their business models.

Obvious abuses we have all seen include doctors "shilling" for companies or their products at national meetings; clinical guidelines committees seeded with biased members; unbelievable amounts of money (well above "fair market value") being paid to key doctors for consulting services; long advertisements disguised as continuing medical education events; and ghost-writing scientific papers, then recruiting prominent physicians to sign on as "authors" after the fact. There are many others.

Such ongoing abuses of their fiduciary duties ought to be deeply embarrassing to anyone in the medical profession.

And if it's not embarrassing, it is at least becoming painful. In the United States, physicians who are discovered doing some of these things are being called out publicly, are being investigated by Congress if not the Justice Department, are losing their prestigious academic positions, and are having their reputations destroyed. It is hard to be sympathetic toward them.

Despite all the negative attention – both public and legal – that such conflicts of interest have brought to the medical profession in recent years, many doctors continue to have tin ears. Self-policing apparently does not work with doctors any more than it does with other varieties of the human species.

Accordingly, a number of groups – most prominently the Institute Of Medicine – have recently made formal, and tough, recommendations regarding physician-industry relationships. The final "rules" under which doctors will all have to live are still being negotiated. But it is highly likely that they will include many if not all of the following:

- Doctors should not accept any gifts, no matter how small, from industry. These include trivialities such as pens and notepads, and more substantial gifts such as meals and travel.

- Doctors should not give presentations in which content is controlled or influenced by industry.

- Doctors should not consult for industry without a written contract, nor should they receive more than "fair market value" for consulting activities.

- Doctors should not accept drug samples from industry.

- Doctors who have a financial interest in a product or company should not participate in clinical trials in any capacity that involve that product or company, including patient enrollment, data collection, analysis or reporting.

- Doctors who have industry ties should not participate in the development of clinical guidelines.

- Medical schools and professional organizations should not accept direct funding, or attributable funding, for continuing medical education.

- Any interaction with industry will be fully disclosed, and made publicly available.

What this "full disclosure" will look like can be seen in the Physician Payment Sunshine Act, a Federal law which is pending. Under this act, all "transfers of value" totaling $100 or more in a year to any physician will be reported by each company to the government annually, along with each physician's identifying information. Such "TOV" includes food, trinkets, entertainment or gifts; travel; consulting fees or honoraria; funding for research or education; stocks or stock options; ownership or investment interest, and any other economic benefit. This information will be posted on a public, searchable government website. Companies will be fined $10,000 for each incident of an unreported TOV.

Activities that have been acceptable, and even encouraged, will now be strongly discouraged – and companies and physicians that allow these activities to happen will be punished. Doctors need to choose their interactions with industry very carefully, and very circumspectly.

Everything I have just discussed assumes that the real issue regarding doctor-industry relationships is the issue that people are talking about, i.e., conflicts of interest. Indeed, everything I have discussed assumes a particular way of looking at industry relationships, which I will call Theory A. Theory A goes as follows:

Theory A:

- Medical progress is Good, and benefits mankind.
- Industry is responsible for a high proportion of medical progress.
- Industry-driven progress requires the active participation of physicians.
- Therefore, a well-managed cooperation between industry and physicians is beneficial to mankind, and ought to be encouraged.

If you subscribe to Theory A you believe that, because well-managed physician-industry relationships benefit mankind, these relationships are good. So, fundamentally, it's the management of these relationships which is at issue. These beneficial relationships produce unavoidable conflicts of interest, which we must manage by strictly limiting their extent, and fully disclosing the ones that are left.

And on the surface, at least, that's what the debate is about – where to draw the necessary limits. But just below the surface, the debate is about something else entirely. Beneath the surface, Theory A is rejected outright.

Today we hear prominent voices telling us that merely managing conflicts of interest does not go far enough. No amount of conflict of interest is acceptable, and all physician-industry ties should be prohibited. Among these is Jerome Kassirer, former editor of the *New England Journal of Medicine*, who says, "The ideal handling of conflicts of interest is not to have them at all." For these voices, Theory A simply does not apply. Rather, (I submit) they subscribe to Theory B, which is a natural extension of the anti-progress aims of the Progressives, as articulated in the commentaries of Brooks and Callahan:

Theory B:

- *Medical progress creates excessive costs, and produces far more harm to society than good.*

- *Physician-industry alliances strengthen the biotech industry's research and development efforts, and thus increase the harm.*

- *Therefore, crippling these unholy alliances is critical to the interests of society.*

Most proponents of Theory B do not present their case publicly as an anti-progress argument. Rather, they generally claim to be working under Theory A: It's not progress itself they are against, it's the greed of the biomedical industry. De-legitimizing any practical relationships whatsoever between industry and physicians will help to stem this greed; and as a bonus it is a useful way to suppress, if not cripple, the research and development efforts of the biomedical industry.

Physicians who cooperate with industry to advance medical progress are now to be stigmatized. This is something new. Until now, for doctors to work with industry has been encouraged, since it helps to advance medical progress in a practical and more clinically useful direction. Physicians who have done so have been regarded as doing good, since their work with industry allows them to bring their clinical perspective to the biomedical engineers developing new products. Industry itself thrives on the participation of knowledgeable physicians, since developing products that actually help patients is what ultimately produces success.

But now doctors who cooperate with greedy industry will be viewed as tainted, and their names will be posted on public websites as being in the pockets of these forces of evil. As a result, clearly, nothing they say and nothing they write henceforth ought to carry any credibility whatsoever. Academic promotions will become harder to come by. And worst of all, they will become ineligible for participation in the government's expert panels – panels which will have more authority over life and death than that enjoyed by most kings, and participation on which is destined to become the ultimate determinant of power and prestige in the medical community.

In addition to stifling medical progress, Theory B also advances the Progressives' goal of controlling the flow of information, that is, of preventing profit-drunk industry – and its greedy physician spokespersons – from expressing their opinions, to either doctors or to the public, regarding the appropriate use of medical technology.

That kind of information can only be managed by unbiased sources. Theory B relies on those government-appointed expert panels not only to determine which products of industry are good and which are bad, but also to manage the flow of information about them. Information coming from anywhere else is to be regarded as being charged with bias and greed, and should be ignored, or even suppressed.

Inherent in this viewpoint is the notion that the Central Authority is an honest broker, with no bias of its own, except to do what is best for the population. The State, in its disinterested beneficence, is the only civil entity which can pass judgment on which medical information is suitable for general consumption.

Even as a general proposition no government is an unbiased and honest broker. Government officials do not cancel their own human nature when they put on a government name tag. As they go about the business of determining who gets what, when and how, they inevitably – and most often intentionally – create various favored constituencies, fiefdoms, and clienteles to suit their own goal. That goal is to consolidate and expand their own authority. In this way, in the exercise of its political mandate the government always creates co-dependencies, and determines winners and losers. So even in the general case, the government cannot be an honest broker.

But with regard to healthcare, as we have seen, the bias of the Central Authority goes far beyond the general case. To agents of the Central Authority, controlling healthcare spending is an existential problem, an issue that justifies any solution that has even a slight chance of working. This is why they cannot restrain themselves from demonizing the obese, or of trying to "lower the expectations" of the elderly, to the point of encouraging suicide. And this is why they cannot restrain themselves from trying to stifle medical progress.

Yes, industry is biased, and industry will act on that bias whenever they can get away with it. Industry just can't help itself. That's just the way it is.

But the Central Authority is also biased. And the Central Authority will also act on that bias whenever they can get away with it. The government can't help itself. That's just the way it is.

Industry will try to exercise its influence over doctors by data-driven persuasion, and when that fails they will try to sweeten the persuasion, perhaps even with subtle or not-so-subtle bribes.

But the exercise of persuasion is even more dangerous when done by the government. While the government may also try to influence doctors with data-driven persuasion, it is very quick to resort instead to propaganda (i.e., the art of information-control by which people are told only what the expert classes have determined is best for them), and when that fails, the Central Authority will resort to its ultimate form of persuasion – the enforcement of new and suppressive regulations at the point of a gun.

Medical progress driven by industry-physician collaboration is good for mankind. But that collaboration inevitably creates conflicts. Physicians need to control those conflicts, or the collaboration will be forcibly terminated altogether. Physicians' professional history to date is bleak in this regard, and they only have one chance left to get it right, if that.

But in controlling their conflicts of interest, physicians should not allow themselves to be pushed too far. They should agree to reasonable limits on conflicts, and on full disclosure of any conflicts that remain. But they should draw the line when they are urged to forgo all relationships with industry altogether. They must recognize that industry and its selfish goals provide a necessary counterbalance to even more powerful forces whose own selfish goal is to stifle medical progress altogether.

IS THE BIOMEDICAL INDUSTRY REALLY EVIL?

Of course, nobody needs to remind us that the biomedical industry is evil. We have all observed as the pharmaceutical industry has fired off a never-ending parade of wasteful "me too" drugs, mainly aimed at keeping the joints, bowels, bladders and genitalia of Old Farts nicely lubed up, then running a steady stream (so to speak) of television commercials regarding same, which renders prime time TV far too embarrassing to watch with preadolescents.

Other evil behaviors abound. We can all see the biotech industry systematically fail to publish research that makes their products look less than spectacular; routinely over-hype research that suggests a modicum of effectiveness; callously corrupt doctors with plastic, logo'd ink pens; and likewise corrupt legislators with huge campaign contributions, rides on private jets equipped with plenty of booze and bimbos, and $150 million advertising campaigns to support their favorite legislation (after which the indignant legislators propose laws against plastic logo'd ink pens); and most annoying of all, gouge American citizens with astronomical prices for their new drugs, while selling those same drugs to Canadians and other undeserving foreigners at greatly discounted prices.

But still, most objective observers must reluctantly admit that, every now and then, and probably by mistake, a medical company will do something worthwhile. Here and there they manage to come up with a real breakthrough product that cures a disease, prolongs survival, restores functionality, or relieves suffering. That is, the biotech industry (in spite of all its evil behavior), has done a lot of good over the years. Ask a parent whose child has survived acute leukemia, or the person who has survived a life-threatening infection, or the woman whose heart attack or stroke was aborted with clot-busting drugs, or – yes, this too – the aging Lothario who once again can enjoy fine and durable erections upon demand. Such individuals, even if today they would join the Progressives in promoting the demise of the biotech industry, have undeniably had their lives improved by that industry.

So the question we must address before we allow the Central Authority to cause the biotech industry to roll itself into a ball and hide in the shadows for the duration, is not, "What have you done for me lately?" (since their inventions will live on even if they do not), but rather, "What can you do for me tomorrow?" Some of us in the boomer generation, for instance, would like to think that current research in the areas of Alzheimer's, Parkinson disease, kidney disease, heart attack, stroke, arthritis, osteoporosis and cancer will allow us to remain healthy and functional for a few extra years. And judging from the massive amounts of money American citizens of all ages donate to medical research of all types, it is apparently not held among the whole of the populace that medical progress has already gone as far as it should. Many of us would not be entirely pleased to stand pat right here. Many of us would like to see more improvements.

And while it may not seem obvious to many of us, we stand at a threshold of truly amazing medical innovations. These innovations are made possible by a convergence of several divergent technologies including wireless communication, social networks, physiologic sensing technology, new knowledge regarding the human genome, and ubiquitous personal computing/analysis/communication devices (known as smartphones). These convergent technologies make possible – today – healthcare products and services that were unimaginable just a few years ago. A key feature of these new products and services will be their decentralization of critical and actionable knowledge – that is, they will empower individuals to manage their own healthcare.

Such advances will collapse the centralized, top-down, command-and-control structure of any Progressive healthcare system. Therefore, such innovation poses an existential threat to Progressives. And the drive to stifle medical progress is largely the drive to prevent any of this from actually happening.

I will discuss these emerging medical advances in more detail in Part 3 of this book, and consider what we must do to allow such advances to proceed. The Progressives – who for the most part control the Central Authority with all its power and all its enforcement muscle – mean to stop it in its tracks.

This is why Progressives are beginning to say out loud what they have long been thinking – that medical progress is a bad thing, and must be suppressed. It is a difficult message to sell – but they have a lot of resources. And in the meantime, whether they can sell the message or not, they are pulling out the stops to actually accomplish it.

As a result, we in the huddled masses have only a limited window of opportunity to set medical progress solidly along the path to individualized healthcare. Unfortunately, in contrast to the Progressives, most of us don't realize that there's a fight going on, or even that there's anything to fight for, or that time is wasting.

PART 3 - WHAT WE CAN DO ABOUT IT

CHAPTER 15 – THE CRITICAL IMPORTANCE OF INDIVIDUAL AUTONOMY

"We prefer self-government with danger to servitude in tranquility."
- Kwame Nkrumah

A few months before the 2012 election, Chief Justice Roberts revealed his decision to stand with the Progressive wing of the Supreme Court, and declare Obamacare constitutional. Why he (supposedly a Conservative) did so has become a matter of widespread conjecture. I believe that Justice Roberts found a way (convoluted as it may have been) to let the law stand precisely because this law represented a pivotal moment in American history, and he believed, therefore, that whether the law stands or not ought to depend on the will of the people as expressed by their elected representatives, and should not rest on one swing voter on a 9-person panel. With a critical election only four months away, and with the bulk of Obamacare not yet implemented, Roberts (I maintain) manufactured a way to turn it back to the people. Let the people decide whether they want this law, and all it implies about the kind of country we will have. (And now that they have done so, I can only offer an opinion from another famous Jurist: "Forgive them, for they know not what they do.")

The actual constitutional question turned on whether the federal government had the authority to invoke the "individual mandate" (i.e., the mandate under the law that all Americans must acquire an approved health insurance product by 2014, or pay a penalty). The Obama administration argued that the authority to do so is granted by the Commerce Clause. Opponents countered that the Commerce Clause cannot possibly give the government the power to force individuals to buy a specific product (or, more precisely, to enter into a specific contract) against their will, since, if the government had that power, it would necessarily also have the power to force individuals to do anything else the government wanted them to do.

The argument that the government ought to have such power goes to the very heart of Progressivism. In order for the Progressive Program to work, that is, in order to move toward a perfect society, individuals simply must behave according to the dictates of all those designated experts, who will determine what is best for society. Ideally, people will voluntarily follow such dictates because it's the right thing to do. But for recalcitrants who do not agree to follow centralized directives voluntarily, there has to be a mechanism for forcing compliance. The Progressive Program will simply not work without being able to achieve universal cooperation.

So the question of the individual mandate goes to the fundamental problem of Progressivism.

It ought to be obvious to any objective observer that the US Constitution was designed specifically to deny the federal government any such authority over individuals. To have declared the individual mandate constitutional, to have granted that power to the federal government, would not merely have been a misapplication of the Commerce Clause. It would have turned the entire theory behind the Constitution on its head.

Justice Roberts managed to find a way to allow Obamacare to stand, while declaring that the individual mandate is not constitutional under the Commerce Clause. He did this by accepting the government's argument (which had been offered only as a peripheral, back-up, secondary argument before the Court, and that nobody else had taken seriously) that the individual mandate is not actually a mandate, but a tax.

So Obamacare will stand, and in this way the Progressives have won a great victory – but it was by no means everything they were looking for. For Obamacare was allowed to stand in a way that did not finally gut the main idea behind the Constitution.

However, the Progressives are already busily working to rectify this shortcoming. No sooner was the ruling announced than the mainstream media began declaring, "Individual Mandate Found Constitutional." And within minutes the President's surrogates were dispatched to make the rounds on all the TV shows to celebrate the ruling – and at the same time to indignantly deny that the mandate is a tax, but is in fact a mandate as they asserted all along. In other words, the Progressive victors are doing everything they can to create the public perception that it was the individual mandate (and not some bogus tax) that was found to be permissible under the Constitution.

Already, few Americans remember that the individual mandate was actually called unconstitutional by the Court. The conventional wisdom, eventually if not today, is that it is perfectly fine for the federal government to make mandates on individual behavior. So the next time the government decides to mandate that individuals must do this or that, it will not occur to very many people that a court challenge is in order. And the people to whom the notion does occur will be considered troublemakers, and will be dismissed out of hand (or worse).

That the Progressives are loudly denying it's a tax, and insisting that it's a mandate after all, and that the mandate is in fact constitutional, is behavior that ought to further enlighten us as to the true nature of Progressivism. Specifically, true Progressivism is incompatible with the Constitution as it is written, and even with its underlying thesis. The individual autonomy that formed the basis for our constitutional government – the prerogative of individuals to act in their own best interests with an absolute minimum of interference – is fundamentally in opposition to Progressivism. And so the documents that establish the primacy of individual autonomy must be "reinterpreted."

OUR OBAMACARE

Obamacare offers the people several goodies, such as allowing adult children to remain on their parent's insurance for a very long time, guaranteeing that people with preexisting medical conditions can buy insurance, and forbidding insurance companies from cancelling policies when people get sick. From proponents it is only the goodies we hear about.

But what we get along with these well-publicized goodies, while seldom mentioned in any cogent way, is not pretty. We will get a centrally-controlled, top-down, expert-driven healthcare system. Important medical decisions will not be made on the ground, between the doctor and the patient, but rather will be made by distant expert panels under the precepts of herd medicine. The medical actions that are deemed best for the herd will be transmitted down to our physicians, who, acting as agents of the Central Authority instead of as our personal advocates, will let us know what our limited "options" are.

It is inevitable that eventually (if not immediately) the overwhelming fiscal catastrophe that our healthcare spending threatens to bring down upon all of us will cause our Progressive leaders to mandate (now that such mandates are widely acknowledged to be legitimate) that we all must engage in sufficiently healthy lifestyles (since our gluttony, sloth, driving habits, hobbies, and other proclivities are creating an unfair strain on our precious healthcare system). People who allow themselves to become too fat or too old, or who injure too many joints because of carelessness or poor choice of pastimes, or who (by virtue of the fact that they have developed preventable diseases such as cancer, heart attack or stroke) demonstrate that they have paid insufficient attention to proper preventive measures, will (at the very least) have a lesser priority when it comes to receiving healthcare services. Good citizens (the ones who behave themselves, and whose good behavior is manifested by good health) will be taught from an early age to disdain the likes of these lazy, careless, and intemperate individuals who become fat or sick, who care nothing for their fellow citizens, and whose selfish personal choices place those good citizens in unnecessary jeopardy.

Worst of all, full-blown Obamacare means the end of the Great American Experiment.

America is exceptional. But it is not exceptional because we are richer or economically superior to other lands, or that we have been particularly innovative or inventive, or that we have had the strongest military and have won most of our wars, or that we have habitually come to the rescue of Europe and other places threatened by totalitarianism, or that we have been a melting pot of multiple cultures, or that poor immigrants have been able to come here and work their way up to prosperity. America is exceptional because it is the only nation in the history of man that was not founded on the basis of geography, race, culture, language or religion. Rather, it was founded on an idea: the idea of the primacy of the individual, of individual autonomy – the idea that all people have a natural right to live their lives as they see fit, without unnecessary interference.

This idea first developed in Europe nearly 500 years ago, but had trouble taking root there, and really only flowered when Europeans first came to America and had the opportunity to put it to work in an isolated location, where rigid social structures were not already in place. The development of this idea culminated with America's Declaration of Independence, in which our founders declared individual autonomy (life, liberty and the pursuit of happiness) to be an "inalienable" right granted by the Creator, and thus predating and taking precedence over any government created by mankind. And since that time the primacy of the individual in American culture has, more or less, remained our chief operating principle. Individual autonomy – or to put it in more familiar terms, individual freedom – is the foundational principle of our culture. This idea is what has made us great, and why America is exceptional. And until recent years it is an idea that the vast majority of Americans have agreed is worth fighting for.

Whether a nation and a culture founded on such an idea can persist is the Great American Experiment.

Under the Great American Experiment, the only legitimate duties of the government are to protect the citizenry from foreign aggressors, to grease the skids of a free economy, and to allow free Americans to strive as they will as long as they do not infringe on the rights of others. And in so doing, the government may utilize only its very few, explicitly enumerated powers. Otherwise, the government must stay out of our way.

It is inherently true that the Great American Experiment – and thus our founding documents – are entirely incompatible with the perfect, expert-led society envisioned by Progressives. Progressives only rarely say this in public, since most Americans (including the vast majority of Americans who consider themselves to be progressives) still value the American ideal. But every step of the way, the true Progressives have been working for over a century to undermine the fundamental tenets of our Constitution. They have no choice about this, as Progressivism is incompatible with the idea behind the Constitution.

Each time they act to undermine the Great American Experiment, of course, they do it for the benefit of the people. The doctrine of religious freedom can be wrecked, but only so that women can receive free contraceptives. Legal contracts can be abrogated, but only so that union auto workers can retain their benefits. Laws passed by the People's House can be arbitrarily nullified by the chief executive, but only so that young people brought to America illegally through no fault of their own can be given amnesty. Laws can be applied to different groups of Americans in different ways, but only to achieve social justice. Individuals can be forced to enter contracts (heretofore voluntary agreements between co-equal parties) against their will, but only so that 25-year-olds can remain on their parent's health insurance policies.

It is critical to understand that once Obamacare really sinks its roots, the game is about up. When we grant that the government has the authority to establish "healthcare" as a right, and thus has the authority to administer that right to all the people (i.e., to determine who gets what, when and how), then the government will also have the authority – indeed, the responsibility – to control all those choices we make that might affect our utilization of healthcare, which is to say, every choice we make. Obamacare, when fully developed, will cede to the Central Authority, at last, nearly complete control over almost every important aspect of our lives. Such control is the Holy Grail of true Progressives. And this is why controlling our healthcare system is the lynchpin of Progressivism.

Obamacare, along with the individual mandate that (de facto) enabled it, will herald the death throes of the Great American Experiment. We can have Obamacare, or we can have individual freedom. We cannot have both.

And so, for anyone who is not yet ready to declare the Great American Experiment to have failed, repealing Obamacare, despite the long odds against it, has to be the chief priority.

REPEALING OBAMACARE WILL NOT BE ENOUGH

Repealing Obamacare will not be easy. Even if, through some monumental effort, Americans manage to elect a government in the next few years dedicated to its repeal, repeal is anything but assured. To affect a total repeal, Americans will have to hold their representatives' feet to the fire, somehow forcing them to act with totally uncharacteristic resolve against the onslaught of scathing editorials, slanted news reports, threats by the insurance industry to renew their depredations upon the people, and multitudes of human interest stories appearing everywhere, depicting unfortunate souls who will "lose their healthcare" and die if the Republicans go ahead and do what they have been elected to do.

The worst part is that even if by some miracle we should manage to repeal Obamacare in its entirety, as critical as the repeal may be to the Great American Experiment, it will itself not be sufficient to fix the problem. As I have attempted to show, well before anyone ever heard of Obamacare we were a long, long way down the road toward a Progressive healthcare system. Repealing Obamacare, if that's all we do, will merely put us on a somewhat slower trajectory toward that end. That, after all, is what happened after Hillarycare was defeated in 1994.

After the demise of Hillarycare, our healthcare system became steadily and unrelentingly more Progressive, and indeed instituted many of the main ideas embodied in Hillarycare. Chief among these, the control exerted by the Central Authority over the behavior of physicians has grown continuously, to the point that, as early as 2002, the medical profession finally capitulated, and agreed to adopt a new set of medical ethics centered on "social justice." No longer do their ethical standards pledge doctors to concentrate on the needs of their individual patients; the needs of the collective now carries at least equal weight. And so, when doctors find themselves coerced into pleasing the Central Authority instead of doing what's right for their patient, at least they can console themselves with the knowledge that they are behaving "ethically."

Also since the demise of Hillarycare, the prerogatives of the individual patient have steadily eroded. This is because a Progressive healthcare system simply cannot tolerate autonomous, independent patients. There are, of course, the obvious limitations imposed by managed care plans regarding the doctors, drugs, procedures and hospitals that a person is allowed to access. These limitations at least have the virtue of being relatively transparent. But more sinister (and less well known) limitations on individuals have evolved in the intervening years, such as the Medicare patient's inability to purchase healthcare services that are denied to them by Medicare, and the recent court ruling that Medicare patients must remain on Medicare whether they want to or not (unless they are willing to return all past, and forgo all future, Social Security payments). (See Chapter 7.) With virtually no discussion of the implications of doing so, the tenets of herd medicine are being employed to decide which treatments to offer or withhold from specific patients; that is, treatment decisions are being made based on group statistics, even when an individual's own particular situation suggests that an exception ought to be made. For their doctor to attempt to individualize their care would be a grave violation of modern medical ethics, and would likely constitute healthcare fraud. (See Chapter 9.)

Our steady evolution toward a Progressive healthcare system has not depended in any way on Obamacare, and it will continue even if Obamacare should go away. To our political leaders, to the doctors who care to rise to positions of leadership within medical organizations like the AMA, and to younger generations of physicians who have been trained from Day 1 that "stewardship of collective resources" is their primary function, the needs of the individual patient are relegated to a secondary concern, if it is a concern at all. And when collective concerns are primary, the notion that individual patients ought to have real autonomy (instead of "counseling" to help them understand that the options being presented to them are really very good options), simply does not register.

Repealing Obamacare, by itself, would not change any of this. Fundamentally Obamacare does not bring any new ideas to the table; it "merely" takes the things the Progressives have been slowly and relentlessly developing, and bundles them into one great package from which they can all be accomplished at once. Indeed the one great virtue of Obamacare is that it throws the goals of Progressive healthcare into stark relief – and makes the true aims of Progressives plain to anyone who cares to look.

Repealing Obamacare, therefore, will be critical to preserving the Great American Experiment. But it will not be sufficient.

CAN AMERICAN HEALTHCARE REALLY BE FIXED?

The short answer is, yes. If the goal is to bring the healthcare system to a point of fiscal sanity, where it no longer promises to suck us into a fiscal black hole which will wreck our culture, there are actually several ways to accomplish this. I addressed this topic specifically in Chapter 4, where I pointed out that there are as many as four general approaches by which we can finally control healthcare costs.

Unfortunately, none of our political leaders (the ones who are proposing which of these methods we ought to use) have chosen to present the problem to us in the proper way. They act as if our healthcare itself is the chief consideration in deciding how to solve the problem, and they imply that the only thing we need to worry about is which proposed solution will offer us the best deal on healthcare.

This is not true. From the foregoing discussion, it ought to be clear by now that the chief consideration in deciding which kind of healthcare system we should choose is: What kind of country are we going to be? Are we going to continue with the Great American Experiment, and devise a healthcare system that is compatible with it? Or are we going to determine that the Great American Experiment is not worth preserving, and continue with Obamacare or some other Progressive plan?

The fundamental question in deciding how to fix our healthcare system, then, is whether we will choose a system that preserves and protects the primacy of the individual – or not. Whether implicitly or explicitly, we must answer this question before we can decide how to fix American healthcare.

We will settle this question once and for all, implicitly at least, if we allow Obamacare to stand. On the other hand, if we the people see to it that Obamacare is repealed, the question remains open (since a Progressive solution will still be possible, and perhaps even likely). So if Obamacare is repealed we will still have a lot more work to do.

There are plenty of ways of devising a healthcare system that: a) preserves individual autonomy in making healthcare decisions; b) makes sure that everyone has access to at least basic and catastrophic healthcare services, and c) returns public spending on healthcare to fiscal sanity. All of these methods require individuals to make many of their own healthcare choices, and to pay at least a portion of the costs. (One way to tell you are dealing with a Progressive is to suggest such a solution, and watch for the look of utter horror on his/her face at the very idea of individuals being responsible for any of their own healthcare costs.)

The details of which variety of a non-Progressive healthcare system would be the "best" is not something I am going to address in this book*. That, frankly, is of secondary concern. The first question – and the only question that really matters for our children and their children – is whether we are going to preserve the ideal of individual liberty in America, or not. Thanks to Obamacare the choice is stark, and it is upon us now.

_____

* I described my proposal for such a system in detail in my earlier book, *Fixing American Healthcare*.

_____

WHAT CAN WE DO AS INDIVIDUALS?

It is not my intention here to urge readers to engage in whatever political action might be necessary to have Obamacare repealed. I am not a politically active person, and I have no expertise in this area. Besides, the political pathway to getting rid of Obamacare has been tried once already, and it has failed. (Given the results of the 2012 election, it is no longer reasonable to blame the persistence of Obamacare on Justice Roberts.)

Like it or not, we are entering a period in which the prerogatives of individual Americans to purchase the healthcare we want with our own money will be under heavy assault. Progressives can do nothing else.

I understand how inflammatory this statement is. Further, I understand that the large majority of Americans who consider themselves to have progressive leanings will have no such behavior in mind, and will be extremely indignant that they are being accused of wanting to do such a thing. (The large majority of American progressives are mainly interested in doing good; of seeing to it that the disadvantaged are not left to be trampled in the mud; of assuring that a modicum of equity and fairness exists in our culture, and really have no interest in stifling individual autonomy, or undermining our Constitution – except to the extent necessary to achieve these good things.)

The real implications of the Progressive Program are very seldom described in detail by Progressive leaders, even to their progressive followers. They discuss their plans only by describing the near term benefits their efforts will produce (such as providing insurance for the uninsured), benefits which only the heartless can possibly dismiss. (Which immediately brands those of us who oppose their efforts as heartless.) But at its center, the Progressive Program utterly requires that individuals subsume their own "petty" and "selfish" interests for the good of the whole.

And when it comes to healthcare, this means that you will get the healthcare which the experts determine you should have, and no more. For the well-off (or the knowledgeable) to purchase "extra" healthcare outside of the system would not only be horribly unfair, it would also call into question the wisdom of the decisions being made by the experts. It would undermine the whole Program, and so it will need to be stopped. It will need to be stopped only for the best of reasons – for fairness and equity – but it must be stopped.

The right to use your own resources to protect your own well-being, of course, is essential and fundamental to the American idea. Once the

Progressives successfully establish the principle that, in the name of universal fairness, you may not do so, the whole concept of individual freedom evaporates, and with it, the Great American Experiment.

And so, here is the key to the whole mess: A truly Progressive healthcare system cannot exist without completely stifling the foundational American idea of individual autonomy. Conversely, the American idea of individual autonomy cannot persist without making a truly Progressive healthcare system impossible.

What this means is that, in order to prevent the worst of the damage which Obamacare – or any Progressive healthcare system – promises to inflict upon the American idea, and in order to force our leaders to come up with a healthcare system that is compatible with the Great American Experiment, a critical mass of individual Americans will have to stick to their guns, and do whatever it takes to exercise their inherent right to self-preservation. That is, they will have to act as autonomous individuals in the face of Progressivism. They will have to persist in this effort despite coercion, name-calling, demonization, and threats, and as they do so they will have to assert, loudly and often, that they are merely exercising a natural right granted to them by the Creator, a right which no human agency has the authority to take away.

If enough of us do this – whether our relationship to the healthcare system is as a doctor, a patient, or an entrepreneur – we will blaze a trail through the Progressive morass which others can follow. It will be slow going at first. Surveys looking at almost any healthcare system or any health insurance product traditionally show that something like 80% of participants are at least satisfied with what they have. This is because, at any given time, only 20% or so of patients (or citizens or subscribers) have had recent, personal encounters with the healthcare system. And people who have not had personal encounters within recent memory tend to believe all the hype about how wonderful everything is, especially since to believe otherwise would just create unactionable anxiety.

So those of us who refuse to accept what the Central Authority is handing out will not have all that much public sympathy, initially. But as time goes by and more and more people are exposed to the limitations inherent to, and the "misrepresentations" perpetrated by, any Progressive healthcare system, more and more people will be looking for alternatives, for some way to save themselves and their loved ones. And they will begin following the pathways cleared by the pioneers.

Once those pathways become highways, our Progressive healthcare system will no longer be feasible – because individual autonomy cannot persist without rendering a truly Progressive healthcare system impossible. Insisting on our own individual prerogatives is the key, and it is the key no matter what the Progressives do or don't do; no matter what the Republicans do or don't do. And eventually, we might finally be in a position to establish a healthcare system that solves our fiscal crisis, while still remaining compatible with the Great American Experiment.

The critical thing will be for us to invent ways to advance our own individual medical interests within the healthcare system (or outside of it), despite the best efforts of Progressives to stop us from doing so.

CHAPTER 16 - INDIVIDUALIZED MEDICINE - OUR LAST, BEST HOPE

"He is contemptuous of the people and of rule by majority vote, of electoral procedures and of free speech for anyone but himself. When he says that the best political system will come when rulers will become philosophers or when philosophers will rule, he means exactly that: that simple people are unfit to have an opinion about the affairs of state and that only specialists should be allowed to rule."

- Anthony Papadimitriou, Counsel for the prosecution in the New Trial of Socrates, Athens, Greece, May 25, 2012

———

Herd medicine – the top-down, centralized control of medical decisions as handed down by carefully selected panels of experts – is the hallmark of Progressive healthcare in general, and of Obamacare in particular. As we have seen, the entire structure of Obamacare is designed specifically to remove important (i.e., costly) medical decisions from the purview of the individual doctor and patient. The role of the doctor is now to relay expert-guided determinations of what is best for the herd down to the level of the individual patient, and to do it in such a way that their patients do not realize that the doctor's recommendations are population-based, and not tailored to their own needs. (Alternately, the doctors may try to convince their patients that population-based recommendations are in fact always the right recommendation for each individual. All too many doctors seem to have convinced themselves that this is actually the case.)

The role of patients under Obamacare is to trust the wisdom of the experts (as imparted to them by their doctors). They are to behave as Good Citizens, and comply fully and enthusiastically with their doctors' recommendations, for their own good and for the good of the whole. (Those old Soviet propaganda films accurately depict how Progressives view the ideal citizen: Happy, hearty peasants jauntily marching along to the tune of uplifting anthems, to their patriotic work in the collectivized fields.)

If everyone would simply behave in the prescribed manner, we would be one giant step closer to achieving the perfect society, and all would be well.

In this light, individualized medicine – using science and technology to tailor medical care to the best interest of the individual instead of the best interest of the herd – ought rightly to be seen as an existential threat to Progressive healthcare. Individualized medicine is the antithesis of herd medicine. If medical decisions are to be carefully tailored to the needs of each individual, centralizing the control of those decisions becomes impossible. Individual decision-making (and the individual autonomy that goes along with it) becomes necessarily predominant. It is hard to see how any truly Progressive healthcare system – and therefore, any truly Progressive system of government – can survive under a paradigm of individualized medicine.

For those of us who still value the Great American Experiment, and who see Obamacare as its death knell, individualized medicine may be our last best hope. For Progressives, it is something that must be nipped in the bud.

WHAT IS INDIVIDUALIZED MEDICINE, AND WHY IS IT SO IMPORTANT?

For the purposes of this discussion, individualized medicine means gathering specific physiological information pertaining to individuals, compiling that information into a digestible and actionable form, and presenting that compiled information to the individuals themselves (and to their doctors or other designated agents), in order that they may decide what action to take on behalf of their own well-being.

Today, individualized medicine, as I have just defined it, is feasible for the first time in history. It is feasible because of the fortuitous convergence of several technologies, including the Internet, ubiquitous wireless communication, massive data processing power, new physiologic sensors, the power of genomics, social networking, and smartphones (i.e., personal information and communication systems). These kinds of technologies are being brought to bear to provide individuals with the resources they need to manage almost every aspect of their lives – except their healthcare. I will describe later in this chapter why healthcare is lagging behind. But despite the lag, this remarkable technological convergence has made it possible to devise systems with which people can control their own healthcare in ways that were unimaginable a decade or two ago.

If these technologies are permitted to develop "naturally," over time they promise to render impossible a healthcare system built around top-down, centralized medical decision-making. By so doing they threaten to wreck Progressive healthcare.

Obviously, then, Progressives will do whatever they must to prevent these technologies from developing freely. So, whether individualized medicine ultimately overwhelms Progressive healthcare, or whether instead the Progressives manage to poison the whole thing before it ever really gets started, may very well turn out to be the main event, the battle that will determine where our healthcare system, and our society, ultimately will go.

WHAT WILL INDIVIDUALIZED MEDICINE LOOK LIKE?

It is always risky to try to predict the long-term results of emerging technologies. When the Wright brothers first launched themselves to the lofty height of 20 feet over the sands of Kitty Hawk, who would have predicted that a few decades later flying machines would be routinely transporting 300 people at a time from coast-to-coast in four hours – or that before boarding these machines all 300 of those people would have to remove their shoes and belts, raise their arms above their heads, and submit to intimate fondling by bored government agents? When Gutenberg printed his first Bible in the vernacular, who could have known that he had just launched an era of individual empowerment that eventually would result in the Declaration of Independence – but only after Western civilization first spent a couple of hundred years killing off its citizens in religious wars?

Trying to predict what individualized medicine will look like in ten years is a fool's errand. I will stipulate up front that nobody can know the directions which individualized medicine will take (if it is permitted to develop at all). Indeed, the possibilities seem almost endless. So I am going to limit myself to briefly reviewing the two general areas in which individualized medicine is poised to take off – personal biosensors and genomics.

PERSONAL BIOSENSORS

Numerous sensors exist or are being developed that can measure various interesting aspects of our physiology that can reflect the status of our health, help us detect acute illness, or assist us in managing chronic medical conditions. These biosensors can be worn on clothing or jewelry, held against the skin by a Band-aid-like adhesive patch, or inserted beneath the skin. They can be coupled with wireless technology that will allow them to communicate with a smartphone, a smart wristwatch, or the Internet. The data transmitted by these sensors can then be processed either locally (by a smartphone, for instance) or distantly (by powerful computers in communication with the Internet), and then presented to our doctor – or back to us – in a usable form.

Many uses for biosensors like these immediately come to mind. Indeed, the uses I am about to list are not the product of my fertile imagination, but are things that are being actively explored today, generally by small start-up companies nobody has ever heard of. Many of these technologies currently exist in one form or another, and have already been used, at least experimentally, in actual patients. The deployment of these things into general clinical usage does not depend on any new scientific breakthroughs, but only on our interest in having them.

Diabetes. A key to preventing many of the complications of diabetes is to keep the blood glucose levels within a relatively narrow range at all times – or as close to "at all times" as one can manage. New sensors are being developed that can measure blood glucose levels nearly continuously, which will allow insulin doses to be titrated much more precisely than current systems permit. These glucose sensors can even be coupled with a wearable, automatic insulin pump, to create a "closed-loop" system that automatically controls glucose levels – a virtual artificial pancreas.

Heart failure. Sensors that measure the resting heart rate, the rate of breathing, activity levels, the "angle of repose" (whether one is able to sleep flat, or must sleep with the head elevated), and body fluid levels can be used to monitor patients with chronic heart failure. Keeping track of these parameters can help medical personnel, or the patients themselves, more tightly manage the treatment of heart failure, to prevent symptoms from developing and reduce the need for hospitalization.

Asthma and chronic lung disease. Similarly, sensors can measure the rate of breathing, resting heart rate, the relative degree of obstruction of the airways, body temperature, and blood oxygen saturation, to help patients with asthma and chronic lung disease manage their conditions.

Neurological disorders. Sensors can be used to monitor balance, tremors, activity levels, and even mood changes in patients with neurological disorders such as Parkinson's disease.

Cardiac arrhythmias. Sensors deployed on a Band-aid-like patch can be worn comfortably for weeks at a time to check for known or suspected cardiac arrhythmias, such as atrial fibrillation. Knowing that certain arrhythmias are occurring can lead to treatment to prevent severe consequences (such as sudden death, or stroke).

Home care for the elderly or disabled. Sensors can be used to make the home environment safer for elderly people or people with disabilities, and thus can make living at home feasible for these people when it otherwise might not be. These sensors can monitor activity levels, changes in balance, sleep quality, medication compliance, the state of hydration, and changes in vital signs.

Sleep disorders. Unobtrusive biosensors can monitor sleep apnea, as well as general sleep quality (by tracking the duration of total sleep, and of REM sleep). Formal sleep studies, which today require an expensive, in-hospital, ungainly, uncomfortable process which can only be done for special indications, could be conducted routinely and cheaply at home, as often as might be desired.

Blood pressure monitors. Sensors that can measure blood pressure either continuously or frequently can revolutionize the therapy of hypertension, which today is all too often done poorly.

Heart attack detectors and stroke detectors. Sensors that can detect acute heart attacks or acute strokes (conditions in which rapid treatment can prevent permanent disability or death) do not yet exist, but are conceptually possible. Such sensors could reduce the delays in treatment that are often seen today with these acute conditions.

Dysautonomia. The dysautonomias are a family of often-disabling disorders which include vasomotor syncope, inappropriate sinus tachycardia, postural orthostatic tachycardia syndrome, and post-traumatic stress disorder, among several others. These conditions are commonly characterized by rapid, unexplained fluctuations in heart rate, blood pressure, breathing rate, and skin temperature. The dysautonomia disorders are very often misdiagnosed by doctors as "anxiety." Biosensors could help to pin down the diagnosis, and help in the management of these often very frustrating conditions.

Miniaturization and personalization of sophisticated diagnostics. Current technology would allow the SIM cards inserted into a smartphone to rapidly analyze a drop of blood, urine, or saliva for electrolyte disturbances or chemical imbalances. A transducer plugged into a smartphone could convert the device to a portable echocardiogram machine, so that the heart, blood vessels, and certain other organs could be visualized.

The possibilities abound, and I have only scratched the surface.

All the technologies I have listed (most of which exist today, and all of which are entirely feasible) are very threatening to any healthcare system which is built around the centralization of every important medical decision. Deploying these sensors will inherently individualize medical care – by providing specific, actionable physiological information, on an as-needed basis, to the affected individuals themselves. Judgments must necessarily be made locally (either by the doctor and patient working together, or – heaven forbid! – by the patient him-or-herself) on how to respond to this information, in order to optimize medical care according to the often-fluid needs of the individual. The centralized decision-makers are cut out altogether.

Under Obamacare this will never do.

HUMAN GENOMICS

If you have not been paying attention, you may have missed some of the remarkable things we have learned about human genetics since the completion of the Human Genome Project in 2000. This would be understandable, since the common wisdom is that we really haven't gotten much out of it. This general perception was well illustrated on its 10-year anniversary, when numerous publications (such as the *New York Times* and the *Wall Street Journal*) offered postmortems on the Human Genome Project with titles like, "The Failed Promise of Genomics."

It is true that scientists haven't yet cured cancer or stopped the aging process, as we were all promised. But we have nonetheless learned a lot.

The human genome turns out to be much more complex than anyone had predicted. The basics haven't changed, of course. DNA still consists of long, paired polymer strands of four different bases, with every three base pairs coding for one amino acid. At appropriate times the code is translated, and the appropriate amino acids are assembled into proteins. Each gene codes for one protein.

Given the six billion bases contained in the 23 paired chromosomes of the human genome, everyone was expecting that the human genome would contain at least 100,000 distinct genes. But that's not the case. It turns out that the entire human genome codes for only 23,000 genes. Indeed, researchers now tell us, nearly 99% of the DNA in the human genome does not code for any genes at all.

So what is all that "extra" DNA doing? It seems that most of our DNA actually codes for various species of RNA, and that the RNA serves a regulatory function. Our genome, it appears, is an extraordinarily highly-regulated system. All of that regulatory RNA helps to determine when a gene will code for a protein and when it will not, under various times and circumstances, and in various organs and cells – and even helps to determine the function of that protein once it is coded. The amazingly complex regulatory influences, tugging this way and that on every gene, makes it relatively unlikely that a single mutation in a single gene will result in that gene having a runaway influence over some important physiological function. Indeed, it appears that the remarkable regulatory complex that is our genome has evolved, over many millennia, specifically to keep things from changing radically should a gene go awry.

The human genome thus resembles what a Progressive society would look like if human nature could be perfectly controlled, and society could thus develop as Progressives have envisioned. That is, for every worker who is actually producing a product, there are 99 experts and regulators telling him or her what to do. They are busily making sure the worker is doing precisely the assigned task, at the right time and place, without a nanosecond or a millimeter of variation. In other words, the huge majority of what the human genome appears to be doing is the biologic equivalent of paperwork.

Another thing we have learned is that only a very few diseases can be tied to the simple, single-gene mutations of classic Mendelian genetics. Rather, it appears, most genetically-influenced diseases are related to the summation of the behaviors of many different genes. Furthermore, thanks to the extremely tight regulation inherent in our genome, most of the genetic variants that have been identified seem to merely influence, rather than to determine, whether a person develops a disease. So the odds that an individual will develop most kinds of genetic-related diseases is not definitively determined just by knowing what is in the genome. In most cases, the odds of developing most genetic-based diseases is a probabilistic function rather than a deterministic one.

Therefore, every person's genome is a cauldron of probabilities. And researchers are rapidly assembling a database of specific combinations of genetic variants, along with the probabilities these genetic variants yield for the specific diseases with which they are associated. This database is growing monthly.

It is now possible for you to send a DNA sample to one of a few companies for a GWAS analysis – a Genome Wide Association Study. The GWAS will yield your lifetime probabilities of developing a whole series of various diseases. A GWAS does not sequence every one of your base pairs (that kind of study is called whole genome sequencing). Rather, it uses a catalog of known single-nucleotide polymorphisms (SNPs) to map various known regions of your genome for variants known to be associated with particular diseases.

If you were to have a GWAS done, for instance, you might find out that you have a 75% lifetime probability of developing prostate cancer. This knowledge might cause you to decide to have that PSA screening test (or to wish you could have one, since the United States Preventive Services Task Force now says you may not). A 10% probability of developing prostate cancer, on the other hand, might make you OK with the recent USPSTF directive prohibiting the PSA testing.

An area where GWAS appears to offer a particularly tangible benefit is in pharmacogenetics – associating genetic variants with the response to drug therapy. It looks like genetic variations are quite deterministic (as opposed to probabilistic) when it comes to a person's response to drugs. This is likely because we humans have not had time to evolve the regulatory RNA necessary to mitigate drug-related issues, so single-gene variations affecting the response to drugs are much more likely to be expressed.

For instance, GWAS has allowed researchers to predict, with a high degree of accuracy, which patients with hepatitis C will respond to interferon therapy. GWAS can also tell doctors which patients will fail to respond to Plavix – a blood thinner which is important in patients who receive stents for coronary artery disease. Perhaps more importantly, it looks like GWAS may be able to predict which people are likely to have specific side effects from specific drugs, for instance, to have muscle or liver toxicity from statins.

GWAS, then, may turn out to be important for drug therapy, both to predict the likelihood of a response in an individual, and to predict the likelihood of specific side effects. GWAS may even help to "resurrect" drugs that have been removed from the market because of side effects – drugs like Vioxx, which relieved painful symptoms in many patients who were not helped by other anti-inflammatory agents. If we are able to say ahead of time which individuals will have side effects and which will not, we can target drug therapy only to the people who can take them safely.

Some day, all of us may routinely choose to have GWAS performed. Then, as the database of genetic associations grows, each person would have an ever-expanding list of specific lifetime probabilities of developing various diseases, and, more importantly, an expanding list of likely responses (favorable and unfavorable) to specific drugs. This latter benefit is likely to turn out to be the most practical use for GWAS.

Whole Genome Sequencing (WGS) – mapping out every single one of the 6 billion bases in a person's chromosomes – so far is prohibitively expensive to do routinely, but the cost is coming down exponentially. WGS has proven useful, in several cases, in identifying a specific genetic abnormality that is causing a disease that has been difficult to diagnose or treat. Knowing the precise genetic abnormality can help to target therapy to the specific protein with which it is associated.

The most obvious use of WGS is in the treatment of cancer. Cancer, by definition, is caused by a mutation in the human genome. By comparing the genome of a patient's cancer cells with the genome of the patient's non-cancer cells (a process that requires doing two full WGS analyses, and then painstakingly comparing the two results), it has been possible to target therapy at the root cause of a patient's specific cancer. So, instead of using chemotherapy aimed at "breast cancer," therapy can be aimed instead at the specific genetic abnormality being displayed by the patient's actual breast cancer cells. This optimal therapy may turn out to be treatment that is typically used for leukemia or prostate cancer, for instance, instead of for breast cancer. By specifically targeting therapy at the individual's own cancer cells, the probability of a favorable response can be greatly increased.

Today, the great expense and severe impracticality of doing WGS for cancer, or for other diseases, precludes using this method except in a very few exceptional cases. But in those cases, early results have been quite encouraging. I will give just one example.

On July 12, 2012, the *New York Times* reported on the case of Dr. Lucas Wartman, a young physician who developed adult acute lymphoblastic leukemia, a disease that is usually rapidly fatal, and for which there is no effective treatment. Dr. Wartman's colleagues at Washington University performed WGS on his cancer cells, and on his normal cell line. The job required round-the clock work for many days by the University's 26 sequencing machines, a supercomputer, and several senior scientists. But after making this monumental effort they discovered a single gene mutation in his cancer cells that was producing a protein that appeared to be stimulating the cancer's growth. It turned out that a new drug existed that was targeted specifically at shutting down the offending protein, a drug that to that point had been used only for kidney cancer. When they administered the drug to Dr. Wartman, his cancer went into complete remission.

Discovering the "right" treatment for Dr. Wartman's specific cancer would not have been possible without WGS. The cost of doing routine WGS is currently prohibitive, but the cost has come down remarkably in just a few years, and in a few more years is likely to be within the range of costs we typically see in the healthcare system.

So, while the aging process has not been halted, and while cancer has not been cured, the mapping of the human genome has opened up a whole new field of endeavor for understanding, preventing and treating a host of diseases.

By definition, using a person's genetic makeup to guide their medical care is individualized medicine. It is not herd medicine. As in the case of Dr. Wartman, genome-based therapy will require gathering specific genetic information about an individual, and puzzling out a unique solution for the individual's medical problem. Genome-guided medicine cannot be dictated or controlled by a centralized panel of experts handing down generalized directives. It utterly undermines the underlying operating principle of a Progressive healthcare system.

Therefore, we should expect our Progressive healthcare system to make every effort to stifle it.

How Will Individualized Medicine Be Stifled?

If it turns out I am wrong about all this, that I am being unreasonably paranoid about what the Progressives will do in response to individualized medicine, all the better. For, if Progressives fail to take steps to stop individualized medicine and instead allow it to evolve naturally, then the Progressive healthcare system which I described in Part 2 of this book is doomed to fail, and all will be well. So I hope that, as many readers undoubtedly believe, I am simply being paranoid.

Unfortunately I do not see how this is possible. I assert that Progressives, eventually and one way or another, will have to pull out all the stops to cut off individualized medicine. They will have no choice in the matter, because individualized medicine fundamentally undermines their entire program. It is a simple issue of survival for the Progressives.

Inhibiting the Development of Biosensors

When it comes to inhibiting the development of personal biosensors, it is unfortunately true that Progressives will have to do very little additional work. The healthcare system as it currently exists, even before Obamacare takes effect in any major way, makes it extremely difficult to make much progress on this front.

I have had a fair amount of personal experience in this area. When I left medicine in 2000 (after 25 years of hands-on medical practice), I was recruited by the CEO of a major medical device company to serve on a 5-person "skunk-works" team he was assembling, that was charged with advising the company on (and I quote) "what to do about the Internet."

Uninitiated readers might blanch at the idea that a major biotech company took so long to figure out that the Internet was more than just a flash in the pan, and was, in fact, something that ought to be considered in long-term business plans. Consider this startling fact to be an introduction to the idea that the healthcare system – from top to bottom – tends to be fundamentally conservative and sclerotic in outlook. This is what happens when you function in a system where every step you take is massively regulated – once you learn to survive in such a dystopian environment, then anything really new that comes along tends to be viewed as a major threat to your modestly satisfactory existence. Fundamental innovation is to be avoided, and if it cannot be avoided, then it is adopted as slowly (and painfully) as possible. This is a hallmark of heavily regulated systems – you get stability of a sort, but not innovation. (Again, the similarity to the human genome is striking.) If you doubt my words, ask yourself why the healthcare system has had to be dragged, kicking and screaming, to adopt electronic medical records, or why doctors still have not discovered e-mail.

Our skunk-works team consisted of myself (serving in the role of grizzled clinician) and four brilliant bioengineers, who were young enough and low enough in the company hierarchy to still maintain their air of excitement at the idea of innovation as a way of improving peoples' lives. Remarkably, as it turned out all five of us had been independently thinking about the application of the Internet to modern medicine, and when we began brainstorming together our thoughts dovetailed. Within a few hours we had agreed on the broad outline of our plan.

Our thinking went like this: The company (a manufacturer of pacemakers and implantable defibrillators) already had their products positioned inside patients' bodies. Those products contained sophisticated, battery-driven microprocessors that took electrical signals from the heart, processed those signals with complex algorithms, and accurately decided to deliver or withhold therapy (a pacing impulse, or a defibrillating shock) on a moment to moment basis. Why not take advantage of: a) the inside-the-body location, b) the microprocessor, and c) the existing expertise with algorithm development, to deploy biosensors in these devices, biosensors that could detect useful information about a patient's physiology? Such information could easily be transmitted outside the body by inserting, say, a Bluetooth radio in these devices to send data to some sort of external relay, which could then send it on to the Internet. (Smartphones did not exist in those days.) In this way the data gathered by the biosensors could be passed on to more powerful computers at the server level, and applied to more sophisticated algorithms, and even combined with data from other sources (the patient's medical history or medication list, for instance), in order to turn it into actionable information. This information could then be distributed to whoever ought to see it – the patient, the doctor, the patient's family, etc.

We then spent time compiling a list of biosensors that either existed or could be rapidly developed, and with that list devised another list consisting of the medical conditions that could benefit from monitoring these biosensors. (The list we devised looked remarkably like the list I produced earlier in this chapter. Many would-be innovators have come up with similar lists.)

Our value proposition was this: By using targeted biosensors to monitor a patient's physiology, we could enable the precise titration of therapy for chronic medical conditions, thus preventing acute exacerbations of those conditions. Expensive hospitalizations could be avoided; patients would remain healthier and happier; and lots of money could be saved. Since the healthcare system would save so much money, we figured naively, a mechanism could easily be devised to return a portion of those cost savings to the company that was producing them.

Because a relatively high proportion of patients who received the company's products had chronic heart failure, we recommended that heart failure should be the initial focus for the company. Accordingly, we devised a first-pass algorithm which incorporated several readily-available biosensors to assist in the management of heart failure. After working diligently for three months, we had a business proposal ready, and a formal presentation before the company's top management was scheduled.

After listening to our presentation with increasing dismay, management tossed us out of the board room on our respective ears. To say that our proposal was ill-received would be to understate the matter significantly. They more than hated it; they were horrified by it.

There were several reasons the top executives were horrified. A few of those reasons were bogus, and can be attributed to a general fear of embarking on a major change in the company's direction. But two of those reasons were quite legitimate, and made their decision to banish our skunkworks team into the wilderness the correct call.

First, despite our naive assumption that surely the healthcare system would be willing to spend a little money in order to save a lot of money, this is not the case. The healthcare system does not reason like this. It reasons like a bureaucracy. For practical purposes, the only things a company (or a doctor) can get paid for in our modern healthcare system are healthcare services for which a Medicare billing code already exists. If you devise a new kind of medical service for which there is no code, you have only two pathways to payment. You can petition Medicare to create a new billing code, and then ask them to assign to the new code a reasonable reimbursement value. This two-step process typically takes several years, and there is no guarantee of success – in fact, odds are that you will fail. Or, you can rationalize a way to shoehorn your new medical service into an existing code, and convince Medicare that your rationalization is justifiable. This pathway has a higher probability of succeeding in a reasonable period of time (say, a year or so) – but then you must accept the reimbursement that is already in place for that pre-existing code, and you must accept it, essentially, forever.

No billing code existed for our biosensor proposal, and the company's management understandably expressed no interest in embarking on the lengthy and difficult process of pursuing a new billing code. And any existing billing codes into which we might conceivably have shoehorned our new service reimbursed only a pittance – not nearly enough to cover our costs, let alone to make the endeavor profitable.

The bottom line was that the only conceivable way for the company to profit from our proposal was to add our proposed heart failure management system as a new "feature" to their pacemakers and implantable defibrillators, essentially at no extra charge. The company would have to rely on this new feature enticing doctors to select its implantable devices over some other company's devices. In other words, it would have to be a pure market-share play.

And this brings us to the second very legitimate reason top management was right to send our team to the woodshed. Far from enticing doctors to choose this company's devices over the devices of other companies, our heart failure management system would have doctors avoiding this product in droves. The V.P. of Marketing said it best: "The last thing our doctors want is a data dump, especially data they never asked for in the first place, but which is dumped on them at the whim of some defibrillator they implanted in some patient two years ago. You say it won't be a data dump, but a reporting of pre-digested, actionable information. Did the doctor ask for that actionable information? Did he ask for it at 3 AM? What is his liability if he fails to act on it within 24 hours, within an hour, within a minute? And does he even remember who the hell this patient is? And how is he supposed to get paid to do this job he never asked for in the first place? Just as there are no billing codes for our company to be reimbursed, there are equally no billing codes for the doctor to be reimbursed for interpreting and acting upon the unsolicited data we are foisting off on him. We will have just placed this doctor on-call, 24/7, for every patient he's ever implanted a device in, forever, and without pay. And you think the threat of doing this to doctors is going to entice them to select our devices over the devices of our competitors? And finally, if we do this thing, even if the doctor never ever uses one of our defibrillators ever again — as you must admit seems likely — we will have created an expectation out in the world. This product will exist, and doctors who choose to avoid it will be seen as bad doctors, and potentially will be liable for failing to use available technology in patients who might benefit. Not only will doctors avoid our devices, but we will be creating an actual, visceral, permanent hatred for our company among our customers for unleashing such a travesty upon the world. And then our company will cease to exist — and with just cause."

These, one must admit, are pretty good arguments.

Like the residue from an actual skunk, however, our team proved pretty persistent, and a couple of years later we managed to convince the company to make implantable devices that talked to the Internet — but only to transmit data about the device's own functionality, and not the patient's. This feature proved to be very useful and very popular, in that it enabled any device malfunction to be quickly detected and dealt with. Because there was still no viable alternative, it was indeed added to devices as a pure "feature" without additional charge, as a market-share strategy. And, as is almost always the case with market-share strategies, the advantage to the company was temporary. The competition soon added their own similar features. So at the end of the day, the cost of doing business went up for all the companies in this space, and their profit margins went down — without much net change in market share for anyone. This kind of experience does not encourage similar innovations in the future.

Never one to give up easily on what I consider to be a good idea, five years ago I signed on as the chief medical officer for a start-up company which aimed to devise wearable biosensors to help manage medical conditions. We designed an adhesive patch that contained several biosensors and which communicated with the Internet, that could be worn comfortably (including during sleep, showers, and vigorous exercise) for up to two weeks at a time. We decided to focus initially (again) on heart failure, since the healthcare system by this time had explicitly identified heart failure hospitalizations as a major financial drain, and healthcare bureaucrats were making a lot of noise about employing (and paying for) systems that would reduce these hospitalizations. Also, it looked to us as if doctors – having by now been made wards of the state – would soon have to use such systems whether they liked it or not, once they were ordered to do so.

We actually accomplished quite a bit. We built the devices, derived an algorithm based on several biosensors to monitor the status of heart failure, did a large clinical trial in patients with heart failure to prove that the algorithm worked, and saw a peer-reviewed paper published that documented the effectiveness of the biosensor-based algorithm. Things were looking up.

That's when the regulators noticed that several entrepreneurs were doing similar things – developing systems for chronically monitoring the physiology of patients with sundry medical conditions – and they became very concerned about it. I am willing to concede to skeptics that their concern may only have been subliminally about individualized healthcare. Their more proximate concern, likely, was the fact that an entirely new area of medical service was being invented right under their feet, and they were worried that (despite the claims of the inventors) it was going to increase the cost of healthcare. In any case, regulatory action was required to suppress it.

And so regulators, without issuing any formal change in policy, began quietly relating to these companies that from now on, before any such "diagnostic" could be approved, it was very likely that the company would no longer merely have to demonstrate that their product accurately measured exactly what it said it was measuring (such as, in our case, that when we said a person's heart failure was slipping out of control, the heart failure was actually slipping out of control). Rather, companies would have to prove, in a long-term, randomized clinical trial, that using their product would significantly improve the actual clinical outcome of the patients enrolled.

This new sub rosa regulatory requirement essentially blew us out of the water. Randomized clinical trials proving that a therapy changes clinical outcomes are difficult and expensive enough to operate. But when you are testing a diagnostic instead of a therapy, the proposition becomes an order of magnitude more difficult. This is because when testing a diagnostic, the clinical outcome does not merely depend on your product (as it generally does in a therapy trial), but also on the decisions the doctor and patient make in response to the information your product is giving them. How a doctor may act in response to actionable clinical information is extremely variable. And how a patient accepts the doctor's recommendations, and follows them, is also variable. Such clinical actions are entirely out of the control of the company, and are entirely unrelated to the accuracy of the information the product is providing the doctor and patient.

A quick back-of-the-envelope calculation revealed to us that conducting such a clinical trial would probably cost more than the estimated valuation of the entire company. Not only could we not afford it, but also it was impossible to consider going to outside investors for that magnitude of additional funding. (Only the government is routinely bone-headed enough to "invest" far more money in a favored company than that company could ever be worth.) At that point the company's leadership made an executive decision to put heart failure on the shelf. Fortunately, they have been able to redirect their technology to a much more mundane, less exciting, less useful-to-mankind – but reimbursable – application, so at the moment the company is actually doing pretty well. And maybe – when it becomes as flush as Apple and can afford to take the risk – heart failure will be taken up again.

But for at least the foreseeable future this company has stopped attempting to advance the management of heart failure, or any of the other chronic or acute medical conditions which biosensors can address – and consequently it is no longer advancing the cause of individualized healthcare in any substantial way. That effort has been successfully suppressed.

So my personal experience has taught me that the roadblocks to applying personal biosensors to advance individualized medicine are substantial. There are roadblocks regarding reimbursement. (How can you get paid in a timely manner for a new medical service for which billing codes do not exist?) There are roadblocks regarding the willingness of physicians to change the way they practice. (Individualized medicine, in which doctors might have to react at any time to information that might pop up about one of their patients, without any pathway for receiving payment for such services, is far from an attractive proposition for doctors.) And the regulatory pathway for gaining approval for biosensor-based products has rapidly become virtually prohibitive for any but the largest enterprises.

So, while personal biosensors, in theory, pose a major threat to a Progressive healthcare system, in practice it is going to be a huge challenge to advance these biosensors to the point where they can truly enable individualized healthcare. In fact, to have any chance of getting there some creative strategies will need to be developed, because the traditional pathways have been all but blocked.

THE COMING BATTLE OVER HUMAN GENOMICS

Nothing in the material world defines us as individuals as much as our own personal genome. And while the last decade has taught us that the manner in which our genetic makeup is expressed is far more complex than we had ever dreamed, we have also learned – through occasional blinding new insights – that genomics is the key toward targeting therapy, in previously unimagined ways, to the specific cause of a specific disease in a specific individual. If we allow this line of investigation to continue to its logical outcome, very much of medical care, if not all, will eventually be tailored to the individual.

And nothing I can think of poses a more dire threat to herd medicine.

Since the top-down, centralized control of all important medical decisions is the fundamental organizational structure of Progressive healthcare, genomics-based healthcare ought to be seen as an existential threat by Progressives. They should, one might think, be taking steps to stifle it.

While admittedly I do not have the sort of "inside scoop" regarding genomics that I might have with biosensors, I find it striking that few such stifling efforts by Progressives seem visible. Indeed, far from stifling it Progressives seem happy to let genomic science develop – for now, at least. The Human Genome Project was funded by the government, after all. And the efforts of the government-funded NIH are instrumental in continuing the development of knowledge based on the human genome. I see no signs that government funding for these efforts is going to be slackened any time soon.

How can it be that a Progressive healthcare system, if anything, seems to be encouraging genomic research, when individualized healthcare is such a threat to the Progressives' entire program? There are several possible answers to this question, and we should consider all of them.

Perhaps I have the entire thesis of this book wrong. Perhaps centralizing the control of all healthcare decisions is not the fundamental tenet of Progressive healthcare. But I submit that the contents of this book, explaining the behaviors we see in our Progressive healthcare system in light of this fundamental tenet, strongly mitigate against this possibility. Readers, of course, must consider the strength of this argument for themselves.

Perhaps Progressives are so excited by the possibilities for curing terrible diseases, cures made conceivable by genomics research, that it has overwhelmed the natural enmity they would otherwise feel for such an individualized approach to healthcare. Indeed, it is very likely that your typical, run-of-the-mill progressive, the ones who join you around the dinner table at Thanksgiving, are overtaken with this kind of enthusiasm (if they have actually looked into the implications – either positive or negative – of genomic research at all). I am skeptical, on the other hand, that Progressive leaders – the ones who are making the decisions, and who, for instance, undermine the Constitution every chance they get – have let their enthusiasm for medical cures overwhelm their animosity for anything that returns the control of medical decisions to individuals.

The final possibility, the one that is most disturbing, but unfortunately the one that appears most probable, is that Progressives have no intention of stifling genomics research, because instead they intend to control it.

People tend to get very angry when you accuse them of espousing eugenics. So I hasten to assert that I am not accusing Progressives of espousing eugenics – yet. I am merely advising prudence.

When you have a known, convicted sex offender living down the street, even if you have met him and he seems at the moment to be an entirely reasonable and steady person, if your eight-year-old daughter must walk past his house on her way to the school bus it is likely you will take every precaution to make sure nothing untoward happens to her. This is because, as a general rule, something in the makeup of sex offenders makes them likely recidivists. You should never quite trust them around your kids, no matter how normal they may appear at the moment.

In a similar way, eugenics is not merely a prominent facet of the history of Progressivism, it is in the DNA of Progressivism. And while their regulatory RNA seems to have kept it in check for the past several decades, their past history alone ought to give us great pause. We should no more give Progressives control over genomics than we should give our ex-alcoholic brother-in-law control over our liquor cabinet. If they, or our brother-in-law, should become indignant about our refusal to trust them completely, we should not bend. Their past actions have placed us in this position. We should only explain that we love them very much, and for that reason will not willingly allow temptation to get in their way.

The history of the eugenics movement among American Progressives is remarkable, and equally remarkable is the relative success with which that history has been expunged from popular memory. I submit that this is a form of amnesia in which, at this moment in our history, we cannot afford to indulge.

I will not go into a detailed description of the late eugenics movement. I will merely point out that for a half-century it was openly and enthusiastically espoused by the cream of the Progressive crop, and it was more than merely a point of discussion. Involuntary sterilizations were conducted on "undesirables" across the country, and doctors were encouraged to let "defective" babies die. The *New York Times* encouraged at least the passive euthanasia of defective individuals, urging its readers to look upon such "medical care" "without the horrified exclamations of unenlightened sentimentality."

I could go on, but I will just make one more point to illustrate the prominence of eugenics in the early 20th century. In 1927, the United States Supreme Court heard the case of *Buck v. Bell*, which challenged the constitutionality of the involuntary sterilization program then in operation in Virginia. The Court ruled eight to one that the sterilization program was entirely constitutional, and furthermore, Chief Justice Oliver Wendell Holmes in his opinion made the case that involuntary sterilization of undesirables was a natural and useful thing to do, and is well supported by objective science. Holmes wrote: "It is better for all the world, if instead of waiting to execute degenerate offspring for crime, or let them starve for their imbecility, society can prevent those who are manifestly unfit from breeding their kind. The principle that sustains compulsory vaccination is broad enough to cover cutting Fallopian tubes." Then, addressing the case of the unfortunate young woman whose proposed sterilization had brought the issue before the Court, "Three generations of imbeciles are enough."

And there we see, starkly revealed, what really underlies Progressive compassion. (As one who has been called an imbecile, and far worse, by Progressives who have stumbled upon my blog, such sentimentalities must give me pause.)

The point I am making here is that for many decades eugenics was mainstream. Proudly, enthusiastically, loudly, and assertively mainstream.

The second point I want to make about the American eugenics movement is that it was no fluke. The conditions that led Progressives to embrace it still exist. They will always exist.

Progressives started out, as they invariably do, with the best of intentions, that is, they deeply desired to help the downtrodden. So in the late 19th century they instituted all manner of reforms aimed to lift up the poor, the disabled, and the criminals (who, they believed, were criminals only because they acted in ways that displeased the rich). Unfortunately, as will always be the case, the objects of their sympathetic efforts did not respond in the manner predicted by Progressive dogma – many of them did not become ideal citizens. Far from it.

Because it could not possibly be the Progressive Program that was mistaken, the fault could only lie with the inherently defective natures of the people they were trying to help. It followed, then, that the real fault must be in the genes of these unfortunates. And so, it became clear that in order for the Progressive Program to advance as it would benefit all mankind for it to advance, something had to be done about the gene pool. And hence, eugenics.

Here's the thing. It seems unlikely to me that human nature has changed very much during the past century. And it seems just as unlikely today as it was a hundred years ago that the citizenry will simply comply, fully and uncomplainingly, with the Progressive Program.

Progressives always begin the same way. They assume that, because their system is so inherently logical and scientific, any reasonable person will immediately see the benefits of submitting to the expert-driven system (whichever one they are pushing at any given time) they have prescribed for us. And when human nature compels many of us to fail to subsume our own individual interests to the interests of the whole, Progressives begin to get frustrated.

At first, they attribute the failure of their program to insufficiently educating the public about the great and wonderful benefits of it. As I write this, President Obama has just allowed that the greatest failure of his Presidency, so far, is the failure to "tell the right story." That is, it's his failure to sufficiently educate us, the great unwashed, on the righteousness of his historical journey to a fundamentally different society. This is the classical first-pass Progressive reaction to the people's mule-like refusal to submit.

When we still refuse to behave as prescribed, even after efforts at educating us have been redoubled, the Progressives invariably come to the conclusion that the actual problem is something other than their suboptimal explanations of benefits. The only other possibility, of course, is that they are dealing with substandard material. We in the unwashed – many of us, at least – just don't stack up.

Anyone who does not accept the pure logic and scientific correctness of the Progressives, even after all efforts have been made to teach us the right path, can only be evil, stupid or crazy. One is justified, of course, in simply doing away with the evil ones. The ones who are stupid or crazy may deserve a bit more compassion – but still, they need to be dealt with.

And sooner or later it occurs to Progressives that, at the very least, these people need to be kept from propagating, lest their recalcitrance be passed on down through the generations. The Progressive Program requires – absolutely requires – a citizenry that understands the overall goodness of what Progressives are attempting to do. And how can such a thing be achieved if the people who don't get it – who can never get it, through their own inherent shortcomings – keep perpetuating their genetic material?

Look. I am not saying that today's progressives are engaging in eugenics, or openly espousing it, or even secretly espousing it. I am merely pointing out that the same circumstances that led them to adopt eugenics in the past – to a remarkable and stomach-churning extent, to such an extent that only the atrocities of the Nazis at last made them back off – still exist today.

The general population, forever slaves to human nature, will still be as recalcitrant to the prescribed program as they have been in the past, and Progressives will become no less frustrated by it. Medical ethicists are already beginning to broach the idea of a kinder, gentler form of eugenics – a type they refer to as "positive eugenics," in which people with undesirable traits are "discouraged" from propagating. Most Progressives, I'll stipulate, are not thinking about eugenics today. But the ethical groundwork is being laid for them and will be ready when they get around to it.

And today, thanks to genomics research, the ever objective and scientific Progressives will be more likely than ever to convince themselves that they've got the tools they need for determining which genetic traits can be considered positive and which are negative.

While the notion of eugenics may remain subliminal at the moment for most Progressives, I am arguing that the very nature of the Progressive program will almost inevitably – if it hasn't already – bring the consideration of eugenics (doubtless renamed to something with less negative historical implications) to the fore. We have placed that ex-alcoholic brother-in-law in charge of our liquor cabinet.

If I am correct, the Progressives will be doing something of a balancing act. They will need to allow genomics research to proceed, but while somehow discouraging the development of individualized medicine that would naturally result from it.

In this effort they will have the support of their ever-vigilant allies, the medical ethicists. In reporting on the Wartman case, the *New York Times* also dug up several medical ethicists for suitable comment. And of course their remarks indicate that it is indeed unethical to offer such avant-garde therapy to the well-connected. The ethicists question "whether those with money and connections should have options far out of reach for most patients before such treatments become a normal part of medicine." The chair of the department of bioethics at the University of Washington asks, "If we say we need research because this is a new idea, then why is it that rich people can even access it?"

This is the usual Progressive "fairness" argument, in which we are to achieve equity not by raising up the have-nots, but by tearing down the haves. By the same ethical argument, no major advance in medicine would be able to proceed. Most radical, ground-breaking advances initially require expensive equipment, hundreds of expert man-hours, or procedures that by their very natures can be used, at first, in only a few patients. By this ethical standard we would never have had things like organ transplants, robotic surgery, implantable medical devices, or even coronary artery bypass surgery or MRI scans.

This is a fine argument for stifling medical progress in general, but it is particularly suited for stifling individualized medicine. It is an argument that, if accepted, will permit genomic research to continue, but will simultaneously preclude the application of genomics to solve the unique disorders of specific individuals, as in the case of Dr. Wartman.

So What Now?

Individualized medicine, fully developed, would completely undermine the fundamental paradigm of Progressive healthcare, and would require us to reform the healthcare system in different way – in a way that is compatible with the Great American Experiment, that is, with the primacy of the individual as its organizing principle.

It is therefore inevitable that Progressives will try to smother individualized medicine in its crib. They have made an excellent start at it, with a rigid government-controlled payment system that does not easily recognize new kinds of medical services, onerous regulatory policies that make it extraordinarily difficult to bring this type of product to market, and the enervated sclerosis of a medical profession struggling just to keep its head above water. This "excellent start" merely reflects the long-term results of a gradual shift to a Progressive healthcare system. Obamacare merely accelerates that trend, and makes the real intent of Progressive healthcare quite stark for anyone who cares to see. The question of repealing Obamacare, given the current state of things, is likely to determine not whether we will have a Progressive healthcare system, but merely what trajectory we will take in getting there.

Yet, the tools for individualized medicine are right there before us, tantalizingly close. And whether Obamacare is repealed or not, individualized medicine, threatened as it is, remains our last, best hope for reasserting individual autonomy in our healthcare system.

A critical mass of people who insist on asserting their inalienable rights despite the Progressives, a few entrepreneurs who find creative ways to supply them with the tools they need, and a few brave doctors who rededicate themselves to the traditional doctor-patient relationship, can allow individualized healthcare to progress to the point where everyone will demand it. Indeed, as long as enough Americans refuse to surrender their individual autonomy, it is difficult to see how a Progressive healthcare system can persist in the long run.

In the next chapter, the last chapter of this book, I will address what we each should do if we want to preserve individual autonomy in American healthcare, and in our culture.

CHAPTER 17 - WHAT WE NEED TO DO

"You are not only responsible for what you say, but also for what you do not say."
- Martin Luther

"The buck stops with you."
- Barack Obama

Whatever Conservatives do in their efforts to overturn Obamacare, whatever Progressives do to uphold it, whether Republicans win at the polls, or whether Democrats do, herd medicine can only work if we citizens agree to become bovines.

This is the key.

As we have seen, Obamacare – and any Progressive healthcare system – absolutely requires centralizing major healthcare decisions; it requires removing those decisions away from the doctors and the patients who are immediately affected by them. Hence, Obamacare is constructed to utterly control the behavior of physicians. And this is why so much has been done already to prevent individuals from being able to bypass the official healthcare system, to purchase medical services the Central Authority thinks they should not have. The reason Progressives must suffocate individual prerogatives is not, as many claim, because they are power-hungry. While many of them (being human) do indeed become power hungry, that is not their primary motivation. Their primary motivation is to achieve the perfect society envisioned by the Progressive Program, a goal that requires society to be directed by enlightened experts. There is simply no room to allow individuals – imperfect, self-interested individuals with nothing grander on their minds than their own comfort and happiness – to make their own decisions in areas that are critical to the Progressive Program.

And healthcare is critical to the Program.

It is thus necessary for the sake of the Program for the people to sacrifice certain of their individual prerogatives. Progressives invariably begin with enticement; they attempt to induce the people to make this sacrifice not with force, but with persuasion. In this case, they offer healthcare security – insurance for the uninsured, access for the disenfranchised, equal care for everyone. And because our healthcare system is indeed rife with injustices, absurd practices, abuses and waste, when Progressives proclaim with supreme confidence that they know the only way to fix all these problems, they invariably gain a lot of support*.

---

*Progressives never allow that there are actually four ways to fix our healthcare problems – they simply present Method Two as the only possible solution, without any further discussion. (See Chapter 4.)

Those of us who are not persuaded by simple enticements are subjected to other persuasions. We are told that when we insist on our autonomous right to make our own choices – to exercise healthcare options beyond those prescribed by the Central Authority's expert panels – we are really advocating for a two-tiered system, one in which we (likely being successful or rich, or otherwise "other"), will have access to better stuff. Therefore, we are pointed to – and pointed out – as being "unethical." We want something other than the Progressive solution of a perfectly fair, perfectly efficient, and perfectly affordable healthcare system – and this makes what we want inherently unfair, inefficient, and wasteful. It makes us evil. This ethical argument is the chief method by which we are to be "dissuaded" from using our own resources to make healthcare decisions for ourselves. The threat, should we persist in our beliefs, may eventually become more than just implied. After all, taking the necessary steps to keep unethical, evil elitists from bringing down the system would be entirely justifiable, and no more than prudent.

To say it another way, for people to insist on their individual autonomy, when it comes to something as important to society as healthcare, is unrealistic, counterproductive, and ultimately, just plain selfish. It's unethical, and we who think this way should be ashamed of ourselves.

THE ETHICS OF INDIVIDUAL AUTONOMY

Individual autonomy is the bedrock of the Great American Experiment. Our founders believed – and asserted – that we are all equally endowed by our Creator with certain inalienable rights that, added together, amounted to an inalienable right to individual autonomy. This belief is the bedrock of our founding.

What Progressives and their forebears noticed was that when you have a society where millions of people are each striving for their own best interests, even if you allow that, over time, those societies (occasionally or often) make improvements that benefit everybody, if you look at the details you see a lot of inequity, failure, cheating, cruelty, poverty and all other manner of suffering. And so, the proto-Progressives concluded, whatever the (occasional or frequent) successes you'll see in societies where individual autonomy is predominant, nobody can possibly argue that all the human suffering that goes along with it is ethical. It follows, then, that there has got to be a better way, and that whatever the best solution turns out to be, individual autonomy cannot possibly be the primary ethical imperative of the perfect society.

This is a foundational belief of Progressivism, just as the opposite is a foundational belief of Conservatism. (And this is why I personally do not understand what it means to be a "moderate," or what moderates mean when they implore Progressives and Conservatives to compromise with one another on issues of fundamental importance.)

So the impasse is over whether the right to individual autonomy is, or ought to be, the highest ethical imperative. In trying to resolve this impasse, it is instructive to notice what the Nuremberg tribunal concluded about it when they wrote the Nuremberg Code in 1947.

The Nuremberg Code was a statement of ethics which the tribunal felt obligated to promulgate after it passed judgment upon the Nazi doctors following World War II. The Nazi doctors had conducted horrifying medical experiments on people who were held in concentration camps, justifying their actions by the fact that these people were going to die anyway, so for the sake of humanity one might as well use their already forfeit bodies to advance medical knowledge. (This species of thinking ought to be recognizable to anyone familiar with the utilitarian ethics espoused by many prominent medical ethicists today.)

The Nuremberg tribunal was interested not only in punishing the Nazi doctors, but also in laying out some universal principles of ethics that (if followed) would prevent such a travesty from ever happening again. In searching for such principles, they took note of the fact that when the decisions were made to conduct these experiments, neither society as a whole, nor the central government, nor the local authorities, nor religious authorities, nor the medical profession, took any steps to prevent or to stop them from happening, and indeed, many of these institutions (including the medical profession) found ways to rationalize these experiments. So any ethical precept that would rely on society, governments, organized religion, or the medical profession to prevent similar atrocities in the future was demonstrably insufficient. Somewhat reluctantly, the tribunal concluded that the only ethical precept that ultimately could be relied upon in this regard is the precept of individual autonomy; that is, on the idea that no human experimentation can be performed ethically without the explicit, fully-informed, free consent of the human subject him-or-herself. This irreducible, primary ethical precept – ultimate respect for the autonomy of the individual – therefore became the bedrock ethical precept upon which the Nuremberg Code relied. And the Nuremberg Code became the foundation for the Declaration of Helsinki, a statement of medical ethics in human research that has been adopted by virtually every country around the world.

What is particularly noteworthy about this formulation of ethics is that individual autonomy was recognized as primary not for any positive reason – not because individual autonomy represents the highest state of human existence, or because it is a God-given natural right. Rather, individual autonomy was declared primary for a negative reason – there really is no other choice. No entity – no institution, organization, government, or panel – can be trusted, under duress, to do the right thing. Individual autonomy must be the primary ethical precept because it is a line in the sand, a backstop, the only ethical precept that, at the end of the day, can offer to prevent the official abuse of individuals in service to a purported higher cause.

Progressivism inherently subsumes individual autonomy to the needs of the whole, and thereby inherently defeats this ethical line in the sand. Progressivism removes that ethical barrier, the only possible ethical barrier, and exposes individuals to official – and officially "ethical" – abuse in advancement of the higher collective cause of the day.

Even people who object to the primacy of individual autonomy as formulated in the Declaration of Independence, on the grounds that they do not believe in a Creator, or that they have discovered a truth that is even more inalienable than the one stated therein, cannot argue with the formulation of the Nuremberg Code. That latter formulation was not based on some lofty ideal, or on an assertion of some pinnacle of Western philosophy, but was a simple statement of cold, hard, sad, scientific logic, derived from painfully objective evidence, evidence paid for in human blood, tears, suffering and untold anguish. It is as evidence-based an ethical precept as is ever possible to have.

We now know two things. First, Obamacare cannot work if enough of us refuse to acquiesce to herd medicine. And second, whatever vituperations, innuendos, accusations and castigations are thrown at us, our non-cooperation with herd medicine is not only ethically justifiable, but for the sake of our progeny it is the only truly ethical path we can take.

HOW CAN WE ASSERT OUR INDIVIDUAL AUTONOMY IN HEALTHCARE?

There are two general strategies for reversing herd medicine and restoring the rights of individuals within our healthcare system. The first is the political strategy – collective action aimed at electing political leaders who are dedicated to overturning Obamacare, undoing the restrictions to individual prerogatives already present in our pre-Obamacare healthcare system, and establishing a healthcare system that recognizes freedom of individual action as a foundational principle. I believe such a system would be based on a "Method 3" model, as described in Chapter 4.

I, for one, hope very much that this happens.

But I think it is likely that, no matter what happens politically, we will need to use the second general strategy for reversing herd medicine. Even politicians who truly "get it" will find it difficult to reverse the Progressive tide. Any dedication they express in support of individual prerogatives (and its necessary partner, individual responsibility) will be loudly advertised by their political opponents and the American media as having proven themselves to be elitist, selfish, hard-hearted caterers to the rich, and oppressors of the poor. They will be painted as evil, stupid, and/or crazy. Politicians generally cannot survive such attacks, and realistically we should not expect them to try.

This leaves us with the strategy of individual action. We, as individuals, need to understand the "bargain" which Obamacare represents – an assurance (ultimately false) of healthcare security in exchange for our individual prerogatives – and then act in our own, enlightened self-interest. In the battle for individual autonomy, individual action is a fitting and proper strategy.

In adopting this strategy, we will need to rely on the bedrock precept of individual autonomy the same way the Nuremberg tribunal did – as the last possible bulwark against tyranny. And it is this ethical precept, so derived, upon which we must stand. We must draw our own line in the sand, and declare: "I assert my right to act in my own best interests, in any way that does not infringe on the rights of others to do the same. Accordingly, I will not allow any human authority to restrict my right to protect my own well-being, as long as I am using my own resources to do so."

If enough of us make this simple declaration, and act aggressively upon it, and if we make it clear that by doing so we are merely asserting humanity's primary ethical right, Obamacare cannot stand, any Progressive healthcare system cannot stand, and the Progressive Program itself cannot prevail.

Unfortunately, Obamacare is carefully designed to utterly suffocate individual prerogatives. Every step we or our doctors attempt to take that is not officially sanctioned by the Central Authority will be snuffed. This means that we may ultimately have to operate largely outside the official healthcare system, in the places where the grasping tentacles of Obamacare do not yet quite reach.

WHAT DOCTORS SHOULD DO

The medical profession is in a truly sorry state. As far back as 2002, under exceeding duress for more than a decade to place the interests of the payers ahead of the interests of their patients, and "guided" by their Progressive-minded leaders, the medical profession abandoned over two thousand years of tradition, law and ethics, and formally adopted a New Age medical ethics that obligates them to work for "social justice." That is, doctors have charged themselves with an ethical obligation to distribute medical resources equitably. They have accepted the task of covertly rationing healthcare at the bedside. (See Chapter 3.)

New Age medical ethics renders the classic doctor-patient relationship entirely moot, and leaves sick people – as they attempt to navigate an increasingly hostile and parsimonious healthcare system – without the dedicated professional who, until now, has been obligated to act as their personal agent. Worse, doctors have not made explicit to patients their new mixed (at best) loyalties. Indeed, doctors are trained to hide that fact. When young doctors today learn about the doctor-patient relationship, they are no longer learning classic medical ethics. Rather, they are learning techniques for fruitful communication and subtle manipulation, in order to better induce patients to "comply" with the expert-guided medical recommendations they are handing out these days.

By abandoning their sacred fiduciary obligation to their patients – the one ethical precept that renders the practice of medicine a true profession in the first place – doctors have committed the original sin. They are now professionals only in the sense that master plumbers are professionals – that is, by virtue of their special training in some field of work. They are no longer members of a true Profession, as attorneys are, for instance. (While doctors may disparage lawyers as ambulance chasers, at least lawyers have not abandoned their sacred fiduciary obligation to their clients.)

In the perpetual struggle over the use of resources, doctors have officially thrown in with the payers. It should be obvious that this leaves their abandoned patients in a bad place. But for the purposes of the immediate discussion, we should note that by this capitulation doctors have set themselves adrift. As a profession they have no moral anchor. And because they have abandoned their sacred professional obligations, they find themselves at the mercy of the payers who induced their capitulation.

While this change has profoundly affected every American doctor, the doctors who are most directly and severely affected, so far at least, have been the primary care physicians.

THIS IS YOUR PCP ON OBAMACARE

For most Americans, the most important person in the healthcare system is our primary care physician. These are the doctors we see first if we have a new medical problem, who (theoretically, at least) stick with us through the ups and downs of our chronic medical conditions, and who direct traffic for us if we need to see a specialist. Our PCPs are the doctors we know the best, and who care about us the most (which, admittedly, might not be saying much today). It is our PCPs, more than anyone else, who will determine how well we are going to fare in our encounters with the American healthcare system.

PCPs are equally important to the Central Authority. To a large extent PCPs drive the overall cost of healthcare, and decide how much of the Central Authority's healthcare dollars are spent, and on whom, and when, and how. Among other things, PCPs are the gatekeepers who determine to a very large extent which patients will see specialists, how aggressively and how well patients' chronic and acute illnesses are to be managed, and which patients receive which preventive services. To control healthcare costs, therefore, it is absolutely essential for the Central Authority to control the behavior of PCPs.

In Chapter 8, we saw how Obamacare's infrastructure is designed specifically to control the behavior of physicians. And while this control will greatly affect every American doctor, it is primarily the PCP upon whom the screws of oversight will be urgently turned. Every move they make on our behalf will be carefully monitored, measured, scrutinized, analyzed, and compared against the lists of guidelines, processes, procedures, rules and dictates under which they must operate. Even locally they will no longer be independent agents, whose medical knowledge and ethical precepts must guide their decisions. Rather, they will be just one member of a "healthcare team," consisting largely of non-physicians, which will make decisions jointly. They will no longer be primarily accountable to their patients for their actions. Rather, their patients will become merely objects of their accountability. PCPs will be held accountable first to their teams, then to the Accountable Care Organizations which employ their teams, and, ultimately, to the Central Authority itself.

When it comes to independent thinking, much less to independent action, our PCPs will be on a very short leash. Their real jobs will be to act as the most proximate agent of the Central Authority.

However, I don't want to give the impression that it is Obamacare which has wrecked primary care medicine. That job had been pretty much completed before anyone had ever heard of Obamacare. For many years now PCPs have been a downtrodden and beleaguered lot, unhappy, dissatisfied and demoralized. Large numbers of them can think only about retiring at the earliest possible date, or if retirement is too far away, changing careers – perhaps becoming corporate executives, or deep-sea fishermen. And even though a majority of entering medical students claim that they aspire to become PCPs, only a tiny minority actually end up doing so.

It is instructive to have a look at why all those medical students are changing their minds. Part of the reason, of course, is the relatively low pay of PCPs. But PCPs have always made substantially less money than specialists, and in the past a lot of doctors still chose primary care. The larger part of the reason is that today, when motivated and idealistic medical students spend a little time interacting with actual PCPs during the course of their training, they are horrified at what they see.

There are numerous reasons why few doctors in their right minds would choose primary care medicine as a career today.

- The pay of PCPs is determined arbitrarily (and literally) by Acts of Congress, not by what they're worth to their patients or to the market, and indeed in this way PCPs have a lot in common with workers in the old Soviet collectives.

- While all doctors these days are directed to "practice medicine" by guidelines and directives which are handed down from On High, the centralized control is particularly focused on PCPs. They have as little latitude in making medical decisions as the Central Authority can possibly arrange. Indeed, it is the unspoken policy of the Central Authority to dumb-down the practice of primary care medicine, to reduce it to a series of reproducible and robotic activities that almost anyone with a modicum of training can do.

- PCPs are forcibly limited to between 7.5 and 12.5 minutes per patient encounter, and the specific content of what must occur during those 7.5 minutes is strictly determined by sundry Pay for Performance checklists, so as to severely limit any ad hoc discussions that might occur between doctor and patient, discussions which might introduce new spending opportunities, and which do not meet the approved agenda for such encounters.

- Everything a PCP does must be carefully documented according to incomprehensible rules, on innumerable forms and documents, that confound patient care but that greatly further the convenience of healthcare accountants and other stone-witted bureaucrats who are employed specifically to second-guess every clinical decision and every action the PCP takes.

- PCPs are expected to operate flawlessly under a system of federal rules, regulations and guidelines that cover hundreds of thousands of pages in immeasurable volumes that are never available in any readily accessible form. If they do not operate flawlessly according to those rules, regulations and guidelines, they are guilty of the federal crime of healthcare fraud. Furthermore, the specific meanings of these rules, regulations and guidelines are not merely opaque and difficult to ascertain, but indeed they are fundamentally indeterminate – that is, no individual or group of individuals in existence can say what they mean. So, PCPs operate under a massive quantum cloud of rules as best they can, but their actual status (regarding healthcare fraud) is, like Schrodinger's cat, fundamentally unknowable – until the "box is opened" (perhaps through criminal prosecution), whereupon the meaning of the rules is finally crystallized in a court of law, and doctors who had been practicing in good faith find that they have at least a 50- 50 chance (like the cat) of learning that they are actually professionally dead.

- Worst of all, PCPs have been charged with the duty of covertly rationing their patients' healthcare at the bedside, and they have been pressed to nullify the classic doctor-patient relationship by the healthcare bureaucracy that determines their professional viability, by the United States Supreme Court (*Pegram et al. vs Herdrich*, 2000), and by the bankrupt, new-age ethics of their own profession.

It is small wonder that few young doctors are anxious to sign up for this duty, or that our existing PCPs are demoralized and are desperately seeking the nearest exit. Any of us who are lucky enough to have a PCP who remains dedicated to our welfare, despite the heavy bureaucratic burden under which they are all struggling, should regard them with the same sense of awe and wonder with which we would regard the nun who chooses to live and serve in a leper colony.

HOW OBAMACARE "FIXES" THE PCP SHORTAGE

During the Obamacare debate in 2009, the President and his supporters repeatedly proclaimed that their new law would solve the PCP shortage. The legislation provides two explicit methods for doing so – and one less-explicit method.

First, Obamacare promises to address some of the pay discrepancy which punishes doctors for going into primary care specialties. And second, it proposes to fund new training opportunities for PCPs.

Regarding the modest pay increase, I will merely repeat that over a period of years the Central Authority has intentionally rendered primary care medicine such a soul-wrenching, personally and professionally demeaning endeavor that it has pushed most PCPs beyond mere anger, frustration, or resignation. Since it is not primarily their relatively low pay that has caused all this anguish, a modest boost in pay cannot overcome it. Indeed, tossing this bone to PCPs, in light of what the payers have done to their profession, constitutes no more than a grave insult.

And while increasing training slots for PCPs may sound nice, one must wonder what effect it will have, when existing training programs cannot come close to filling the slots that exist today.

It should be clear to everyone that these proposed "fixes" cannot possibly provide anything approaching an actual solution to the PCP shortage. I for one cannot accept that the authors of Obamacare can possibly believe they will.

To find out what our leaders are really up to with regard to our PCPs, we must look a little deeper.

And sure enough, the real answer to the PCP shortage – at least, the answer our political leaders are actually relying upon – is revealed deep within the bill, buried in Section 5501 (which I believe very few humans have ever read), where the definition of "Primary Care Practitioner" is actually provided. Note, first of all, that Obamacare now being the law of the land, "PCP" no longer means "primary care physician," but rather, indicates "primary care practitioner."

And here's how the new law defines Primary Care Practitioners:

> *The term 'primary care practitioner' means an individual who —*
>
> *(I) is a physician (as described in section 1861(r)(1)) who has a primary specialty designation of family medicine, internal medicine, geriatric medicine, or pediatric medicine; or*
>
> *(II) is a nurse practitioner, clinical nurse specialist, or physician assistant (as those terms are defined in 9 section 1861(aa)(5))*

And so it is my sad duty to report to American PCPs that the real "fix" our political leaders have devised for the shortage of people who practice primary care medicine is to declare you and nurses to be functionally (and legally) equivalent.

This, I submit, is all a PCP really needs to know about Obamacare. What this means is that today there are two pathways to becoming a PCP. You can spend four years in college, four years in medical school and three years in a clinical residency – or you can go to nursing school and do another year or two of clinical training. Given this established fact, one can hardly fault the wisdom of medical students for choosing another career.

All this should be expected. Having painstakingly reduced you unfortunate practitioners of primary care medicine to tools of the state, to people whose job is to rotely follow checklists of centralized directives, it is only natural for the Central Authority to eventually notice that you really don't need all that training to do the kind of job they have invented for you. Nurses – who can be "trained up" much more rapidly than you, who will work for much less money than you, and who (they think) will be much less recalcitrant about following handed-down directives than you – will fill the gap.

And the reason so much effort has been taken to render primary care medicine such an excruciatingly frustrating and enervating profession now becomes entirely clear. The Central Authority does not really want its PCPs to be physicians at all. It wants the people functioning as the critical gateway to the American healthcare system to be people it believes will be easier to control than physicians.*

_____

*This statement is not intended to be an insult to nurses, but only reflects what I have concluded is the Central Authority's intention. I have worked along side a great many nurses in my career, and I find them to be at least as dedicated to the welfare of patients as any doctor. Perhaps more so, since to the best of my knowledge the nursing profession has yet to water down its ethical standards in the way that doctors have done. I believe that at the end of the day our Progressive leadership will find nurses far more difficult to "manage" than they seem to believe.

_____

But I have even more bad news for primary care doctors. Even if doctors had perfect control of the healthcare system and the political realities, primary care medicine (as we know it) would still be in trouble.

This is because of an axiomatic truth revealed by the annals of human progress, to wit: As knowledge increases and technology improves, activities that used to require the services of highly-trained experts become available to non-experts who have much less training. A lot of what PCPs have traditionally done – check-ups of well patients, screening for occult disease, controlling cholesterol, advising on diet, weight loss and exercise, managing routine hypertension and diabetes – really can be reduced to a series of guidelines and checklists, which can be adequately followed by individuals with much less training than these doctors receive.

When any area of expertise evolves to this level, it is inevitable (in a free economy) that lesser-trained individuals will inherit it. This event greatly increases productivity, makes the services in question more readily available to many people at lower cost, and (ideally) frees up the experts to take on more challenging endeavors. While this kind of transition is nearly inevitable, it is often painful and disruptive. The pain and disruption are being experienced by PCPs today.

Primary care medicine has advanced to the point where it really would make sense to turn over many of the routine, mundane, and reducible-to-checklist tasks that PCPs typically perform to non-physicians. PCPs who are fighting against this inevitability are wasting their time and energy. They are fighting not only Obamacare, but also both history and the laws of economics, so in the end it is a losing battle. It is time for PCPs to move on.

So, in this way of looking at it, it was really only a formality for the Obamacare legislation to make the death of primary care medicine official.

WHAT ENLIGHTENED PCPs SHOULD DO

It is time for PCPs to abandon what has become "primary care medicine" altogether. It is time to move on.

Walking away from primary care should not be a loss, because actually, primary care has long since abandoned you. Whatever "primary care" may have once been, it has now been reduced to something that, by law, can be done by a lot of people who are not physicians. Primary care has been dumbed down to the point where abandoning it is no loss; indeed, it ought to be liberating to walk away from it.

So walk away from it.

The beauty is that to survive and flourish, you don't really need to change your medical ideals or even your medical behavior (unless, of course, you have bought in to the New Age ethics, and the strict adherence to guidelines, checklists, etc.) You simply need to practice medicine exactly as you were trained to practice it all those years ago – taking all the time needed for careful, thoughtful attention to detail; seeking out the meaningful nuances in your patients' medical conditions; personalizing both diagnostic and therapeutic recommendations not only for your patient's medical problems, but also for their psychosocial and economic circumstances; relishing the challenge of making the difficult diagnoses, and managing the complex medical disorders that so often break from the designated norm; and treating guidelines as just that, as often-helpful guideposts, rather than mandates; and most important of all, embracing the classic doctor-patient relationship in all its particulars, and having the latitude to become a true advocate for your individual patients within a hostile healthcare system. In short, you can go back to being a real doctor, and not a cipher in some bureaucrat's database.

There are only two things you need to do to move in this direction.

First, abandon the "primary care" label. Remember, primary care is now the standards-based, checklist-driven, one-size-fits all, "high-quality" system of practice imposed by government bureaucrats, a practice which is now open to both doctors and nurses (and, in the future, most likely to others). That's not what you do any more. So find a new name for yourself.

The choice of nomenclature is yours, of course, but I humbly suggest "Advanced Care Physician."

What you do is not primary care; it's far more advanced than that, and nobody could do it without the sort of extensive training you have. "Advanced Care" captures that notion. This name also opens the possibility of referrals from the new-style, government-sanctioned "PCPs," some of whom undoubtedly will come to recognize that at least 20% of their patients will present as clinical puzzles that do not fit very well with any of the standard medical diagnoses with which they are familiar, and another 20% will not respond to the recommended therapy as the guidelines say they must. These patients obviously will need advanced management, management beyond what a modern primary care practitioner is able (or allowed) to offer. Why not refer them to an ACP?

Second, you need to establish practices whereby you are paid directly by your patients. You need to do this because it is the only method available for avoiding the bureaucratic nightmare that wrecked your former profession of primary care in the first place. Payment models can be established that will allow most patients – anyone, say, who can afford a cell phone contract or cable TV – to participate. (Making your services readily available to the masses may help blunt the obligatory attacks of "elitist!" which will be aimed your way in the attempt to shame you back into the primary care gulag). There really ought to be nothing particularly revolutionary about this kind of practice, since it was the norm throughout most of the history of medicine until 40 years ago. It is likely that many patients who today would never consider paying any doctor out of pocket will eventually change their minds, once it becomes apparent to them the depths to which primary care medicine has fallen in the United States, and that as a result their lives are on the line.

In any case, when you are paid by your patients, you answer to your patients (not some hostile bureaucrat), and the quality of the care you deliver is measured by your patients (and not some other hostile bureaucrat). There are no externally imposed time-limits to your office visits, no checklists you must complete, no bizarre documentation rules you must follow for reimbursement, no guidelines you must obey even if it makes no sense for your patient. Those things are for the modern, government-approved "PCPs" to concern themselves with, poor souls, and you do not dwell among these unfortunates anymore.

And happy it is that primary care medicine is killed off now, at this time – because time is of the essence. I have described (Chapter 7) how an essential feature of our new Progressive healthcare system will be to make it illegal (in the name of fairness) for individuals to spend their own money on their own healthcare. For Advanced Care Medicine to become a viable path, you've got to begin immediately to make it a fait accompli – to establish it as something patients value, and which they fully expect as a personal healthcare option, and furthermore, as an indispensable referral resource for those sad souls – physicians, nurses and others – who retain the label "PCP," and who will be powerless (if not clueless) when it comes to providing complex medical care to patients who come in with a difficult diagnosis, or more than one diagnosis, or who otherwise display guideline-unfriendliness.

So at the end of the day, the fact that Obamacare has formally brought primary care medicine to a merciful end may turn out to be a positive thing.

How Advanced Care Physicians Should Answer the Whiners

Precisely because ACPs will gravely threaten the whole paradigm of Progressive healthcare, these new-style physicians will need to be ready to answer the complaints and accusations that will rise up against them. Progressives will be extremely threatened by the idea that the physicians formerly known as PCPs are dropping out of the dysfunctional healthcare system altogether (the system that has, purposefully and with malice aforethought, wrecked their chosen careers), and are striking out on their own, establishing private practices in which they are paid directly by their patients.

Great and loud protests will be raised, in an attempt to create a general public hatred toward these physicians, to label what they are doing unethical, and finally to render it illegal.

The general proposition opponents will be arguing, with far more vituperation than employed here, can be reduced to this: For doctors to demand that patients pay them directly is elitist and unethical; only the rich will be able to afford this kind of care; a two-tiered healthcare system will develop, and public health will suffer.

ACPs need to be prepared with a compelling answer, an answer that does not offer any apologies, but that boldly explains why what they are doing is the ONLY ethical way for them to practice their profession. What ACPs need is a John Galt speech.

A John Galt Speech for Direct-Pay Physicians*

"You demand to know what has happened to us, the primary care physicians you thought you controlled. You have cried that our sins are destroying the world and you have cursed us for our unwillingness to practice the virtues you demanded. Since virtue, to you, consists of sacrifice, you have demanded more sacrifices at every turn. You have sacrificed all those evils which you held as the cause of your plight. You have sacrificed justice to mercy. You have sacrificed independence to unity. You have sacrificed wealth to need. You have sacrificed self-esteem to self-denial. You have sacrificed happiness to duty.

"While you were dragging us to your sacrificial altars, we physicians who value justice, independence, reason, and self-esteem — we finally came to see the nature of the game you were playing, which we had previously been too innocently generous to grasp. And we have chosen to play no longer.

"All the physicians who have vanished from your system, the doctors you hated, yet dreaded to lose, we are gone from you. Do not cry that it is our duty to serve you. We do not recognize such duty. Do not cry that you need us. We do

not consider your need a claim. Do not cry that you own us. You don't. Do not beg us to return. We are making our own way, apart from you.

"In your cynical attempt to control the healthcare system, you have coerced us — with your threats to our livelihood, threats of massive fines, threats of jail — to abandon our sacred obligation to our patients. Society must come first, you say. The needs of the collective are paramount, you insist. We must do what the experts tell us to do, you demand. And in the process you have destroyed the doctor-patient relationship which is the backbone of our profession. You have reduced physicians to ciphers, to puppets. And you have reduced our patients — the living, loving, hoping, striving people who come to us, who place their trust in us and their lives in our hands — to interchangeable members of a vast herd. You have demanded that we guard society's interests, and abandon our sick to their own devices in your cruel and parsimonious healthcare system.

"Your process is now firmly established. Your methods have been legislated by Congress, embodied in volumes of rules, regulations and "guidelines" (strictly and ruthlessly enforced), upheld by the courts, and finally (and most tellingly) sanctioned as being entirely "ethical" by your allies, the leadership of our own professional organizations. You have made the healthcare system untenable for doctors who value true medical ethics.

"You have placed us into a position where we must either resign ourselves to an unethical, demeaning, health-destroying style of practice, or get out. We have gotten out.

"We have gotten out. We have left your Program. We refuse to sacrifice ourselves for you any longer. We will not sacrifice our livelihoods, our morals, our independence, our minds, or our patients for your bastardized idea of virtue.

"We will practice medicine in the only manner that still permits us to behave ethically toward our patients, in the only way that we can honor the true doctor-patient relationship, in the only way we can legitimately regain the title of professional. We have chosen to be paid directly by the people to whom we provide our services, by the people to whom we dedicate ourselves as professionals. We have chosen to cut you out.

"To argue that direct-pay practices are unethical — to argue that any innovation that would somehow restore both our professional integrity and the patient's rightful advocate is unethical — is completely upside down. This argument only reveals your own inner corruption. We are taking the only pathway that remains to us to restore the true foundation of medical ethics, to restore our profession — to always place the patient first.

"To argue that direct-pay practices threaten the general welfare completely ignores reality. We are doing the only thing we can do to begin restoring protections that people are supposed to have when they are sick and facing a healthcare system that is utterly bent on withholding their care whenever it can be gotten away with.

"To argue that direct-pay medicine will create a two-tiered healthcare system is absurd on its face. It provides a mechanism by which at least some of your intended victims can escape the deadly obstacles you have laid before them. Saying that it amounts to a two-tiered healthcare system is as absurd as arguing that slaveholders were wrong to free their slaves before Emancipation, because doing so would create an elite subpopulation of former slaves; that until all slaves are freed, no slaves should be freed. But when a few slaves were freed and walked the earth as free men, that action was not only ethical, but it also showed others what was possible. Over time, it created a widespread expectation for freedom that eventually could no longer be ignored, and that, at huge cost, was finally fulfilled.

"You wouldn't understand this – you who already know everything, you whose experts already have all the answers – but any innovation that can potentially spare patients from some of the harm you have in store for them will necessarily be applicable to only a few patients at first. That is how disruptive processes work. In your proposed perfect system, of course, disruptive processes are anathema – because they disrupt. But in the real world disruptive processes are creative processes, processes of growth, processes of rejuvenation, processes that create opportunity. This is why you always try to suffocate disruptive processes, with your cries of "unfair!"

"Disruptive processes always begin as niche products or services, attractive only to a few high-end users; too expensive or too marginal for the vast majority; ignored, ridiculed or castigated by current providers. But if at their core they are offering something fundamentally useful, they will slowly demonstrate their worth – and eventually all the potential users will see the light, and demand for the product will become explosive. At this stage the means are invariably found to make the new product affordable and available to meet the demand, while preserving the core benefits. And when that happens, the traditional providers (who never saw it coming) are suddenly out of business.

" We are a disruptive process, and the process we are disrupting is yours.

"We are not playing your game any longer. We will no longer be victims; we will no longer subject ourselves to your attempts to make us guilty. We will no longer walk, heads bent down, to your altar of sacrifice.

"You no longer have any hold on us. We have done our time. We are getting out. If we decided to leave medicine and open a road-side fruit stand, or become lumberjacks, or just spend our time puttering around in the basement, you would have no objection to that. So by what right do you object if we hang out our shingles, and see a few patients who voluntarily come to us, using their own resources to do so? You can have no rightful objection to such a thing. So be quiet about it, or admit to your own corruption."

------

*To put this speech into the correct frame of mind, I have liberally borrowed parts of the first three paragraphs from the actual John Galt speech in *Atlas Shrugged*. The blame for the rest of it falls solely upon your faithful author.

——

To this final argument Progressives will either have to withdraw from the field, or reveal the true extent of their aims. For, if they reply that PCPs not only must not become direct-pay practitioners, but also they "owe" society a duty not to change careers at all, then they are admitting that they consider physicians to be their captives, people who, in exchange for a government-issued license to practice medicine, have signed up for a lifetime of indentured servitude. This, in fact, is the only logical conclusion one can reach when listening to Progressives' angry indignation over the idea of direct-pay practitioners.

I would urge PCPs who decide on the direct-pay, ACP route to explicitly offer a new pact with their patients. They need to do this. They cannot succeed on their own, as their enemies will be terrible. But if they offer, as part of their service, a new doctor-patient compact – based on traditional medical ethics, where the patient agrees to hold nothing important back from their physician, and the physician agrees to place the interest of the individual patient above all other considerations, and fight for the patient's well-being against all the hostile forces aligned against them – they and their patients, together, will become invulnerable.

There is a limited window of opportunity to establish direct-pay practices. The vociferousness of the complaints we are already hearing against them indicates just how threatening these are to the Progressive program. Unless this practice model gains a sufficient toehold, and quickly, it will be made illegal. Because Americans cannot be permitted to spend their own money on their own healthcare.

And so, on behalf of my children and projected grandchildren, and on behalf of the Great American Experiment, I implore American PCPs to consider these arguments.

What about Specialist Physicians?

I have addressed my comments to PCPs because their plight is most acute, and the means of escape and redemption is more readily available to them than it is for most specialists. Specialists, to a great extent, rely on the entire healthcare system not only for their referrals, but also for the expensive equipment and the armies of support personnel necessary to do their sophisticated procedures. It is much more difficult for you who are specialists to leave the system.

But there are probably things you can do. Remember that the key to saving your profession is to individualize the healthcare your patients receive, and, perhaps more importantly, to create an expectation among your patients for individualized care. So at the very least, tell your patients the truth. "I think that in your case the best thing to do would be X. But the IPAB says I can't offer X to men over the age of 75. So in my judgment the next best thing is Y. Let's hope for the best." You will only be telling them the truth, and at the very least your patient has a right to the truth. If you can't practice medicine exactly the way you think is right, at least let the patient know the reason this is the case – that under Obamacare they are interchangeable members of a herd. If enough patients hear that message perhaps someday they will insist that something be done about it.

Whenever possible, consider suggesting to your patients who have complex medical problems that they should think about seeing a direct-pay, advanced care physician, a doctor who will be able to spend the time necessary to help them to manage their conditions as they should be managed. Many patients, of course, will be unwilling to pay out of their own pockets for this service, at least at first. But you will still do them a favor by notifying them that such a service is out there, and that Obamacare does not have to be the only variety of care. Further, you will be helping to create an expectation for this kind of care. It will help re-introduce people to the idea that, even in healthcare, you get what you pay for.

Particularly creative specialists undoubtedly will be able to imagine ways of advancing individualized healthcare with new products or services that address a particular need, and in so doing may gain themselves a large dollop of independence, and perhaps even extricate themselves from the healthcare morass. While there is little chance that such an escape route will be realized by more than a handful of specialists, the ones who are successful can have a big impact on the general direction of our healthcare system.

In general, however, the more specialized you are, the fewer options you have in regaining your prerogatives for independent action without making a substantial change in your field of practice.

What Biomedical Entrepreneurs Should Do

The American healthcare system as it has operated since World War II has been a tremendous boon to the biomedical industry, since, as long as its products promised some measurable (or perceived) benefit to patients, the Tooth Fairy would pay for them. This "if you build it, they will come" paradigm led to explosive growth within the biomedical industry over the last 50 years, and to remarkable progress in our understanding and management of a host of diseases. Unfortunately, it also led to one of the most convoluted business models that capitalism has ever produced.

The biomedical industry is unlike any other. To successfully sell a medical product within the American healthcare system, a business must: a) invent, develop and build the product; b) convince the FDA, often with evidence from randomized clinical trials (each one at a cost of $100 million or so and several years of effort), that the product is sufficiently safe and effective; c) once FDA approval is gained, convince insurance carriers and Medicare that they ought to pay for it; and finally, d) convince doctors to prescribe it.

Each one of these steps is immensely costly and complicated. Both the business risk and the cost of overhead involved in operating within such a business model are massive, and these costs guarantee that any products this industry sells, even if the "unit cost" of manufacturing an item is quite small, will be very expensive.

Nobody would design a business model like this on purpose. But a few score of large biomedical companies have adapted to it, and over the decades successful companies have developed all the processes and subsystems necessary to function within this complex model. Companies that have learned to operate under this model are often not anxious to change it, since it creates a huge barrier to entry for new competitors.

THREATS TO THE BIOMEDICAL INDUSTRY

We have seen how, ironically, the entire idea of medical progress is a threat to Progressives, and needs to be stifled. (Chapter 14.) But of all the threats posed by medical progress, none is greater than that posed by innovations that advance individualized healthcare. It is virtually axiomatic that, one way or another, our Progressive leaders will have to act to suppress companies that aim with their technology to enable the individualized care of patients.

The biomedical industry as it now exists is particularly vulnerable. The built-in complexity of their business model, combined with their utter dependence on hostile third-party payers, makes these companies highly susceptible targets for suppression. Even a small tweak in regulatory requirements can delay a new product for years, or cause management to remove it from the product map, or, in the case of smaller entities, cause a company to go belly-up. And since the tweaks in regulatory requirements – small and large – that lead to such results are common and unpredictable, investors are already extremely reluctant to bet on new categories of products, whose pathway to market has not been traveled many times before.

Another vulnerability is that these businesses usually have little or no direct contact with those who actually reap the benefits of their products – the patients. Their chief potential allies in any efforts to develop products that would empower individual decision making, therefore, are largely indifferent to them.

Biomedical companies often have great difficulty articulating exactly who their customers are. This is because they have, out of necessity, very many customers, including the FDA, Medicare, other federal agencies, insurance companies, HMOs, professional organizations and societies, and, most especially, the prescribing doctors. But patients have very little to do with the decision to purchase the products these companies make, and so (while virtually every biomedical company's mission statement, to be sure, solemnly proclaim that patients are their primary reason for existence), in general patients are no more the customers of the biomedical industry than al Qaeda terrorists are of the companies that make unmanned drones.

The distance between the industry and the patients who benefit from their products is not merely an accident. Biomedical companies have found it in their best interests to avoid a close relationship with patients. Keeping patients at a distance has been an essential part of their business because doctors (their chief customers) have traditionally insisted on it. (In insisting that everyone else keep their hands off their patients, that is, to stop telling their patients things, doctors ironically invoke the sanctity of the doctor-patient relationship that their own profession has made defunct.) Partly as a result of the companies' arm's-length relationship with their end-users, the public is at best indifferent toward them, and are often more than ready to become quite angry at them.

This, unfortunately, leaves the biomedical industry extremely vulnerable to efforts at demonization. Many executives in this industry are taking note of this growing and disturbing phenomenon. Drug companies especially, but increasingly others as well, are no longer spoken of as good corporate citizens, or as the institutions whose dedicated efforts provide ever-improved methods of curing disease and alleviating suffering. Instead, they are increasingly painted as evil and corrupt, as all too willing to satisfy their own greed by means of graft, double-dealing, lying, cheating, stealing, animal abuse, and even manslaughter.

Demonizing the biomedical industry (whether they deserve it or not) is a key strategy of the Progressives and of their allies in the American press. This strategy seems to have great traction with the public, and creates support for new laws and regulations ostensibly aimed at bringing the out-of-control biomedical industry to heel, but is actually aimed at making the business so risky that few would be stupid enough to enter it.

In the battle over its future, the biomedical industry has few allies. Many of its customers – especially the federal government and insurance companies – are customers only reluctantly and resentfully, and are indeed chief among its demonizers. The industry's other main customers, the doctors, may not be actively hostile toward the industry, but are engaged in a battle for survival themselves, and are not likely to be effective or focused allies.

The industry's only natural allies in this fight are those who are directly helped by its products, and who ought to have good cause to defend it from destruction. It is the patients. Patients would be extremely powerful allies, indeed almost invincible, if they rose up in the industry's defense. But, as we have seen, the public in general and patients in particular do not usually have warm feelings for the industry, and are all too happy to line up with its persecutors.

For the most part, the biomedical industry just doesn't get it yet. They don't realize that they are in a battle for survival, one that will determine whether they are to continue as innovating enterprises, or instead as mere assembly lines, churning out government-approved quotas of government-approved widgets and pills. While the industry continues playing under the old rules, keeping patients at arm's length, the Progressives and their allies are filling the public's head with horror stories, trying to work the public into a frenzied cry for those in the greedy and callous biomedical industry to be tossed to the lions – or at least regulated into utter docility.

The outcome looks quite inevitable. Unless the biomedical industry wakes up and figures out how to get the public on its side, it faces something like ruin.

HOW CAN THE BIOMEDICAL INDUSTRY RECRUIT PATIENTS TO ITS CAUSE?

This is not something that can be accomplished with multi-million dollar public relations campaigns. The public is already convinced that biomedical companies are routinely engaged in price gouging, in withholding vital information to keep their unsafe products on the market, in lying about the supposed benefits of their products, and in bribing doctors. The public is being fed this story every day in a hundred ways by prestigious newspapers, medical journals, politicians, medical experts, cable news channels, and talk show hosts. (Admittedly, by their actions companies often enough provide plenty of fodder for this story.) Against this unrelenting attack, even the slickest advertising campaign seems pretty futile. Battling the press in the press is rarely a winning strategy.

A better way to win patients over would be to provide them with something they desperately want and need, and cannot easily get. That something is empowerment.

EMPOWERING PATIENTS

Biomedical companies that want to assure their long-term survival as fully independent and self-directed enterprises should strongly consider partnering with patients in their quest. They need to work with the growing minority of patients who understand the dangers of herd medicine, and whose goal is to become self-empowered. Simply put, businesses that learn how to enable patient empowerment will be effectively immunizing themselves against subjugation by the Progressives. Empowered patients will not stand by and watch the destruction of the entities that make their empowerment possible.

Many companies in the biomedical industry will find this hard to do. They don't sell products directly to patients, or know how to interact with patients. They don't know what patients want. Instead, they are fully geared up for the much more complicated task of selling things to the healthcare system. They are intimidated by actual patients.

Even the remote contacts they do sometimes have with patients, such as producing educational materials or running TV commercials, are viewed as controversial or inappropriate (since the doctors reserve the authority to determine what patients ought to know, and the Central Authority – which now has the doctors under its thrall – supports them strongly in this). Avoiding direct contact with patients is often deeply embedded into their corporate cultures, and many companies will find the idea of starting a "patient empowerment" business counter to their core values.

Still, successful companies that want to remain successful over the long term will have to find ways to work around this barrier. There is a huge and untapped demand for empowerment tools among the public, and therefore a massive business opportunity exists.

I am not suggesting here that biomedical companies should abandon their current businesses altogether in order to concentrate on patient empowerment. Rather, I am suggesting they should engage in patient empowerment so they have a better chance of continuing their core businesses. In many cases this might require establishing "spin-off" enterprises that can develop and market patient empowerment tools without "contaminating" the core business. But they should take this effort seriously, as if some day, the patient empowerment side of the business might be their chief source of revenue. Because some day it might just come to that.

WHAT WILL PATIENT EMPOWERMENT LOOK LIKE?

Nobody knows what patient empowerment will actually look like, of course, because it hasn't been invented yet. Like most entries into new markets, this one will probably begin with a few relatively tentative and primitive forays, exploring the landscape, and seeing what patients will respond to and not respond to. When they recognize the possibilities, patients will begin asking for specific products, services, and features – that is, the customers will begin to better "define" the market. And, seeing the growing demand, more and more entrepreneurs will jump into the fray, testing an increasing array of ideas. Sooner or later, there may come a "killer app," a VisiCalc of patient empowerment, that forever changes expectations and makes the empowered patient as common as the smartphone. If we reach this stage, herd medicine will be doomed.

We already know some of the things patients want. Older people want tools to keep themselves independent and out of institutions. Patients with chronic illnesses that need a lot of management – diabetes, heart failure, and difficult-to-control hypertension immediately come to mind – want the tools to help them do most of that management themselves. And those at high risk for treatable cardiovascular emergencies – heart attack and stroke – want to prevent these emergencies, and, if they cannot be prevented, to immediately detect and treat them whenever and wherever they occur. These are among the things that people will pay for themselves (admittedly only a few high-end users at first, but eventually, as expectations change, large numbers of people).

There are diagnostic tools that can be miniaturized and reduced to a smartphone app, that will make the lives of direct-pay physicians and their patients easier and more convenient. Indeed, partnering with direct-pay physicians, and working to fulfill their needs as they work to re-establish the classic doctor-patient relationship outside the "real" healthcare system, will be a fruitful area for innovation.

A lot of tools can be brought to bear to begin meeting these needs, including a multitude of technologies, sophisticated communication systems, and data management and decision support systems, all aimed at providing remote monitoring, self-monitoring, effective diagnostics, and novel therapies and services. I described many of these in Chapter 15. But the possibilities are endless, and as the market defines itself those possibilities will come to seem obvious.

How to Start?

In Chapter 15, I described the ways in which the Central Authority, wielding its regulatory muscle, seems to have all but stopped the development of personal biosensors, a key technology for individualized healthcare. It is now extremely difficult, bordering on completely impracticable, for companies to introduce products based on personal biosensors into the healthcare market place. If you are such a company, your future does not appear bright.

And so, I humbly suggest, companies who are working with these sensors should not even try bringing them into the healthcare market place. Instead, they should bring them into the consumer market place.

Develop these products for non-medical use, and sell them to regular people. You will have the huge advantage of not having to jump through all the regulatory hoops; the advantage of being able to sell your product without having to convince two different third parties (doctors and payers) that its purchase is absolutely necessary and cannot be avoided; the advantage of typical, normal, understandable and predictable market forces determining the success or failure of your product; the advantage of selling your product without government-imposed pricing, so that you can discover the optimal price-point in the normal way; the advantage of a potentially huge and unrestricted market; the advantage of being able to iterate multiple successive versions of your product, based on customer response, without having to repeat all the regulatory hoops with each iteration; and the advantage of introducing your technology directly to the broad public, and making it seem commonplace and normal for people to use it. Pretty soon, people will be asking: "Say! Why can't we just use this stuff to help us manage our (fill in the blank here with your chronic illness of choice)?"

Imagination is called for here, but I will give you two obvious ideas just to get you started.

Elder care. More than increased longevity, we Old Farts want to remain healthy and independent into our old age. We want to avoid disability and institutionalization. Our kids, members of the "sandwich generation," want the tools to help keep their aging parents out of institutions, without neglecting their own young families. So think of ways to make it feasible for old people to continue living at home.

Wearable biosensors can be adapted to monitor the activity levels of the elderly – the amount of time they spend up and about versus sitting or lying down, the level of activity they perform, and when and how often they are active. Trends of such activity parameters may alert a family member that a loved one may be going downhill, early enough that something can still be done about it. Biosensors can also detect episodes of falling, and can send out an alert if a person does not get up in a specified period of time after they have fallen. Degrees of tremulousness can be measured. In many cases – far more often than doctors know – the medications which elderly people are taking can disrupt their sleep, leading to general deterioration. Biosensors can easily monitor sleep quality on an ongoing basis. Biosensors can also help detect whether the elderly person is taking his or her medications regularly – at least whether they unscrew the pill bottle or open the medication dispenser.

Athletics. Athletes are vitally concerned about their performance. Are they overtraining? Undertraining? Are they allowing themselves to break down? Are they pushing themselves into dehydration, heat cramps or heat stroke? Are they developing potentially dangerous heart rhythm problems? All these things can be monitored in real time in active athletes – under the rubric of athletic performance aids, and not medical products.

For instance, sensors can monitor specific levels of activity, and correlate these with heart rate and breathing rate. The "slope" of the change in heart rate and/or breathing rate as a function of activity is a reflection of cardiovascular efficiency, and thus, of the level of training. Deteriorations in that slope can indicate overtraining. In summer football camp, or in endurance events such as a marathon, a dehydration sensor and core body temperature sensor (both of which can be implemented in an adhesive skin patch) can monitor for early signs of impending collapse – and a trainer or the athlete him/herself can intervene in time to prevent a potentially dangerous event.

All of the sensors that you would use to make products for athletes or elder care can be easily adapted for use in patients with heart failure and other chronic medical conditions. Putting them into formal medical products today would be nearly out of the question. But putting them into medical products would become an obvious step after they have become commonplace in applications people encounter every day. And, since the sensors are the same ones that would be used in medical applications, smart patients will figure out how to apply them to help manage their own illnesses – and social networks will take care of disseminating that knowledge.

Indeed, when people begin asking you why you haven't adapted these sensors for obvious medical conditions, you can simply tell the truth – the Progressive healthcare system has erected insurmountable obstacles to your doing so. This is something people have a right to know.

So: learn about the needs of your true end-users, and design to their needs, and market your products directly to them. You may find the consumer market so dynamic and lucrative and welcoming of innovation that you may decide to abandon medical products altogether. In any case, the pathways you establish can always be employed, should our healthcare system regain its sanity, to devise products that will directly benefit patients.

WHAT THE GOOD CITIZEN SHOULD DO

Ultimately, the viability of Obamacare depends entirely on a credulous public, and on "well-behaved" patients. Maintaining a Progressive healthcare system requires citizens to ignore the necessity and the reality of covert rationing imbedded in herd medicine, and to believe that any apparent limits on healthcare result from corruption, waste, and inefficiency, which, thanks to the efforts of the Progressives, are slowly being rooted out. More importantly, when citizens become patients themselves, Obamacare requires them to rely serenely and without further question on the information their doctors give them, and on the treatments their doctors say are right for them.

This requirement is the Achilles' heel of Progressive healthcare. When you think about it, it is actually astounding that Progressives expect Good Citizens to limit their scope in this way, in our present era, where information about everything is ubiquitous and readily available. The majority of Americans who receive a new diagnosis today will immediately go to the Internet to learn what they can about it. And once Americans understand the personal dangers to which herd medicine exposes them, they will be especially interested in learning whatever they can about their medical conditions. For, once you become a patient, behaving as Obamacare expects you to behave will produce an immediate threat to your own life and limb. Complete acquiescence with the dictates of herd medicine, without questioning whether what's good for the collective herd is actually good for you, requires that citizens act in a manner that is clearly against their own best interests. It simply does not comport with human nature.

People who understand this – that it is probably not in their best interests to rely entirely on the advice of their Obamadocs – can take immediate steps to protect themselves. Instead of passively accepting at face value the diagnoses and treatment recommendations that are presented to them, these individuals will check things out for themselves, and seek independent confirmation that nothing is being overlooked, missed, ignored or "forgotten." If individual citizens begin confronting their "providers" with objective evidence that the recommendations they are receiving are dangerous to their well-being, it will become very difficult indeed for Obamacare to work the way it is designed to.

If enough people acted this way, the infrastructure of Obamacare would collapse under the weight of tens of thousands of self-empowered individuals, acting independently in their own enlightened self-interest. And when that happens we would be presented with another opportunity to reform our healthcare system.

Those new reforms will have a far different foundation than the reforms of Obamacare. This is because Obamacare will have failed specifically thanks to a new multitude of self-empowered Americans. The American populace will fit even less than it does today the profile necessary to establish a paternalistic, top-down, government-controlled healthcare system. Whatever system we would establish at that point to replace Obamacare, whether or not it resembled the system I discussed in Chapter 4, it would have to honor the now self-actualized, self-empowered, autonomous American patient. It would have to be compatible with the Great American Experiment.

The catalyst to a uniquely American solution to the problem of Obamacare, then, is the empowered patient. Americans – not all Americans, not even necessarily a majority of Americans, but simply a critical mass of Americans – are going to have to begin taking their healthcare matters into their own hands. For this to become possible, a sufficient number of doctors will have to recognize that empowered patients are their last hope for salvaging their profession, and they will have to take the difficult and risky steps necessary to support those patients. And entrepreneurs in the American biomedical industry will have to understand that their own survival may depend on their finding ways of helping patients to become self-empowered.

But the ultimate catalyst is the average American citizen – enough of them at any rate – refusing to subject themselves to herd medicine, and taking the steps necessary to protect themselves and their loved ones from it.

How Do You Get The Information You Will Need?

There is a tremendous amount of information on the Internet on just about any medical disorder you can think of. And the information ranges in quality from solid to absolutely ridiculous. So it is very easy to be misled. Still, gaining the right kind of knowledge is the indispensable key to empowering yourself within the healthcare system.

It shouldn't be this way. Individuals shouldn't have to figure out the best approach to their medical conditions themselves. That's what your doctor is supposed to be for. Your doctor is supposed to have enough basic medical knowledge – which options are available, what works and what doesn't, which information is over-hyped or quackery and which is solid and proven – to make recommendations that are particularly suited to your own individual needs. But under Obamacare your doctor cannot – must not, if he knows what's good for him – do that any more.

And so it behooves you to learn what you can about the medical conditions you or your loved ones have. You may have devised your own methods for doing this, or you may come up with your own method as you work through a topic you are researching. But here are some general thoughts I have on the matter.

First, get a good, general grounding on the medical condition you are researching. For this step, instead of just Googling the topic, go to a few sources that you can be pretty sure are reasonably objective and which generally provide useful information.

One site I personally find useful is the Merck Manual site (merckmanuals.com). The Merck Manuals cover most topics in medicine very well, are very readable, and to my eye are quite objective. There are manuals written for patients, and manuals written for physicians. You should read both. The manuals are free on the Internet. (The Merck Manuals are supported by Merck & Co, Inc., which is said to be one of those evil biomedical outfits. So keep that in mind.)

Other sites that are often helpful for grounding yourself include Wikipedia (which has obvious shortcomings, but whose coverage of medical topics usually – but not always – turn out to be reasonably straightforward and objective), WebMD, mayoclinic.org, and health.nih.gov.

Be skeptical of everything you read on the Internet, including information on these sites. But if you read about your topic on several of these sites, you will usually be able to discern without too much trouble the kind of basic information that is universally accepted, and therefore, which information appears likely to be correct.

Second, after you have a good, general grounding, then look for sites that might have more specific information regarding your area of interest. You might try the sites of specialty organizations, like the American Heart Association website, or the website of the American Cancer Society. Organizations dedicated to general consumer advocacy, like the Consumers Union (consumersunion.org) can also be helpful.

In recent years focused patient advocacy groups have launched websites that can offer valuable information that is difficult for non-specialist physicians to find anywhere else. Websites like KnowBreastCancer.org, the Michael J. Fox Foundation for Parkinson's Research (michaeljfox.org), and the National Dysautonomia Research Foundation (ndrf.org) not only provide insights on the basics, but also keep up with – and help you interpret – the latest research on the medical disorder you're researching. They also provide resources for advocacy and policy, and (perhaps most importantly) can connect you with a community of people who are also vitally concerned with the same disease you or a loved one are dealing with.

Third, look for social networking sites that deal with the medical disorder you are researching. In a recent article* appearing in the Huffington Post, Riva Greenburg described a host of social media websites dedicated to various medical conditions, and the advantages they provide – including information, support, community, and advice. Greenburg took particular note of the rise of new "patient-experts" who are emerging from these social media sites, and pointed out how social media is helping patients move from a "tell and instruct" paradigm to an "explore and partner" model.

_____

*http://www.huffingtonpost.com/riva-greenberg/are-doctors-losing-their_b_596060.html

_____

Social media health sites are still in their infancy, but they have the potential to drastically reduce the knowledge gap between patients and their doctors, and to remove patients from the role of a mere supplicant, a mere receiver of instructions, in their encounters with their doctors. It is difficult to envision patients equipped with such knowledge simply opening wide and saying moo.

Fourth, learn to recognize the really crazy stuff. Once you branch away from trusted sources on the Internet, you will have entered the Wild West, where anything goes. Here is a tip on how to recognize much of the quackery and charlatanism on Internet health sites: Such sites typically claim that the great medical-industrial complex is intentionally withholding vital – usually curative – information from the public; the writer/company/organization publishing the site exclusively knows the real cure; the same writer/company/organization offers exclusively to sell you the secret cure. Now, I'll have to admit that this system smacks at least a little of what I've been saying in this book – that the Central Authority and insurance companies have coerced doctors into withholding information that may be vital to their patient's care. The difference is that the information which the Central Authority wants withheld at the bedside is usually readily available from reputable sources on the Internet (like the ones I've mentioned), and the information which doctors are coerced to withhold would, if divulged, lead to some form of expensive medical service that the entire healthcare system would be expected to provide and to pay for. The secret cures offered by the shills, in contrast, can only be provided by the shills themselves.

So, finding the information you need is not entirely straightforward, but it is most often do-able with effort, patience, and care.

FIND ALLIES

No matter how knowledgeable you are, empowering yourself as an individual under Obamacare will be very difficult without allies.

The best "ally" you could have when you are sick, of course, is a good doctor. It is entirely possible that, despite the coercions placed upon him or her by the Progressive healthcare system, your own doctor is still able to function as your personal advocate. If so, nurture that doctor with every means at your disposal. Because even if this doctor has managed to hold onto the classic ethical standards of the medical profession, it is very likely he or she will be able to really go to bat only for a few selected patients who really need the help. So try to be the patient for whom the doctor would be willing to go out on a limb. This is not a book on nurturing relationships, so I hope you know how to do that already. If not, here's a tip: brownies help.

A better bet – since the unfortunate truth is that doctors as a group have been completely cowed by the Central Authority – is to find yourself a direct-pay physician. These are the only doctors remaining who have at least the inherent capacity to become a personal advocate for every one of his or her patients. They depend for their livelihood on doing right by you – not on doing right by the Central Authority or health insurance companies. Their stock in trade is to tell you the truth about your medical conditions, to describe all the options that exist for addressing your health problems, and to help you sort through the options to pick the one that is best for you. They can treat guidelines as guidelines – as helpful general guidance in managing a particular kind of medical problem – and not as an absolute directive whose violation will lead to punishment. A direct-pay physician is really the only kind of doctor today you can reasonably trust, as a matter of course, to honor the classic doctor-patient relationship.

When your legislators or the executive branch move to render direct-pay medical practices illegal or unfeasible – as they are already beginning to do – take it personally. They are moving to rob you of the only kind of physician left who can routinely try to do what is right for you as an individual, instead of treating you as an interchangeable member of the herd. Let your political leaders know that you will not take kindly to this sort of life-threatening action.

If you cannot find a direct-pay physician, or if the day arrives when direct-pay physicians can only ply their trade to fellow inmates while serving their life sentences, you still might be able to find a professional advocate who can help you navigate through the healthcare system. Two organizations that provide such services are My Nurse First (http://www.mynursefirst.com) and AdvoConnections (http://www.advoconnection.com). A professional advocate does not practice medicine, but can give you guidance when you need it, and can even go to bat for you with recalcitrant providers or insurance companies.

BE WILLING TO PAY FOR EMPOWERMENT

Commerce is a wonderful thing. If some people have a strong desire to acquire an item, and some other people have a strong desire to sell that item, nothing on the face of the earth can keep the transaction from occurring. This is why Prohibition did not work, why marijuana is California's biggest cash crop, why the Orthodox Church re-emerged in Russia even after several generations of Soviet-sponsored suppression, and why there will always be pornography on the Internet.

And it is why, if people demonstrate their willingness to pay for the means to control their own healthcare destiny, entrepreneurs (sooner or later) will trip over themselves to provide the products and services that enable them to do so.

People who understand just how vulnerable they are within a healthcare system that will do almost anything to avoid having to spend money on them, and who understand that placing all their trust in such a system is dangerous to their health and survival, will also understand that it might be necessary to invest some of their own funds to safeguard their medical welfare. The demand for products and services that provide these safeguards will grow in direct proportion to the public's awareness of just how vulnerable they are.

This awareness is increasing daily.

We are just seeing the beginnings of the "self-empowerment" industry, and most of it is still below the radar at this point. It is critical to know two rules that are necessary to make real self-empowerment possible. We will need to remember these rules when our Progressive leaders notice what is going on and then, recognizing the greatest threat they can ever face, stop at nothing to put an end to it.

The first rule of empowerment: Only you can pay for your own empowerment. In our entitlement society, whenever anything "good" shows up that is in any way related to healthcare, people expect it to be provided for "free." This will no doubt be true for products and services that are developed that advance patient empowerment. No sooner will such things appear than people will start calling for it to be "covered." I am very sorry, but this cannot be allowed to happen. When the central authorities agree to pay for empowerment services and technologies, they will control them. And when they control the means to empowerment, they will destroy their usefulness. They will have to destroy it – because individual empowerment wrecks Progressive healthcare.

The most obvious example of this is physician services. Doctors are designated by tradition, ethics, and law to be the patient's advocate. In other words, they are the original empowerment tool for patients. But not only has the Central Authority strangled the advocacy role of physicians, it has actually converted doctors from a tool for patient empowerment into a tool for centrally-directed covert rationing.

If we allow the new empowerment tools that are just now being invented to be co-opted by the government or third-party payers, the same thing will happen. Indeed, how they will co-opt the new empowerment tools is readily predictable. When the Progressives notice the swelling movement toward individual empowerment, they will initially try to stifle it altogether by making it illegal or unfeasible. Should these stifling efforts prove ineffective, they will shortly change tactics. "You are right," they will say, "these methods for improving individual empowerment are vitally important. They're so important, in fact, that it would be unfair of us not to provide them, so as to guarantee equal access to everyone."

We simply cannot allow this to happen, or patient empowerment will go the way of the doctor-patient relationship – to the dust bin of medical history. Individuals must be responsible for their own empowerment.

The second rule of empowerment: Self-empowerment is not a sin. You will be told that by using the tools of self-empowerment, by going "outside" the designated and approved pathways for your own healthcare, you are contributing to societal discord; that you are an elitist, helping to create a two-tiered healthcare system; that you are broadening the gulf between the haves and the have-nots, between the privileged and the underclass; that you are joining with the cigar-smoking, brandy-quaffing, expense-account-consuming, numb-hearted oppressors of the masses. You and your kind will be the subject of news articles in the *New York Times* and exposés on 60 Minutes. There is no way around it – you are evil.

Do not listen to these aspersions. They are not genuine; they are desperate attempts to bring you back into the herd. Remember: You are spending your own money to protect yourself and your loved ones from people who are trying to kill you (or, to be less unkind, who are at least willing to let you die).

And remember something else: While the primary reason you're empowering yourself is (and should be) self-preservation, by doing so you are also taking up a higher cause. You are joining an army that is fighting with the only weapon at its disposal against an opponent that is choking the life out of patients, the public, and the principle of individual autonomy. By fighting for your own individual prerogatives you are not leaving others behind – you are showing them the way, clearing a path to safety, and helping to preserve the Great American Experiment for future generations.

AND IF IT ALL GOES SOUTH

There is a realistic chance, of course, that Obamacare will not be repealed; that direct-pay physicians will be driven out of practice; that biomedical entrepreneurs who want to advance individualized healthcare will be driven out of business; and that for citizens to empower themselves with medical knowledge will lead only to increased frustration, and not to improved healthcare. This, after all, is the plan. It's the Progressive Program.

Critics of my writings on Progressive healthcare have always insisted that I am simply making too much of the Central Authority's aversion to individual autonomy. Our government, they insist, whatever its tendencies, will not really act to curb individuals from their freedom of action within the healthcare system, for the simple reason that Americans would never put up with such limitations. And in fact, I fundamentally agree with these critics, at least to this extent: Americans – many of us, anyhow – just won't put up with it.

Where I quibble is in the specifics. Most moderates will insist that our government (presumably, taking the American character in which they so deeply believe into account) would never actually try to limit the freedom of Americans in such egregious ways as I have described. But I have attempted to carefully demonstrate that the government has already begun using every means at its disposal to make it illegal, infeasible, or both, for Americans to spend their own money on their own healthcare. (Chapter 7). And I fear, sadly, that the many Americans who "won't put up with it" will eventually find themselves having to act counter to the wishes (and laws and regulations) of their government. That is, Americans who insist on exercising their natural right to become "the proper guardians of their own health," may have to do so extra-legally.

To say it even more bluntly, Americans wishing to enjoy the individual liberties which our Constitution promises us will, in this instance, need to engage in black market healthcare.

BLACK MARKET HEALTHCARE

Black markets develop naturally whenever a society's controlling authority attempts to prevent its citizens from acquiring an otherwise available good or service which they very much want (or need). In fact, as we have noted it is a law of nature that, wherever a group of people exists who badly desire a certain product, and another group of people exists who very much want to provide that product, there is no force in the universe – governmental or divine – which can keep those two groups from engaging in commerce.

To see what is likely to happen when the government institutes its prohibitions on individual prerogatives in healthcare, we ought to think about what happened when that same government instituted its alcohol prohibition (i.e., Prohibition). The 18th Amendment (one of the big triumphs of the Progressive Era, and one which, quite typically, relied for its ultimate success entirely on a fundamental change in human nature), went into effect at midnight, January 1, 1920. By noon that day, an entirely new industry had sprung up. This industry – the alcohol black market – eventually employed hundreds of thousands of Americans in various capacities, such as distillers, alcohol "re-naturizers," bootleggers, rum-runners, speakeasy proprietors, accountants, individuals who today might be called "lobbyists," and various species of "muscle."

My own dear grandfather, who had only recently arrived from Eastern Europe to work in the steel mills, found more profitable employment instead, through the 1920's and into the Great Depression, as a distiller of spirits and a gun-toting rum-runner. Each weekend he filled the hidden tank under the back seat of his big Buick sedan with 100 gallons of his prime home-made spirits, and would place my young grandmother (as documented in photos, wearing an impressive hat) next to him, and their three innocent little children (among them my toddler mother) would be perched over the hidden contraband in the back – the very picture of a happy young family out for a Sunday drive – and in this guise would make his deliveries across northeastern Ohio. I will never understand why, at the end of Prohibition, Grandpa ended up as a laborer for the city street department, instead of the filthy-rich Ambassador to England like his fellow bootlegger, Joe Kennedy. (But on second thought perhaps it is better this way. If Grandpa had ended up like Ambassador Kennedy, I today would be spouting the Progressive mantra, like all those other guilt-ridden souls burdened by unearned wealth.)

In any case, the government took great issue with the new bootleg industry that its Prohibition policy had created overnight, and attempted to end this black market by employing the ultimate expression of any sovereign authority – the legal exertion of violence. (The enforcers, it happens, were Treasury Agents, the very same enforcers who now will be ensuring compliance with certain mandates being imposed by our new healthcare system.) This effort on the government's part led to an organized response, and resulted in the maturation of American organized crime. (Interestingly, this organized crime effort happened to be centered in Chicago, a happenstance which arguably resulted in a persistent and evolving thugocracy within that city, whose ultimate ramifications – some say – are today influencing current events on a much broader scale).

When its concerted application of force against the bootleggers failed to end the black market, our government turned to applying a different kind of force, this time against the consumers. The recalcitrant consumers of illicit alcohol were, after all, guilty of failing to change their behavior, despite all the heroic efforts which were being made to educate them about the pitfalls of demon rum. The understandable frustration this caused finally led our government to resort to deadly force against the obstinate public itself. Author Deborah Blum has recently documented* how the U. S. government caused poisonous substances to be added to the alcohol supply, an act that is estimated to have eventually killed 10,000 American citizens. The chief medical examiner of New York City at the time called this action "our national experiment in extermination." And in 1927 the *Chicago Tribune* said, "It is only in the curious fanaticism of Prohibition that any means, however barbarous, are considered justified." (The "curious fanaticism of Prohibition," of course, is merely a particular embodiment of the curious fanaticism of Progressivism.) It was partly the revulsion against such official atrocities that forced the end of Prohibition in 1933.

*http://www.slate.com/articles/health_and_science/medical_exami ner/2010/02/the_chemists_war.html

I relate this little-remembered tragic episode merely to illustrate the lengths to which our Central Authority will go when its attempts to control human nature through legislation fail. This is worth keeping in mind as we conjure up ways to establish what I hope we will not need, but fear we'll not be able to avoid, namely, a black market in healthcare.

Black market healthcare will not be for the faint of heart. But then, no great human endeavor ever is. Let us consider some specifics.

First, however, I must first assure readers (and any government officials who may inadvertently stumble upon this book) that I am a strictly a law-abiding citizen, and do not condone illegal activities. So I will suggest here only activities for black market healthcare which, strictly speaking, will not be illegal under American law; though not so much by complying with the law, but by avoiding it.

I have complete trust in my readers that they can think up the more illegal kinds of black market activities for themselves, and thus they do not need my help with this aspect of the endeavor. Many of these more obvious illegal forms of black market healthcare (e.g., "medical speakeasies," located in back alleys for the proletariat, and in swanky office buildings for public officials; rolling surgical suites hidden in semi-trucks; smuggling rings for drugs and medical equipment; an "underground-railroad-style" transport system for itinerant physicians who need to ply their illicit trade while on the move; etc.), can be established by individuals, or by relatively small groups of entrepreneurs, and with relatively little up-front capital or lead time – and with no coaching necessary from your humble author.

But the varieties of black market healthcare which I have in mind – certain "less illegal" activities, which will drive the US government into states of apoplexy but over which it will have little legal jurisdiction – will require a much larger scale, and a significant investment in time and energy. So anyone who is interested ought to get started with the necessary organizational activities right away.

I have three such suggestions. With all three of them, I envision that implementation would be driven by a major private healthcare organization (or a consortium of them) which has a record of innovative thinking, as well as access to significant financial resources through their own holdings, or through their connections with rich benefactors from around the world. I am thinking of organizations like the Cleveland Clinic, the Mayo Clinic, or the Kaiser system.

For the sake of mankind, I offer these suggestions free and clear. They may be taken up, with my blessings, by any institution or organization that wishes to employ them, with no obligations or strings attached whatsoever.

1) Floating Off-Shore Medical Centers. In this scenario, the Cleveland Clinic (say), with the help of their friends in Abu Dhabi, buys or leases a mothballed former Soviet aircraft carrier (nuclear power preferred), and refurbishes it into a floating, world-class medical center. The ship will ply the international waters off the American coasts, providing regular helicopter transport to and from major cities. There's a lot you could do with an aircraft carrier, of course, to make it an attractive destination aside from medical care, including (for instance) establishing a world class hotel, food services, casinos and other entertainments. But the chief attraction would be that Americans will be able to buy the best healthcare services in the world, without fear of being arrested.

The fact that this floating medical center will be based on a former warship may turn out to be an advantage. Obviously, it would be useful to maintain at least some weaponry on board, if only to repel "pirates." But given the anger this ship will generate among American government officials, the Cleveland Clinic (or whoever) might be wise to remain intentionally ambiguous about just how much firepower the ship has retained.

2) Native American Medical Centers. There are two things about the current state of Native American culture which make this approach to black market healthcare at least feasible, if not compelling. First is the recognized "sovereign status" of Native American reservations, the same status which has allowed various tribes across the land to open gambling casinos, even in states which otherwise do not allow such establishments. If their sovereign status justifies casinos (establishments of mere entertainment, which, in fact, encourage bad behaviors of all sorts such as alcoholism, prostitution, smoking and – gasp!- obesity), then surely the same sovereign status would justify establishing advanced institutions of healing.

Second is the deep guilt that Americans rightly feel about the treatment Native Americans have suffered over the years, much of which was arranged by the US government. Note, in particular, that one of the ongoing claims which Native Americans have against the larger American culture is the chronically substandard state of the healthcare services they are provided. So, who will dare stand in the way of these oppressed peoples, when they propose to dedicate a portion of their pitiful remaining sovereign lands (with the help of, perhaps, the Mayo Clinic and its benefactors) to the development of world-class medical centers?

One advantage of the "Native American Strategy" for black market healthcare is that it would allow medical centers of various sizes and emphasis to be established in numerous convenient tribal locations around the U.S., as the need and logistics allow. Within a decade or two, if they play their cards right, Native American tribes may even find themselves controlling nearly 20% of the American economy – which would be ultimate justice at its finest.

3) Medical Centers Across the Mexican Border. There are several potential benefits to this suggestion. Converting Tijuana, Nogales, Laredo and Juarez from hotbeds of human and drug smuggling into hotbeds of illicit healthcare would probably be a boon to the local populations on both sides of the border. It would create tens of thousands of good jobs in Mexico, for Mexicans. The heavily-armed gangs of Mexican drug-runners along the border could be hired by the Cleveland Clinic Juarez, or Kaiser Nogales, as security guards, thus absorbing their "talents" into a more legitimate economy. (Being located so close to the border of a powerful nation which will badly want to terminate these medical centers would, one must understand, create a certain need for security.)

If nothing else, world-class medical centers just across the Mexican border would reverse the flow of illicit border crossings. Americans (and Canadians, who, bless them, would now have to travel much farther south for their healthcare) would suddenly be streaming across desert border crossings into Mexico in the dark of night – and Mexicans would be staying put. And its desperate need to get rid of black market healthcare would, at long last, give the US government a compelling reason to control the borders once and for all. We would suddenly see American troops all along the Mexican border, supported by such features as a "no-man's land" seeded with mines, and constant surveillance by drone aircraft armed with cluster bombs.

And before long, Californians wanting to go to the Mayo Clinic Tijuana Medical Center would have to get there by way of Cuba.

A HEALTHCARE REFORMATION

For individualized healthcare to take a firm foothold – a foothold which will inevitably wreck the Progressive model of healthcare – will not be easy. Powerful forces will be brought to bear to stop the creation of a patient-empowering healthcare marketplace, where citizens, direct-pay physicians, professional advocates, and entrepreneurs come together to enable self-directed, individualized healthcare. All the necessary players – those citizens, doctors, advocates and entrepreneurs – will need to persist in their efforts despite increasingly strident, desperate, and threatening attempts by Progressives to stop them, and to have them denounced as elitist, criminal, and immoral.

The Progressive healthcare establishment is at least as entrenched (and corrupt) as the early sixteenth-century Church; the notion of patients becoming self-empowered is at least as frightening as the notion of the teeming masses communicating directly with God; physicians answering only to their patients is at least as threatening as renegade priests answering to parishioners; and empowering technologies are at least as heretical as printing the Bible in the vernacular. The coming fight will resemble nothing, in terms of its intensity and potential for acrimony (and worse), so much as the Reformation.

Most of us "reformers" will enter the fray not in any attempt to become reformers, but rather in the simple attempt to protect ourselves, our families, our professional legitimacy, and our businesses from the perfidies of a broken healthcare system – that is, for ostensibly "selfish" reasons. To survive the vociferous attacks that will undoubtedly come our way, however, we will need to remind ourselves of the higher cause we are serving.

Is what we're doing unfair? It is not. It would be difficult to imagine a healthcare system more fundamentally unfair and inequitable than the one Progressives have in store for us now; in which deceptions, half-truths, outright lies, and coercion are techniques routinely employed by the Central

Authority which manages the healthcare system; in which the interests of doctors have been systematically divorced from the interests of their individual patients; and in which patients are left to fend for themselves, without their rightful advocates, at a time when they are least capable of doing so, within a confusing and dangerous healthcare system. What we are doing – learning to protect our own rights and welfare, and in the process exposing the truth of herd medicine, and establishing the systems and methods for others to follow – is restoring, not destroying, equity.

Is what we're doing immoral? It is not. By insisting on our right to self-determination, we are reestablishing a foundational American principle that has eroded in recent years in large part because of Progressive healthcare. By taking the steps necessary to empower ourselves and to enable that same empowerment for others, we are simply asserting our right to self-determination in matters related to our own personal needs. It is an American birthright. Others are trying to take it away. We are stopping them.

If we allow this attack on our founding ideals to go unanswered, or if we fight back and lose, we will pay a much higher price than merely a bad healthcare system. This is why we owe it to ourselves and to future generations of Americans to vigorously take up the cause.

We need to recognize Obamacare for what it is. We need to shine a bright light into the dark corners where it lurks. We need to point to it, call it by its name, illuminate its methods and reveal its secret language. We need to show what it is afraid of – truth, equity, and the intrinsic worth of the individual.

The shrillness of the cries and the brazenness of the protests against our efforts at self-empowerment should be recognized for what they are – signs of just how far we've already fallen away from those founding ideals, and of how close the idea of individual empowerment strikes at the heart of Progressives. If anything, these protests should steel our resolve. We are fighting for our own rights and welfare, to be sure, but we are also fighting a battle to restore every American's right to self-determination.

It won't be easy. But we are not sinners; we are holy warriors. Here we must stand, for we can do no other.

EPILOGUE

From that newly-discovered fragment (continued):

Socrates: What do you think now about this author's choice for a book title?

Meno: It is less inappropriate than I originally thought. It does, in fact, summarize nicely how these Progressives (as he calls them) expect the common people to respond to their enlightened commands.

Socrates: And, he indicates, by so responding the common people would reveal themselves to have been reduced to a state of mindless compliance.

Meno: Yes.

Socrates: And he believes this state of mindless compliance is a negative thing; that the common man should somehow lift himself up to a state of enlightenment, and take charge of his own affairs.

Meno: That clearly appears to be his thinking.

Socrates: Common women, too?

Meno: Apparently so.

Socrates: You see that this author, then, is a particularly virulent type of democrat, one who has altogether an unrealistic view of the capacity of the masses. He is one who, for instance, would take great offense at our concept of Philosopher Kings.

Meno: Undoubtedly.

Socrates: And he would look upon our current experiment in enlightened government here in Athens, being run by our old friend Critias and his Thirty Tyrants (and which even I must admit has become rather more bloody than I would have predicted), with great disapprobation?

Meno: Yes, certainly. And his book, should it become known, would give false solace and unreasonable encouragement to our opposition.

Socrates: I agree. Remind me. You found this book where?

Meno: Phaedo's Curio Shoppe. Phaedo says It was discovered in an old urn, in a cave, on some remote island, by an illiterate guano collector. Phaedo himself is not much of a reader, and purchased it from this man because he liked the picture on the cover.

Socrates: It is rather nice, as cow pictures go. But what you say is good. It is not too late.

Meno: What must we do?

Socrates: Get rid of every trace. Burn the book. Turn Phaedo in to Critias and his friends for special processing. Then, just to be sure, you must take the hemlock yourself.

Meno: And you?

Socrates: I must remain here as an inspiration to others, at least until I find my Boswell. Oh, and on your way out, my good friend, send in that good-for-nothing scamp Plato with my dinner.

About the Author

Richard N. Fogoros, MD is a former professor of medicine and a longtime medical practitioner, researcher and author in the fields of cardiology and cardiac electrophysiology. He currently makes his living as a consultant with biomedical companies, and as a writer.

Since 2000 he has written a patient-oriented website on heart disease for About.com (http://heartdisease.about.com). In 2012 he was named to the ShareCareNow list of Top 10 Online Influencers On Heart Disease.

As the acerbic DrRich, Fogoros has authored The Covert Rationing Blog (http://covertrationingblog.com) since 2007. His blog won the Medical Blog Award as the Best Health Policy and Ethics Blog in 2011.

His books include *Electrophysiologic Testing* (1990, 1994, 1999, 2006, and 2012), *Antiarrhythmic Drugs: A Practical Guide* (1997 & 2006), and the award-winning *Fixing American Healthcare - Wonkonians, Gekkonians and the Grand Unification Theory of Health Care* (2007).

He lives in Pittsburgh with the lovely woman who has been his wife for 38 years. Grown children show up now and then.

www.ingramcontent.com/pod-product-compliance
Lightning Source LLC
Chambersburg PA
CBHW060837280326
41934CB00007B/819